PERSONALIZED MEDICINE

## BIOPOLITICS: MEDICINE, TECHNOSCIENCE, AND HEALTH IN THE 21ST CENTURY

General Editors: Monica J. Casper and Lisa Jean Moore

*Missing Bodies: The Politics of Visibility*
Monica J. Casper and Lisa Jean Moore

*Against Health: How Health Became the New Morality*
Edited by Jonathan M. Metzl and Anna Kirkland

*Is Breast Best? Taking on the Breastfeeding Experts and the New High Stakes of Motherhood*
Joan B. Wolf

*Biopolitics: An Advanced Introduction*
Thomas Lemke

*The Material Gene: Gender, Race, and Heredity after the Human Genome Project*
Kelly E. Happe

*Cloning Wild Life: Zoos, Captivity, and the Future of Endangered Animals*
Carrie Friese

*Eating Drugs: Psychopharmaceutical Pluralism in India*
Stefan Ecks

*Phantom Limb: Amputation, Embodiment, and Prosthetic Technology*
Cassandra S. Crawford

*Heart-Sick: The Politics of Risk, Inequality, and Heart Disease*
Janet K. Shim

*Plucked: A History of Hair Removal*
Rebecca M. Herzig

*Contesting Intersex: The Dubious Diagnosis*
Georgiann Davis

*Men at Risk: Masculinity, Heterosexuality, and HIV Prevention*
Shari L. Dworkin

*To Fix or To Heal: Patient Care, Public Health, and the Limits of Biomedicine*
Edited by Joseph E. Davis and Ana Marta González

*Mattering: Feminism, Science, and Materialism*
Edited by Victoria Pitts-Taylor

*Are Racists Crazy? How Prejudice, Racism, and Antisemitism Became Markers of Insanity*
Sander L. Gilman and James M. Thomas

*Contraceptive Risk: The FDA, Depo-Provera, and the Politics of Experimental Medicine*
William Green

*Personalized Medicine: Empowered Patients in the 21st Century?*
Barbara Prainsack

# Personalized Medicine

*Empowered Patients in the 21st Century?*

Barbara Prainsack

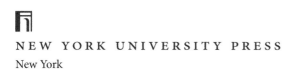

NEW YORK UNIVERSITY PRESS

New York

NEW YORK UNIVERSITY PRESS
New York
www.nyupress.org

References to Internet websites (URLs) were accurate at the time of writing. Neither the author nor New York University Press is responsible for URLs that may have expired or changed since the manuscript was prepared.

Library of Congress Cataloging-in-Publication Data
Names: Prainsack, Barbara, author.
Title: Personalized medicine : empowered patients in the 21st century? / Barbara Prainsack.
Description: New York : New York University Press, [2018] | Includes bibliographical references and index.
Identifiers: LCCN 2017008018| ISBN 9781479814879 (cl : alk. paper) |
ISBN 9781479814589 (pb : alk. paper)
Subjects: LCSH: Personalized medicine—21st century. | Pharmacogenetics.
Classification: LCC RM301.3.G45 P348 2018 | DDC 615.7—dc23
LC record available at https://lccn.loc.gov/2017008018

New York University Press books are printed on acid-free paper, and their binding materials are chosen for strength and durability. We strive to use environmentally responsible suppliers and materials to the greatest extent possible in publishing our books.

Manufactured in the United States of America

10 9 8 7 6 5 4 3 2 1

Also available as an ebook

# CONTENTS

*Preface and Acknowledgments*     vii

*List of Figures, Boxes, and Tables*     xi

*Technical Terms and Acronyms*     xiii

1. Setting the Stage for Personalized Medicine     1

2. The Patient Researcher     15

3. Always On: The Transmitting Patient     46

4. Beyond Empowerment     75

5. Just Profit?     107

6. Beyond Individualism     135

7. The Social Life of Evidence in Personalized Medicine     155

8. Conclusion: Patient Work in the Context of Personalization     187

*Notes*     209

*References*     217

*Index*     259

*About the Author*     271

## PREFACE AND ACKNOWLEDGMENTS

For many years my work has focused on the governance of DNA technologies. From this perspective I saw personalized medicine mostly as a new buzzword, a way of labeling old practices in a different way to open new doors for funding. It was during the European Science Foundation's *Forward Look on Personalised Medicine for the European Citizen* (European Science Foundation 2012), a two-year long scoping and consultation exercise that I had the privilege of helping to lead, that I was convinced of the deeper significance of the idea of personalization. Many practitioners, scientists, and policy makers that I spoke to in those years and the years that followed, from Europe, North America, the Middle East, and other parts of the world, saw personalization as a way to use technological advances to make medicine more "precise." But many of the same people also saw it as an attempt to address the challenges posed by rising health care costs and aging societies. They regarded it as a cost-saving strategy with patients in the driving seat. The role envisioned for patients went far beyond having to manage individual risks: One of the key tenets of personalized medicine is its data-driven nature, including wider ranges of data than clinical or medical ones. Many of personalized medicine's proponents are very open about the fact that patients need to play a key role also in collecting and "sharing" these data.

At the same time that the work required from patients expands, patients' influence over what data and information will be used, how they will be used, and for whose benefit, is waning. The "tapestries of health data" that are envisaged to underpin medical practice and research are prescriptive in what they can include and what they cannot. Narrative, unstructured information and personal meaning have little room in them, and data and information from marginalized populations are often not included at all. This all stands in a clear tension with the pronounced rhetoric of patient empowerment and patient participation. The mission of this book is to address this seeming paradox. Why is it that the work required from patients is becoming more expansive and less self-directed at the same time that the flag of patient empowerment and participation is raised over ever wider territories in medicine and health care?

A lot of people and institutions have supported this book project. I am deeply grateful to the Rockefeller Foundation for inviting me to spend a month at its Bellagio Center in the summer of 2016. I had planned to use that month to try to forget about personalized medicine and start a new project. I ended up doing the opposite: I forgot about my new project and started rewriting the book. The final manuscript has benefited greatly from numerous conversations with my fellow residents, including Isher and Montek Ahluwalia, David Autor, Kate Bredeson, Edith Brown Weiss, Medora Dutton Ebersole, Alec Freund, Matthew Goulish, Ann Hamilton, Ben Hecht, Lin Hinxson, Lynn Leibovitz, Michael Mercil, Pam and Jim Murray, Eric Nordstrom, Auma Obama, Catherine O'Regan, Tania and Antonio Patriota, Sanchita and Somitra Saxena, Stephen Rapp, Donatha Tibuhwa, Charles Weiss, and Karl Zimmerer. I am particularly grateful also to the Center's managing director, Pilar Palacia, and everybody else at the Foundation and the Bellagio Center who has made my time there so special.

Among the colleagues and friends who have helped the arguments in this book take shape are Daphna Birenbaum-Carmeli, Hagai Boas, Marianne Boenink, Alena Buyx, Carlo Caduff, Giulia Cavaliere, Luca Chiapperino, S. D. Noam Cook, Alan Cribb, Peter Dabrock, Lorenzo Del Savio, Edward (Ted) Dove, Sarah Franklin, David Gurwitz, Erica Haimes, Yael Hashiloni-Dolev, Johannes Fellinger, Robert Flanagan, Cesar Enrique, Sahra Gibbon, Torsten Heinemann, Stephen Hilgartner, Giraldo Herrera, Ine van Hoyweghen, Marie-Andrée Jacob, Hanna Kienzler, Puneet Kishor, Lene Koch, Lea R. Lahnstein, Thomas Lemke, Sabina Leonelli, Nadine Levine, Jean Lo, Ilana Löwy, Federica Lucivero, Jeantine E. Lunshof, Claire Marris, Ingrid Metzler, Bronwyn Parry, Maartje Niezen, Mette Nordahl Svendsen, Katharina T. Paul, Manuela Perrotta, Annette Rid, Christoph Rehmann-Sutter, Michael Reinsborough, David Reubi, Nikolas Rose, Amnon Shavo, Robert Smith, Robert K. Smoldt, Tim Spector, Niccolo Tempini, Natali Valdez, Hendrik Vogt, Nicolaas Wagenaar, Ina Wagner and all members of the Data and IT in Health and Medicine Laboratory at King's College London. I wish I could blame them for any errors or omissions, but I am afraid they are solely mine. I thank Sally Eales, Clemence Pinel, and Thomas Palfinger for their research support, and Ilene Kalish and Caelyn Cobb for having made working with NYU Press such a pleasurable experience. To Monica Casper and Lisa Jean Moore, the founders and editors of the NYU Press Biopolitics series, I am grateful not only for their immensely helpful feedback, but also for their enthusiasm for this project and their moral support. Another big thank you goes to the reviewers for NYU Press whose suggestions and constructive criticism have been invaluable.

Adele Clarke, Carrie Friese, Gabriel Krestin, Gisli Palsson, and Tamar Sharon have not only read and commented on several chapters but have also believed in this project at times when I did not; it is not an exaggeration to say that the book would not be here without them.

I dedicate this book to my husband, Hendrik Wagenaar, who I admire for many reasons; one of them is that he understands the world better than I do and has not given up on it. I thank him for his support and inspiration, and for his love.

# LIST OF FIGURES, BOXES, AND TABLES

## Figures

Figure 1.1. Mapping out the Information Commons                6
Figure 4.1. Imaging device quantifying the maximum
    plaque thickness                                           100
Figures 5.1a and 5.1b. Patient information sheet on the
    English care.data initiative                              128

## Boxes

Box 2.1. Criteria for the categorization of participatory
    initiatives and projects                                  27
Box 8.1. "Seven dimensions of contemporary participation"
    by Kelty et al.                                          193
Box 8.2. Characteristics of meaningful participation      201

## Tables

Table 3.1. Types of patient involvement in the creating,
    collecting, or providing of data and information
    in the health domain                                      69
Table 5.1. Three types of prosumption in the context of
    health information                                        120
Table 8.1. Four models of empowerment                     192
Table 8.2. Replacing risk-based data governance with
    new principles for the governance of data use            205

# TECHNICAL TERMS AND ACRONYMS

ALS: *Amyotrophic Lateral Sclerosis,* a rapidly progressive neurological disease that is also called Lou Gehrig's disease, or motor neuron disease.

AMYGDALA (PL. AMYGDALAE): Two almond-shaped parts of the brain that play an important role in decision making, memory, and emotional reactions.

BOP CONSUMERS: *"Bottom of Pyramid"* consumers—the largest but poorest group of people in the world.

CARE.DATA: A program that would have allowed the English NHS to share patient data with health care organizations and commercial companies in the UK and beyond. It led to public resistance due to an alleged lack of transparency about the goals of the program and the plan to have patients opt-out instead of opt-in.

CROWDSOURCING: A composite of the words "crowd" and "outsourcing," that is, the enlisting of large numbers of people (crowds) in a task, often online.

CSR: *Corporate Social Responsibility* refers to programs and strategies that combine profit maximization with the creation of social benefits.

CT: *Computed tomography,* a technology in medical imaging.

DEEP PHENOTYPING: A person's phenotype comprises her actual physical, personal, and behavioral characteristics (to be contrasted with genotype). Deep phenotyping refers to the description of (often disease-related) phenotypes using a data-rich approach.

DTC: *Direct-to-consumer.*

EPIGENETICS: The study of changes in organisms stemming from modifications of gene regulation or expression rather than changes in the DNA sequence.

ESF: The *European Science Foundation* is a nongovernmental nonprofit association of public and private research-related organizations in Europe and beyond.

EU: *European Union.*

FDA: The *Food and Drug Administration* is the U.S. government agency responsible for approving medical products, including pharmaceutical drugs and medical devices.

FTC: The *Federal Trade Commission* is an independent agency of the U.S. government, tasked with consumer protection and anticompetitive business practices.

GBM: *Glioblastoma multiforme,* one of the most aggressive and most common brain tumors.

HIGH-THROUGHPUT TECHNOLOGIES: The computational tools and methods that enable the simultaneous and rapid examination of large amounts of genes, proteins, and other substances.

HIPAA: The *Health Insurance Portability and Accountability Act* was passed by the U.S. Congress in 1996 and established a set of national standards for the protection of certain types of health information.

HIPPOCAMPUS (PL. HIPPOCAMPI): Parts of the brain that play important roles, for example, in memory and special processing.

IOM: The *Institute of Medicine* is a division of the National Academies of Science, Engineering, and Medicine (NAS).

IoT: The term *Internet of Things* refers to connected computing devices (such as sensors) without requiring human-to-human or human-to-computer interaction. Some people expect that our entire physical environment will start to wirelessly "talk to" one another in this way.

IP ADDRESS: *Internet Protocol address,* a numeric label assigned to a device participating in a computer network.

MRI: *Magnetic resonance imaging.*

MS: *Multiple sclerosis.*

NAS: U.S. *National Academies of Science, Engineering, and Medicine* are private nonprofit institutions providing expert advice to policy makers, funders, and similar.

NHS: *National Health Services,* the public health services of England, Scotland, and Wales.

NIH: The *National Institutes of Health* in the United States, a research agency within the U.S. Department of Health and Human Services.

ODL METRICS: Metrics for *observations of daily living.* ODL metrics can be very personal sensory and behavioral indicators for the purpose of health monitoring (and often also for behavior modification).

OMICS: Derived from terms such as biome or genome, "Omics" is an umbrella term for the study of datasets representing different types of molecules in a cell. More recently also disciplines outside of biology have started to use the "Omics" label to denote the analysis of large sets of social or demographic data.

PRIVACY-BY-DEFAULT: An approach that prescribes that only the minimum set of personal data necessary for a purpose should be processed, and that service providers need to offer customers the strictest possible privacy setting by default. It is enshrined in the General Data Protection Regulation in Europe.

PRIVACY-BY-DESIGN: An approach committed to designing privacy-enhancing measures into hardware and software. It was originally developed by Ontario's information and privacy commissioner, Ann Cavoukian, and is now enshrined in a number of laws and regulations, including the General Data Protection Regulation in Europe.

PROM: *Patient-reported outcome measures.*

PROSUMING: A composite of the words "*producing*" and "*consuming*," referring to the practice of users or consumers creating value for corporations by producing some or all of the content or products that they then consume (for example, social media).

REDLINING: Discrimination against specific groups of people on the basis of socioeconomic, behavioral, or other profiling. Redlining is often used to refer to practices that are not illegal (such as not offering certain discounts in specific ZIP codes, or not offering shipment to some regions).

SMART GLASSES: Eyeglasses that are wearable computers.

SOCIAL BIOMARKERS: Information reflecting nonsomatic characteristics of patients that matter to them in connection with their health care.

STS: *Science and Technology Studies,* an interdisciplinary field of studying how scientific knowledge and technologies are produced in conjunction with social and political order.

THERANOSTICS: A composite of the terms "therapeutics" and "diagnostics." It refers to strategies to combine diagnostic and therapeutic capabilities in one single agent or process to tailor both more closely to individual characteristics and needs of patients.

1

# Setting the Stage for Personalized Medicine

## The Changing Meaning of Personalized Medicine

When proponents of personalized medicine explain the concept, they typically tell a story of technological progress. Medicine used to be hit-and-miss, they say. We used to treat all people with a certain disease the same, despite all their differences. With today's technological tools we have become much better at measuring individual difference. Personalized medicine—especially in its iteration of precision medicine, which seeks to include ever wider types of information and monitoring—is the future. It is time to say farewell to "blockbuster medicine."

This future has already started. The idea that medicine and health care should become personalized—in the sense that they should be tailored more closely to individual characteristics of patients—has entered almost every domain of health care. Let us take the example of Type-1 diabetes, which is a relatively common disease. In the United States and in Europe, about two to three in a thousand people are affected by it, most of them at a young age (Menke et al. 2013; Patterson et al. 2009). Historically, the prevalence of diabetes has been highest among European populations, but now it is on the rise also in low- and middle-income countries. In contrast to Type-2 diabetes, which has been known as "adult onset diabetes" and can often be managed by diet and exercise, most Type-1 diabetes patients rely on insulin injections. Before the discovery of insulin treatment in the 1920s, Type-1 diabetes sufferers were put on so-called starvation diets. Fasting and restricted food intake, it was believed, could prolong the lives of patients. Despite this, many patients died within months of the diagnosis.

After the introduction of insulin treatment, the tools required consisted of a simple finger prick set to determine glucose levels, and a syringe to inject insulin. Then, in the late twentieth and early twenty-first century, companies developed more complex monitoring and treatment systems, including microchip sensors, automated insulin pumps, and insulin inhalers. Today, "smart socks" can measure changes in temperature in patients' feet to detect inflammation that could lead to foot ulcers, which affect many diabetes sufferers. And insulin meters can send text messages to parents about their child's glucose levels. Patients in high-income countries are encouraged to use these tools to tailor their diabetes treatment more closely to their individual needs. Every diabetes sufferer is different, so the story goes, and monitoring blood glucose within very narrow ranges with the help of close monitoring leads to better health outcomes—at the cost of five hundred dollars per month or more, with treatment tools and insulin increasing in quality and price.

Another example of the personalization of diagnosis and treatment is the molecular classification of tumors. It is well known by now that the treatment of breast cancer can be improved by looking at the specific characteristics of the tumor. But this practice is not restricted to breast cancer alone. Glioblastoma multiforme (GBM), for example, is a rare but very aggressive brain cancer. Its prevalence is not known exactly because it remains undiagnosed in many resource-poor regions. In high-income countries, it is estimated that GBM makes up about 15 percent of all brain tumors. Once diagnosed, most patients die within three years. GBM tumors are resistant to conventional therapies, and treatment options vary depending on the tumor's location. For a long time, surgery, chemotherapy, radiation, and palliative treatment were the only options available. More recently, gene transfer has been explored as an additional treatment option, and promising results were achieved with the use of a nonpathogenic version of an oral poliovirus type in clinical trials at Duke University (Gromeier 2018). Moreover, factors such as the precise location of the tumor, patient age, and molecular markers such as the concentration of certain growth factors allow probabilistic inferences regarding treatment response and survival rates. The molecular classification of tumors is thus seen as a way to more individualized therapies that "will ideally lead to better outcomes in both the quantity and quality of life" (Choudhry et al. 2013: 303).

Is personalized medicine the crown of the evolution of medicine? Is it a step toward truly individualized medicine, and is the latter something that we should strive for? While many advocates of personalized medicine would answer these questions with a resounding yes, others are less enthusiastic. They remind us that medicine has long been personalized. Physicians, nurses, and carers have always considered the individual characteristics and circumstances of their patients when diagnosing, treating, and caring for them (Hunter 1991). In the days before professionalized medicine, and certainly before medicine's reliance on instruments that only trained professionals could operate, patients played a key role in medical decision making processes: Their stories and descriptions of symptoms were often indispensable for determining diagnosis. Patients and their families have also participated in deciding on and administering care (see also Strauss et al. 1982; 1997). Historically, "bedside medicine," with its close interactions between patients, doctors, and families and with its consideration of the specific circumstances and experiences of the patient, has been the rule, and not the exception.

If we accept that medicine has always been personalized, why is it, then, that the concept of personalized medicine has received so much traction recently? Is there anything new about the kind of personalized and "precision" medicine that is the topic of policy papers, funding calls, and government initiatives today? Although I agree that we should be cautious not to celebrate personalized medicine as an entirely novel phenomenon, it is clear that several developments within the last two decades have changed the institutions, practices, and stakes of medicine. The spread of digital technologies and the "biomarkerization" (Metzler 2010) of medicine—that is, the increasing reliance on objectively measurable somatic markers representing specific stages of physiology and pathology—have changed the meaning of evidence that is used to personalize medicine. In the 1960s, the British novelist Peter Berger portrayed the life of an English country doctor. For decades to come, his book was on the reading list of people training to become doctors. In order to recognize a patient's illness, Berger noted, doctors "must first recognize the patient as a person" (Berger and Mohr 1967: 76). In other words, doctors, when assessing the likely cause and nature of a disease, need to consider wider ranges of factors than the immediate symptoms that a person presents with. This statement is very similar to the slogans of proponents of personalized medicine today: The U.S. Precision Medicine initiative, for example, explores how genes, environment, and lifestyle come together to create a "unique thumbprint" of each patient (National Institutes of Health 2016a). What has changed is thus not the commitment to focus on individual characteristics of patients but the very characteristics that should be considered. When diagnosing and prescribing treatments, Berger's country doctor considered the living circumstances of his patients, their family and social relationships, and their mental state. These were all aspects that doctors who still made house calls used to know—or explore in a dialogue with their patients. Within contemporary personalized medicine, it is a person's genetic predispositions, her lifestyle information, and clinical data that should be brought together into personal health maps informing diagnosis and treatment. It is no longer unstructured narrative information that is seen as the key to personalization, but structured, digital, quantified, and computable data (see also Hartzband and Groopman 2016; de Mul 1999; Nettleton 2004; Webster 2002).

Another push toward such a new understanding of evidence has come from the advance of high-throughput technologies—the devices and computational tools that enable the simultaneous examination of large amounts of genes, proteins, and metabolites. A standard reference in this context is Moore's Law, named after Intel founder Gordon Moore; it predicts that the number of transistors on integrated computer circuits doubles every two years (G. Moore 1965). The cost of sequencing a human genome—the sum of a person's DNA—has decreased faster in the last decade than predicted even by Moore's Law. At the same time, the speed of analysis has increased drastically (National Human Genome Research Institute 2014). Advances in the production of data on gene expression, blood glucose levels, or brain function, for example, have contributed to a situation in which Western biomedicine is now faced with unprecedented amounts of digital data. Finding a way to transform these data into something meaningful and, if possible, clinically actionable, is one of the main challenges that clinicians, patients, enterprises, and health authorities struggle with.

In policy papers, politicians' speeches, and newspaper articles today, personalization appears as the data-intense characterization of individuals at different stages of health and disease in the course of their lifetime. This is different from how the term was understood in the 1990s and early 2000s, when personalized medicine largely meant tailoring drug treatments to genetic characteristics of population sub-groups (Hedgecoe 2004). Today's vision of personalization seeks to make use of much wider ranges of molecular and nonmolecular data and information, including imaging data, information about lifestyle and diet, and records of physical examinations (European Science Foundation 2012; PerMed Consortium 2015; Weber, Mandl and Kohane 2014). This is also how I use the term personalized medicine in this book. I understand precision medicine (National Research Council of the Academies 2011; see also Juengst et al. 2016) and stratified medicine[1] as variants of the idea that I subsume under the generic label of personalization.

## Where Patients Come In: The "Google Maps" of Health Data

Former U.S. President Obama made personalized medicine prime time news when he announced the allocation of $215 million to the study of "individual differences in people's genes, environment and lifestyle" in his State of the Union address in 2015 (White House 2015). He referred to this new type of medicine as precision medicine. The paradigmatic vision of precision medicine was first formulated in a report by the Committee on a Framework for Developing a New Taxonomy of Disease within the U.S. National Academies of Sciences in 2011 (National Research Council of the Academies 2011). The report proposed to replace traditional, symptom-based disease classifications with a new taxonomy based on data-rich characterizations of individuals and disease states. The report used the "Google Maps" feature, with its different layers of data—including data on transportation, land use, and postal codes—as a template for what a new map of patient-centered information could look like. The report's vision was that this map should serve both clinical and research needs (17). In such a system of patient-centered data, genetics may still play the first violin in some contexts, but it is part of a bigger orchestra.

But where do the data for such a personalized health data map come from? Many kinds of nonmolecular data that are envisaged to be part of such a health-data system—including information about the details of a person's lifestyle, mood curves, or data from the daily tracking of functional changes following the start of a new medication—are not readily available from clinical or biomedical research contexts. Some of the data would need to come from other, non-biomedical research contexts, remote sensors, or people's personal domains.

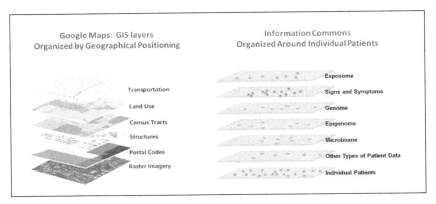

Figure 1.1. An Information Commons might use a GIS-type structure. The proposed, individual-centric Information Commons (right panel) is somewhat analogous to a layered GIS (left panel). In both cases, the bottom layer defines the organization of all the overlays. However, in a GIS, any vertical line through the layers connects related snippets of information since all the layers are organized by geographical position. In contrast, data in each of the higher layers of the Information Commons will overlay on the patient layer in complex ways (e.g., patients with similar microbiomes and symptoms may have very different genome sequences). Source: FPA (Fire Program Analysis) 2011, GIS Overview, FPA Project, Idaho State Office, Bureau of Land Management, Boise, ID, www.fpa.nifc.gov, accessed August 19, 2011 (left panel); screenshot from Insel 2011 (right panel). Reprinted with permission of the National Institute of Mental Health. Original caption was retained.

Since the report was published, the "Google Maps for health" metaphor has become a trope, popularized also by physician researcher and author Eric Topol's use of the comparison between geographical information systems and personal health maps (Topol 2015). Topol argues that in the near future, personal health maps will enable patients to carry out most diagnoses themselves. Even visionaries and practitioners who do not believe that algorithmically supported patients will take over the role of doctors any time soon see the integration of diverse types of data sets as crucial for the realization of personalized medicine. And they agree that this goal, in turn, will depend on the willingness of people to participate in the generation and analysis of data.

Many technologies to help patients with this task are already here. Touch-screen-fitted and portable devices make it technically easier to collect and transfer data and information. Websites and platforms "pull" data from users seeking to access information on the Internet—often without their being aware of what it is they are contributing (Wellcome Trust 2016). In other words, the Internet[2] has ceased to be primarily a provider of information and has become a tool for data collection from patients and citizens (Kallinikos and Tempini 2014; Prainsack 2013; Tempini 2015). Data that were not previously considered relevant in the health care context—such as mood-tracking data stored on smart phones—are now seen as potentially useful resources. Viktor Mayer-Schönberger, an information governance expert, and Kenneth Cukier, an editor at *The Economist,* use the term "datafication" to refer to this process. According to these authors, we are taking "information about all things under the sun—including ones we never used to think of as information at all, such as a person's location, the vibrations of an engine, or the stress on a bridge—and transforming it into a data format to make it quantified" (Mayer-Schönberger and Cukier 2013: 15).

That increasing parts of our lives, bodies, and environments are "datafied" does not mean that these data can always be integrated and interpreted in a meaningful way. Improving the interoperability between different data sets and data repositories, data integration, and quality control at the point of data entry remains a difficult challenge, despite promising attempts of tech developers. But here, too, it is apparent that these challenges cannot be addressed without active participation by patients who are needed to collect, hand over, or help analyze data and information.

The central role of patients in personalized medicine was apparent also in Barack Obama's vision: collaborative health care and "patient-powered" research form central pillars of the U.S. Precision Medicine Initiative (White House 2015). With this emphasis on patient-centered personalized medicine, the United States is not alone: Proponents of personalized medicine around the world believe that it can kill two birds with one stone: to render medicine more effective and, at the same time, "empower" patients.

## Whom Does Personalized Medicine Empower?

But are patients "empowered" by personalized medicine? Social scientists who have been studying twentieth- and twenty-first-century versions of personalization in medicine draw a nuanced picture. Sociologist Richard Tutton, for example, grounds his analysis in the sociology of expectations, which treats speculative claims about the future of a field of science or technology as "fundamental to the dynamic processes that create new socio-technical networks" (Hedgecoe and Martin 2003: 328). In other words, visionary statements about the development of a field often create facts on the ground. In the case of personalized medicine, Tutton argues, the notion serves to overturn the fiction of the *standard patient* (Tutton 2012; 2014). The idea that every disease was marked by a list of specific characteristics and symptoms that all patients in this group would typically display was a central theme within the scientific ideal of Western medicine in the nineteenth century. The current version of personalized medicine, in contrast, draws attention to the innumerable differences between patients and the ways in which their diseases affect them. It highlights the ways in which the same disease develops and expresses itself differently between people, due to differences in lifestyle, diet, genetic makeup, and so forth. In fact, the more we know about differences between people in molecular, lifestyle, and other terms, the farther we get away from the notion that any two people express *the same* disease in the same way (European Science Foundation 2012; Harvey et al. 2012). In its extreme form, personalized medicine means that there are as many diseases as there are people. Diseases could still be bundled together in clusters that display similarities, but the idea of common disease labels would be obsolete (National Research Council of the Academies 2011; Prainsack 2015a).

Tutton argues that this discursive and technological shift draws attention away from social determinants of health toward an illusion of a technological fix for health problems in our societies. In such a context, personalized medicine appears as an overhyped idea that benefits companies and uses the notion of risk to enlist patients in governing themselves more effectively (Tutton 2014; see also Tutton and Prainsack 2011). Similarly, Donna Dickenson, in her book *Me Medicine vs. We Medicine* (2013), sees personalized medicine as a political rhetoric that makes people believe that it is good for them, while it is really driven by corporate interests and fosters questionable values such as ruthless individualism. Also other critical authors consider the main function of the concept of personalized medicine to be a political one: They see it as diverting attention away from the failure of big science and heroic medicine to make a tangible difference for people's health (Nuffield Council on Bioethics 2010). This diversion is achieved by implying a shift "from industrial mass production to targeted fabrication" (Prainsack and Naue 2006: 349), which runs the risk of reiterating racial, gender, and class biases in a more concealed way than ever (Clarke et al. 2010b; see also Prainsack 2015a).

Here, the examples of personalized diabetes management and the molecular classification of brain tumors at the beginning of this chapter are instructive. First of all, in both scenarios, key aspects of personalization are out of reach for people in low-income countries. That the majority of the world's population will be excluded from enjoying the benefits of personalization has indeed been a key concern of critical observers (Khoury and Galea 2016). But it is not only populations in low-income countries that would be deprived of access to personalizing technologies such as blood-monitoring instruments or tumor analysis, but also less-privileged people within high-income countries. Even for people who could have access to technologies and services used to personalize their health care, social circumstances such as the lack of transportation, the fear of missing days from work, or unconscious racial bias represent factual obstacles to accessing health care, or detract from the quality of care received (Brawley and Goldberg 2012; Matthew 2015; Roberts 2011). Moreover, the increasing digitization of tasks and services—ranging from booking doctor's appointments to using video calls for consultations to managing health records electronically—creates new patterns of exclusion. People who cannot or will not do these things risk being disadvantaged. And among those who are happy to do these things online, new divisions are emerging. Although some of us have sufficient skills and bandwidth to assert our needs and interests, and to create content, others are mostly passive data sources whose data help to improve algorithms and services for the more privileged.

Although this problem is not specific to personalized medicine, the current focus on expensive high-tech solutions within personalized medicine is particularly likely to exacerbate existing inequalities. Moreover, while medicine in general is becoming more data-driven, personalized medicine in particular risks increasing inequalities by focusing on populations that are already well researched and characterized. In connection with genomic research, this is a well-known problem: At the time of writing this book, more than 80 percent of the roughly 35 million samples used in genome-wide association studies—a type of study that can help to identify disease-causing genomic markers—came from people of European descent. Taken together, samples from people of African and Latin American descent, and from those belonging to native or indigenous peoples, amounted to less than 4 percent of all samples analyzed (Popejoy and Fullerton 2016). This means that much of the genomic research that underpins personalized medicine uses samples from a small minority of the world's population with, relatively speaking, similar genetic ancestry. Although our genetic makeup is only one of many factors influencing health and disease, it is still important to include people living in different parts of the world, with different genetic ancestry, and different lives, diets, and environments. Although race is not genetic, it is biological: People who suffer racial discrimination, for example, who live in deprived neighborhoods, and who are exposed to high levels of stress and financial worries are more likely to be of poor health than others (Marmot 2015). If such people are missing from genetic and other biomedical databases, their clinical and environmental data is absent as well. Also for this reason, some initiatives, such as the Precision Medicine Initiative introduced by President Obama—the name of which was changed to the "All of Us Research Program" in 2016 (National Institutes of Health 2016b)—make extra efforts to include underserved populations.

Another concern that is frequently voiced in connection with personalized medicine is that patients become enlisted in multi-layered treatment and monitoring regimes that restrict rather than enhance the agency of patients (see also Mol 2000). Instruments that need to be used in particular ways and at particular times, sensors that collect data that patients cannot access and control, or drugs that are offered to patients at a discounted price if patients pay with access to their personal data (Hiltzik 2015) all impose additional tasks and duties on patients. This is quite a contrast to the empowerment rhetoric used by promoters of personalized medicine. Being more active "partners" in their own health care here means that people need to be more alert, do more work, and allow for their lives to be more closely monitored by others. And patients are not the only actors affected in such a manner: Health care

practitioners, carers, and family members all need to slot into personalized disease management plans and other types of digital health surveillance. In addition, with devices and software that are protected by
intellectual property rights, users—including health care professionals—
lose the ability to fix, replace, or modify tools as they wish. They become
part of a complex treatment script that they cannot alter or opt out from
without incurring excessive transaction costs (see also Oudshoorn 2011;
Ratto and Boler 2014). Last but not least, more sophisticated tools to
"personalize" diagnosis or treatment regularly mean higher costs for patients or their insurance providers.

It is at this juncture that the growing popularity of notions such as patient empowerment, patient-centered medicine, or participatory medicine appears in a problematic light. It is not a coincidence that we see a
renewed emphasis on patient participation[3] at a time when medicine is
particularly hungry for data and other contributions from us all.

## Patient Work in the Era of Personalization

Historically, patients have participated in medicine in many ways: by
caring for themselves and for each other, by discussing symptoms, by
contributing to medical research or advocating for new treatments,
research, protocols, or new public and environmental health measures
(see, for example, P. Brown 2013; S. Epstein 1995; 1996; Kickbusch 1989;
Klawiter 2008; Rabeharisoa and Callon 2002; Rabeharisoa, Moreira and
Akrich 2014). Scholarship in the social studies of biomedicine has made
this kind of work more visible (e.g. Clarke et al. 2003; 2010a; Cooper
and Waldby 2014; M. Stacey 1984; 1997; Strauss et al. 1982). The current push toward personalization in medicine, however, increases the
amount and type of work that is required from patients. It also moves
more of this work outside the boundaries of the clinic and includes ever
wider groups of people. Importantly, it includes the witting or unwitting
contributions that many of us make when engaging with online tools,
when using mobile applications, or when "sharing" information. Without patients contributing data, time, effort, and self-care, current visions
of personalized medicine cannot be realized. I call this "personalization
from below." Telling this yet untold story of such personalization from
below is the main objective of this book.

## Overview of the Book

To understand the factors that have created this need for personalization from below, several developments need to be considered in conjunction. I already mentioned the movement toward more data-intensive medicine, both in the domain of research and in the domain of practice (for example, Khoury et al. 2013; Murdoch and Detsky 2013). Data-rich characterizations of people at various stages of health and disease are considered necessary to understand variations in disease biology, which is central to the idea of personalization. Another relevant development is the increasing reliance on web-based tools to collect, process, analyze, and communicate data. Tasks that had to be done face-to-face can now be carried out by people in separate locations. In telemedicine, for example, diagnosis or treatment can be carried out in a different place from where the patient is located (Andersson 2009; Nicolini 2007; Oudshoorn 2009; 2012; Topol 2012). While these developments are often hailed as enhancing health care services in remote areas, or enabling patients to interact with their doctors without leaving their homes, cost reduction is also a driver. In particular, the possibility of sending digital data sets across large distances in real time opens up opportunities for the offshoring of entire tasks or steps of medical service provision to places where they can be done more cheaply: to radiologists in low-wage countries, for example, to call centers on other continents, or to patients themselves.

The first part of this book investigates these developments and organizes them along four main themes: how old and new forms of patient participation in medical practice and research come together in the name of personalization (chapter 2), the new role of patients as continuous data transmitters (chapter 3), the power shifts involved in personalized medicine (chapter 4), and the marriage of health idealism and commercial interest in many of the initiatives and corporations in the field of personalized medicine (chapter 5). In the second part of the book I move from describing and analyzing these developments to addressing the challenges that they pose. Chapter 6 probes the understanding of personhood that underpins Western biomedicine. It argues that we need regulatory and ethical frameworks that overcome an unduly narrow focus on individual autonomy if we want to achieve a kind of personalization that foregrounds aspects that are valuable and meaningful to patients. Chapter 7 discusses concrete ideas and initiatives that serve as guiding examples for this purpose. It also addresses the concern that the reliance of personalized medicine on digital and computable evidence will crowd out human experience and high-touch practices, and proposes ways to prevent this. In the final chapter of this volume (chapter 8) I bring together the different themes discussed in the book. I formulate an answer to the question of what types of participation and empowerment can contribute to a desirable kind of personalized medicine.

## *Data, Methods, and Theory*

Before I start, a note on the data, methods, and theory guiding my analysis is in place. This book is not the result of one single research project. Instead it brings together different strands of research and policy-related work that I have carried out over the last ten years. I have studied policy documents, public discussions, and scholarly research on the governance of databases for health and security purposes (Hindmarsh and Prainsack 2010; Prainsack 2007; Prainsack and Gurwitz 2007). I have worked with identical twins to learn how people with genetically identical others think about similarity and difference (Cherkas et al. 2010; Prainsack and Spector 2006). I have spoken to marginalized people such as prisoners about their views on DNA technologies (Prainsack and Kitzberger 2009; Machado and Prainsack 2012), and I have been involved in exploring the views of research participants on data ownership, consent, and solidarity in the health domain (Kelly et al. 2015) and studied the emergence of governance approaches to biotechnological innovation (for example, Prainsack 2006). In the domain of policy, I have advised governmental bodies on the governance of bioinformation and on other issues pertaining to biomedical research and practice. Most importantly for the topic of this book, I have had the privilege to lead the European Science Foundation's *Forward Look on Personalised Medicine for the European Citizen* (ESF 2012), alongside Stephen Holgate and Aarno Palotie. These explorations and experiences have steered me toward the most interesting, puzzling, and problematic aspects of visions of personalized medicine. On some occasions I will draw upon interviews that I have carried out myself, or that I was involved in analyzing (for example, Harvey et al.

2012). On other occasions I employed interpretive methods to analyze data that are publicly available, such as the content of online platforms, policy documents, or marketing materials. I also often use materials from studies by other colleagues to illustrate my arguments. Empirical studies on "patient work" in the era of personalized medicine are still relatively scarce, as the field is still young, but their number is growing (e.g. Juengst et al. 2016; Noury and Lopez 2016).

My methodological approach is interpretive, focusing on the exploration of what Hendrik Wagenaar called "discursive meaning" (Wagenaar 2011). I look at how actors understand certain terms, developments, and events. In other words, practices of meaning making, and the larger shared and institutionally enacted understandings that are outside of the domain of singular individuals and actors, are the main subject of my analysis. Theoretically I am grounded in critical approaches used in Science and Technology Studies (STS) and policy studies. Like so many others in STS I consider science, technology, and societal order as practices that emerge in connection and interaction with each other (Jasanoff 2004). From critical policy studies—and my training in political science and political theory more broadly—I take a commitment to look at the workings of power—not only when power is exercised in a situation of open conflict but also when it works in more silent ways. Last but not least, and reflected also in my methodological approach, I am inspired by epistemology and hermeneutic traditions that give an important place to meaning in the lives of people, and that are interested in understanding how meaning is made at personal and collective levels.

2

# The Patient Researcher

## What's New? "Activated Patients" as Data Contributors

All visions of personalized medicine, no matter how they are labeled, envisage an active role for patients. As noted in the previous chapter, former President Barack Obama, the initiator of the U.S. Precision Medicine Initiative, was very clear that it can only succeed if patients participate actively. Policy makers in the European Union have been equally explicit about the need for people to contribute time, data, and effort towards the personalization of health care (see, for example, European Commission 2014: 42–43). Mark Britnell, a previous high-level manager within the English National Health Service (NHS) and recent author of a book on health care systems around the world, put it most bluntly: "I do not know of a health system in the world that will not need greater patient activation if it is to become—or remain—sustainable" (Britnell 2015: 216; see also Lupton 2014).

The key message of such statements is not only that personalized medicine specifically requires the active participation of patients to realize its goals but also that health care systems on the whole will only be able to survive if patients become more "activated." But what are "activated patients"? When Anselm Strauss and colleagues coined the term "patient work" in the early 1980s, they focused on the participation of patients in their own care (Strauss et al. 1982; 1997; see also Kerr, Cunningham-Burley, and Amos 1998; M. Stacey 1984). After carrying out extensive fieldwork in hospitals, Strauss and colleagues concluded that:

> Among the people who perform work in [hospitals], contributing directly or indirectly to the care of patients, there is one class of workers which is not so easily recognized. These workers (the patients) have no occupational titles; the tasks which they perform are often unnoted—although paradoxically often assumed and even expected—but their work is certainly not paid for by the hospital. In fact, much of it is quite

invisible to the staff [ . . . ] either because not seen or not defined as work
(Strauss et al. 1982: 977).

This diagnosis still holds true today. Health care continues to rely on the
unpaid work of patients and caregivers—most of the latter are women
(Levitsky 2014; M. Stacey 1984). But in the context of contemporary
personalized medicine, patient work includes a much broader range of
activities. Patients and nonpatients alike are expected to monitor themselves by collecting data on tablets, smartphones, or wearable sensors.
They are asked to help to fill the "data gap" between doctor's visits to
establish baselines of their physiological functioning, or for other purposes of prevention: People at risk for skin cancer, for example, can wear
sensor patches to detect high levels of UV radiation (Gruessner 2015).

Is this a good development? Some authors and practitioners answer
with an unqualified yes. They see every instance of data transfer from a
patient to a doctor, a health care provider, or even a web-based platform
that will analyze patient data as making medicine more democratic. For
some, the fact that people can access previously inaccessible information online, organize themselves on patient platforms, and contribute
to scientific research in novel ways amounts to a participatory turn in
medicine and science (Prainsack 2011b). Others see participatory practices and initiatives in the domain of medicine as unduly romanticizing
patient "empowerment." They believe that the strong emphasis on patient participation conceals some of the other purposes that these initiatives serve, such as shifting tasks that are too expensive or too onerous
for corporate actors to do to patients. For the most disenchanted of observers, the current emphasis on patient empowerment is mostly about
cutting costs.

In this chapter, I will discuss the factors that have led to the understanding that there is a participatory turn in medicine, including the
emergence of so-called lean forward digital technologies. These technologies give information to users but also require that users give information back, thus turning patients into research contributors. This
development, in turn, has consequences on who is empowered and disempowered by these new forms of participation, and it gives rise to new
patterns of exclusion. What happens to those who cannot be, or refuse
to be, "activated"?

## What Is the Participatory Turn in Medicine?

Next to the notion of patient work (Strauss et al. 1982), the concept of self-care is relevant in this context. In the widest sense of the term, "self-care" refers to things that people do to protect or promote their health without formal medical supervision (Dean 1989; DeFriese et al., 1989). In the scholarly literature, self-care often refers to situations where patients decide how they want to manage their own health, free from constraints of institutionalized healthcare. At least in principle, while patient work takes place under the constant presence of the medical gaze, self-care takes any form that people choose. As such, it takes place beyond the boundaries of the clinic, and is as old as humankind.

What, then, is the difference between these older forms of self-care and participation and the kind of patient "activation" and empowerment that is appealed to today? The answer to this question consists of several parts. One is related to the advancement and rapid spread of digital tools. Digital tools and social media have broadened the range of tasks that people can do without the personal guidance of health care professionals. One of the most impactful changes in the doctor-patient relationship has been the ability of patients to access information that was previously inaccessible to most. Even two decades ago, patients searching for medical information had to go to a library and retrieve articles from medical journals. Nowadays, much of this information is available at the click of a mouse.

But this is not the whole story. The participation of patients has also become more visible because it has become individualized. In many regions and contexts it is considered the prime responsibility of individual patients—or their families, if patients cannot do it on their own—to stay healthy or manage their illness (Levitsky 2014; Petersen 1996; Petersen and Bunton 2002; Petersen and Lupton 1996). This focus on the individual is not self-evident. In systems with publicly funded universal health care, for example, patients are part of a collective: They pay into a system and take services out when they need them. They rely on others to pay for services they cannot afford, and collective actors decide what services patients will have access to. In this sense, patients are a group before they are individuals. Absent such solidaristic arrangements, in systems where individual patients must choose what insurance to buy and what preventive measures to spend their money and time on, patients are first and foremost individual actors who are expected to assume responsibility for their supposedly free and autonomous choices. If we see patients in such a way, we will see both their self-care and their patient work as an individual choice too: They decide to be good patients or not, or to be good citizens or not. Such a framing, of course, moves out of sight collective factors such as the social determinants of health (Marmot 2015): Social and economic factors including housing, access to clean water and food, labor rights, income equality, and gender or racial discrimination have been found to be fundamentally important to people's health and disease. Their importance is reflected in the fact that health outcomes do not differ only between high- and low-income countries, but also within one single society or country. Social determinants also shape who *can* participate in their own health care in the first place. They make it easier for some people to "choose" a healthy lifestyle, to "decide" to comply with their doctor's orders, or to agree to participate by contributing data.

## Patients as Research Contributors

Easier access for a greater number of people to wider ranges of information, and better ways to make themselves heard, are clearly positive developments. But when we take a closer look at how people participate in supposedly participatory platforms and groups in the health domain we do not only see empowerment. Sometimes, participatory practices can also make patients more vulnerable. An example of the latter in the offline world is the cooptation of patient groups by pharmaceutical companies, where funding from the latter compromises or even hijacks the agendas of the former (see, for example, Jones 2008). In the online world people can become more vulnerable when their data and information are used for purposes that go against their interests. For example, when a person discloses health information through surveys or website registrations, this information is not protected by the rules that apply to health data in the clinic. It can be sold by the owners of online platforms to data brokers or credit bureaus that provide health care providers or insurance companies with risk scores for individual patients (see Dixon and Gellman 2014: 15). And patients can also be disempowered collectively if, for example, an entire district is redlined on the basis of particular indicators suggesting that people in that area are poorer or sicker or otherwise less desirable clients and consumers. And although discrimination on the basis of racial or ethnic categories is often illegal, online platforms can bypass this prohibition by using proxy information. The social media platform Facebook, for example, has used "ethnic affinity" labels that they calculated on the basis of users' postings and preferences to enable advertisers to exclude certain groups. This has allowed them to use ethnicity as a category without asking users about it, and without technically breaking the law (Hern 2016).

Regardless of whether people are empowered or disempowered by the use of participatory platforms and initiatives, a particular characteristic of online services in the health domain is that they make the difference between patients and research contributors practically obsolete. Personalized online services tailored to serve patient needs, such as PatientsLikeMe (patientslikeme.com), Cure Together (curetogether.com), or online symptom checkers (for example, symptoms.webmd.com), use patient data for medical, marketing, and other research (Merchant 2015). Patients who share information on dedicated online platforms may do this to receive information and support. At the same time, the data of these "empowered" patients are turned into valuable assets for research and profit making by these very platforms and their corporate customers (Kallinikos and Tempini 2014; Tempini 2015). And even those of us who do not use health-specific platforms but use generic search engines or social media or disclose seemingly innocuous information when registering for services can end up having our data used for health-related purposes.

In the following section I will argue that, due to developments such as the proliferation of web-based tools, the roles of patients and contributors to research are converging. I will discuss how the role of the Internet in the health domain has changed since its Bronze Age years of the early 2000s. Using two of the aforementioned online platforms, PatientsLikeMe and CureTogether, I will illustrate how some services that present themselves as support systems for patients are data-collection enterprises at the back end. I will also take a closer look at the notion of participation: What forms of participation do people engage in when using online symptom checkers to self-diagnose health problems, for example (see also Jutel and Lupton 2015; Lupton and Jutel 2015)?

## From Leaning Back to Leaning Forward: The Changing Role of the Internet in the Medical Domain

In 2010, Apple launched a tablet computer, the iPad. It made a splash in the consumer tech market, and other companies soon followed with competitor products. Tablet computers, with their touch screens and their small size, marked a new era in personal computing. Many wondered how the particular characteristics of iPads would affect user behavior. Would tablet computers become another tool for people to passively consume media, or would they be used more actively to search for information, or to upload and edit photos? In other words, would tablet users "lean forward" more when using them, instead of mostly "leaning back"?[1]

Lean-back and lean-forward technologies are two ideal types that should not be seen as denoting a clear dichotomy or reflecting a linear historical development. They overlap in practice. But in a nutshell, lean-back technologies are those that operate without continuous and active input from users. After a person has chosen a clip to watch or a page to read, she can literally lean back. Lean-forward technologies, in contrast, require users to communicate actively through the device and thus continuously input data. Until the second half of the 2000s, online services that targeted patients were providers of information: after typing in search terms or questions, patients were expected to "lean back" and absorb the information. This was not necessarily the case because patients were hesitant to participate more actively, but because these early online health tools did not offer anything different. Social media were not yet widely available, and if patients went online it was presumed to be for the sake of seeking information (see also Cline and Haynes 2001). This also explains why ethical and regulatory debates at that time focused on how users could be protected from incorrect or misleading information, and not yet on other aspects such as privacy (see also Fuchs et al. 2012). At that time, online health resources were seen as competitors to medical professionals, who had until that time been the only group able to provide trustworthy health information.

This situation changed when digital social media entered the scene. What sets digital social media apart from earlier generations of digital media is that they are built for the exchange of user-generated content.[2] File- and photo-sharing sites such as Flickr, social networks such as Facebook, or blogs, including the microblogging service Twitter, are some of the best-known examples of social media. Another important feature of social media is that it is users who both produce and consume content; the medium merely provides the technical infrastructure to do this. This phenomenon is often called "prosuming," a composite of the terms "producing" and "consuming" (Toffler 1980; see also Benkler 2006; Rheingold 2002; Shirky 2008).

Materials that users post on these sites range from the intimate to the trivial to the political. And all of the most successful social media platforms are also heavily used for health-related purposes. Many users of Facebook, for example, discuss health-related issues ranging from diets to the side effects of prescription drugs to the discussion of the most intimate of problems (see, for example, Hawn 2009). Clinical trial participants are recruited via Facebook, and postings on Twitter are mined to discern disease outbreaks: When many people in a certain area tweet about being ill with fever and a sore throat, for example, this can be an advance warning of a flu outbreak in that region. Moreover, sensors on smartphones or smart watches can turn these devices into diagnostic tools (Topol 2015). Although many web-based platforms and services in the health domain still see themselves as information providers, they now do a lot more: They are designed in such a way that users lean forward most of the time. Users are prosumers of health information, sometimes consciously, willingly and happily, and sometimes without being aware what will happen to the data they disclose in this manner. Sometimes they are not even aware that they are contributing data in the first place.

Web-based platforms such as PatientsLikeMe or CureTogether represent archetypical lean forward services. Both platforms integrate the functions of information provision and data collection. They encourage people to contribute data and information about themselves in the process of learning about and from others. This resembles other, offline interactions where people are likely to share and receive information in an iterative manner, such as during a conversation with a colleague or friend over coffee. One key difference between the online and the offline world here, however, is that web-based platforms log and analyze data that are uploaded, and these data can, in principle, also be accessed by or sold to third parties. This does not normally happen in the offline world.

As noted in chapter 1, Viktor Mayer-Schönberger and Kenneth Cukier (2013) use the term "datafication" to signify the representation of ever more aspects of our lives into computable formats, so that these data can be mined for associations. In the context of participatory medicine, the notion of datafication also refers to information previously considered irrelevant for medical purposes that is now being seen as useful. Information on virtually anything that plays a role in people's lives could potentially aid research or medical decision making, such as lifestyle, diet, mood changes, or similar (see also Kish and Topol 2015).

## Leaning Forward for Health

### PatientsLikeMe: Sharing More of You(r Data)

The for-profit company PatientsLikeMe is probably the world's best-known online network for patients. It was founded in Cambridge, Massachusetts, in mid-2002 by three engineers whose brother and friend had been diagnosed with motor neuron disease (also known as amyotrophic lateral sclerosis, ALS, or Lou Gehrig's disease). At the time of writing this book, the network had more than 500,000 users. This is a small number in light of the total numbers of patients in the world, or even those with Internet access. But it is a sizable figure considering that the platform is limited to English-speaking users, and that it is still relatively young.

PatientsLikeMe initially set out to facilitate the sharing of information about their users' experiences with their illnesses and diseases. Members could exchange information about relevant new research, clinical trials, personal experiences, and give and receive support. Via messaging functions, members of the network can contact each other on the basis of any personal characteristics that they are happy to share; most members use nicknames, but they can also use their real name if they prefer. In a way, PatientsLikeMe started out as a platform seeking to simplify what patients have always been doing, namely looking for others who have relevant information or expertise, and pooling knowledge. In the offline world, self-help groups have existed for a long time, and some patients were among the first to use newly emerging technologies for this purpose, such as e-mail lists. From this perspective, PatientsLikeMe did not enable its members to do anything categorically new. Instead it supported them in doing things they were already doing more easily and more effectively. Members could now reach thousands of other patients simultaneously, with only minimal or no marginal cost.

For PatientsLikeMe, it was only a small step from facilitating the sharing of users' experiences and information to using these data for research purposes. In this light, PatientsLikeMe could appear to be a textbook case of successful crowd sourcing of data-collection (Nielsen 2011). If we examine more closely the work that the people running the PatientsLikeMe platform do, however, we see that it amounts to more than merely collecting data from a large number of patients. One of the main tasks for the company is to turn the unstructured conversations and data entries of its members into structured data that can be analyzed and mined (Kallinikos and Tempini 2014). This is also how PatientsLikeMe makes money: It sells data shared by patients to drug companies, device manufacturers, insurers, and medical service providers (PatientsLikeMe 2014). Getting patients to "talk" on its platform is thus one of its key tasks: Users are continuously encouraged to share information on their diseases and lives. In the words of James Heywood, one of the founders of PatientsLikeMe: "Our job is to allow a conversation with the computer that will match a conversation between two patients. [ . . . ] then we capture that dialogue and turn it into useful, clean data" (quoted in Goetz 2008).

Apart from selling patient data to companies, PatientsLikeMe also carries out its own studies. In one famous instance, users of PatientsLikeMe who suffered from motor neuron disease took lithium carbonate—a substance typically used as a mood stabilizer—and recorded dosage, any functional changes, and other relevant metrics in a self-organized study. The study had been initiated by members of PatientsLikeMe after a clinical study had suggested that lithium carbonate could slow down the progression of the disease (Fornai et al. 2008). The patient-led study could, unfortunately, not confirm that lithium carbonate slows down the progression of the disease. But the fact that patients on the platform had organized their own self-experimentation study was seen as a new way of doing disease research (see, for example, Swan 2012), and the platform has since been involved in numerous further studies. It is yet another reason why PatientsLikeMe encourages their users to "lean forward." By participating in the network, users also contribute to experimental groups and studies.

## CureTogether: Quantifying Similarity

CureTogether was founded by two pioneers of the self-tracking movement, Alexandra Carmichael and Daniel Reda, in 2008.[3] At first sight, CureTogether may look very similar to PatientsLikeMe: As with Patients-LikeMe, CureTogether encourages users to quantify and share information about the nature and severity of symptoms, as well as different treatments they have tried. Both platforms aggregate and analyze data generated by users. But in contrast to PatientsLikeMe, CureTogether focuses exclusively on collecting structured, quantified, anonymized data. This means that users are required to enter data in predetermined and computable formats, rather than sharing unstructured narratives. At the same time, the diseases that both platforms include emerge "bottom up" in the sense that users can add conditions that are not yet included. At the time of writing this book, the site had more than thirty thousand registered users.

Users of CureTogether can identify what treatments work for other users who are similar to them: A filter feature on the site allows them to limit comparisons to other users who have similar combinations of symptoms, comorbidities, or demographic characteristics that they do. Once similar users have been found, their data can be used to draw conclusions for one's own situation: For example, if a particular treatment has worked well for women of roughly the same age as my age, who also suffer from migraines and have a combination of symptoms similar to mine, I may be tempted to try this treatment as well. If, in contrast, it turns out that for users very similar to myself a new drug that I have just been prescribed has caused very bad side effects, I may not want to try it, despite my doctor's advice. In countries where access to clinical care is easily accessible for patients, sites such as CureTogether may be used primarily to complement or double-check information that patients receive from their doctors. Patients may consult the website to see what works for other users who are similar to them before they speak to their doctor about possible treatments, or may use the service to replace a clinical second opinion. In countries where access to clinical care is difficult or expensive (or both), sites such as CureTogether may be places that patients turn to *instead of* consulting their doctors. For chronic health problems, and especially in connection with conditions that do not require invasive procedures, such as surgery or chemotherapy, people may feel that learning what kinds of treatments worked for others who are similar to them is all they need to know. Many of the treatments assessed on the CureTogether site are not drug treatments but other remedies and measures such as exercise, or the consumption of specific foods. And even where a treatment with a particular drug is reported as being the most effective remedy, this drug can be bought over the counter or online, in some cases illegally. It is for this reason that concerns have been raised about the potential harm stemming from sites that tempt patients to take medical decision making into their own hands (for example, Vicdan and Dholakia 2013; Haig 2007). In sum, CureTogether turns patients who use the platform not only into contributors to research, but also into data sources for decisions that other patients may make.

In 2012, CureTogether was acquired by the personal genome testing service 23andMe, a California-based genetics company that we will revisit a few more times in this book. For a while after this acquisition, CureTogether encouraged its users to upload their genetic profiles. When sufficient numbers of users have done so, the platform suggested, genetic similarities could become an additional reference point in potential searches for "similar" users. This plan was later dismissed; at the time of writing this book, CureTogether users are merely encouraged to order genetic testing from *23andMe*, not to upload their DNA data.

The acquisition of a nonprofit platform created by self-tracking activists by a powerful commercial player requires further comment: Commercial players often acquire platforms or initiatives that were started by people without profit motives in mind. The new commercial owners sometimes keep the basic services free of charge, as happened also in the case of CureTogether, where users are still not charged anything for signing up or participating. But the sale of user data is now part of the business plan. Many platforms do this without telling users how they make money with their data; PatientsLikeMe is a laudable exception. And most of them retain the rhetoric about participation, democracy, and empowerment. By participating in such platforms, users are given the impression that they not only obtain useful information regarding their own health but also help to make medicine more participatory and democratic.

But do they? In the next section of this chapter I will unpack the notion of participation in more detail. I will explore what forms of participation web-based platforms encourage or require from their users, and against what criteria the "democratic value" of these kinds of participation can be assessed.

## Patient and Public Participation—In What? Categories of Participation in Medicine and Science

Among initiatives that claim the participatory label for themselves, there is great variation in terms of how and what patients and other lay people contribute. So-called citizen scientists—people without professional training in a subject area—can participate by providing funding or participating in data collection and generation, analysis, interpretation, application, dissemination, or evaluation. There are, however, considerable differences in terms of how much influence these nonprofessional participants have. Some initiatives are led by patients or activists in every respect, whereas in others, nonprofessionally trained participants have no decision-making power with regard to core strategies. Instead they merely contribute as data collectors—which often requires expertise, but this expertise does not translate in decision making power about what data will be collected or what will be done with them—or even just as funders. The schema presented in box 2.1 allows us to obtain a better understanding of the type of participation that different projects involve, and the influence that patients or "citizen scientists" have.[4] Taking the aforementioned PatientsLikeMe study on the effect of lithium carbonate as an example, we would first ask about *coordination:* Who was involved in agenda setting, in determining the execution of the main idea, and the procedural aspects of this study? Who decided, and how? What should count as results, and who decided what "good" results were, and what should be done with them? Who decided on intellectual property-related questions?

So, who coordinated PatientsLikeMe's lithium study? According to the authors of the study, the initial idea came from patients registered on the site. The development of the data collection tool was initiated by patients and some friends and family members, and was then developed further by the platform. Data analysis was led by PatientsLikeMe (Wicks et al. 2011). This means that agenda setting was shared between users and employees of the platform. The fact that PatientsLikeMe is a commercial company illustrates the entanglement of health activism and commercial interest that is characteristic of many participatory projects in the medical domain at present (for a more detailed discussion of this aspect see chapter 5).

BOX 2.1. Criteria for the categorization of participatory initiatives and projects (Adapted from Prainsack 2014a)

Coordination: Who has influence in:
1. Agenda setting
2. Determining the terms of the execution of the idea/procedural aspects
3. Deciding what results are (and what "good" results are)
4. Deciding what will be done with results
5. Deciding on intellectual property questions

Participation:
6. Who participates (demographic and social parameters of those who participate)? Why, and how do they participate?
7. How much, and what kind of, training, skill, or expertise is required to participate in this project?
8. Are there cultural, institutional, or other differences in perception and framing of core issues and stakes?

Community:
9. What forms of community precede this project or initiative, if any? Which new communities does the project or initiative facilitate or give rise to? What is the constitutive factor for the feeling of belonging on the side of the participants?

Evaluation:
10. Who decides what good outcomes are? How?
11. What happens to the results of these evaluations?

Openness:
12. Do participants have access to the core data sets?
13. Can participants edit or modify the core data sets?
14. Is the contribution of participants adequately acknowledged in published materials?
15. Are data sets made publicly accessible (open source/open access)?
16. Are main findings made publicly accessible (open source/open access)?

Entrepreneurship:
17. How is the project funded?
18. What is the role of for-profit entities in this project? Are these small, medium-size, or large entities, and where are they located?
19. How are for-profit and other interests aligned in this project (and/or do they conflict, and where?)

The second set of questions in box 2.1 focuses on the practices and modes of *participation:* Who are the participants of an initiative or project, and what characteristics do they have? Why and how do they participate? What are the requirements for participation in terms of technical or language skills, or geographical location? How much and what kind of training, expertise, experience, and skill, and what talents and capabilities, are required to participate in the project? Are there cultural, institutional, or other differences in the perceptions and framings of core issues and stakes among actors at various levels? In our example, the most obvious requirements were that participants in the study had to be registered with the platform, be able to enter data in a sustained and structured manner over a period of several months, have been diagnosed with motor neuron disease, and be able to get hold of lithium carbonate. As data had to be entered by patients—or by family members or caregivers respectively—some level of computer literacy, the ability to read and write in English, and a considerable time investment, were also required. Ironically, one of the very features that makes some web-based studies so successful, namely that they do not require participants to meet face-to-face with researchers, may also contribute to the high drop-out rates.[5] In PatientsLikeMe's lithium carbonate study, of the 348 diagnosed motor neuron disease sufferers who provided sufficient baseline data to be included in the study, only 78 were included in the final analysis. Important reasons for "attrition" were that many patients were unable to take lithium for the full twelve months of the study, and that some patients died during that year.[6]

Notions of *community* are the focus for the third set of questions in box 2.1. Questions to be asked here include: What forms of community preceded a particular project, if any? What do people in these communities have in common? Which new communities does the project facilitate or give rise to? In our example, answers to these questions are relatively straightforward, because the study emerged out of one platform and focused on one relatively specific patient group. If there was a community that preexisted the study, it was a community of patients, family members, and friends around motor neuron disease who contributed time and effort to this trial, hoping that the results would inform their own treatment, or the treatment of others after them. In other projects, however, the question about preexisting communities could be much more difficult to answer, because of the dearth of evidence available on the collective identities and motivations of members of participatory projects in medicine and health (for exceptions, see Hobbs and White 2010; Raddick et al. 2010; Reed et al. 2013).

The fourth set of questions in the box concerns *evaluation:* Who decides what "good" outcomes are, and how is this decision made? Who decides, in turn, what will happen with the outcomes of the evaluation? Outcomes are not the same as results; outcomes include wider societal, educational, and economic impacts, including any unintended consequences. Results are typically the findings of the project or study in the context of the research question or mission. In our example, the people who decided what good outcomes were and how they would be used were the owners of PatientsLikeMe, who led the study, in collaboration with some particularly active patients. There is nothing to suggest that the study was formally evaluated after its conclusion (although PatientsLikeMe says that its projects are regularly evaluated internally).

*Openness* is another relevant aspect in our assessment of participatory projects. It refers to the absence of technical or financial barriers to access. Such barriers include proprietary data that are not available to users at all, or data locked behind pay walls (Suber 2012). When thinking about how open a particular project or initiative is, questions we need to ask include: Do participants have access to core data sets? Can they edit the core data sets? Is the contribution of participants adequately acknowledged in published materials? Are data sets made publicly accessible (open source/open access)? Are the main findings made publicly accessible (open source/open access)? In practice, strongly participatory projects will always entail a certain level of openness, because otherwise active participation by a wide range of nonprofessional contributors would be practically impossible. However, openness is never a *sufficient* condition for a project to be participatory. It is possible, in theory, for a project that publishes all data sets, protocols and other materials online to be run by only one person who makes all decisions by herself. Such a project may meet the criteria for "open science" projects, but it would not be considered participatory. But the openness of such a project would take the edge off autocratic governance here, because if all data collected and generated by this project were available online, anybody could use them for their own purposes. Our example, the lithium study organized by PatientsLikeMe, scores relatively highly in terms of openness. For data protection reasons, however, it would be neither possible nor desirable to make all data sets publicly available. But many useful data sets were published online (see "supplementary data," Wicks et al. 2011).

The sixth and final dimension to be assessed is *entrepreneurship*. Questions to be asked here include: How is the project funded? What is the role of for-profit entities in this project? Are these small, medium-size, or large entities, and where are they located? Finally, how are for-profit, communal, and other interests and stakes aligned in this project? Do they conflict, and if so, where? Answers to these questions may be different for various stages of the project or initiative. This becomes apparent also in the case of PatientsLikeMe, which started out as a patient-led self-help network and is now a powerful commercial player. Although neither the lithium carbonate study nor the platform that hosted it changed their mission significantly during the course of that particular study, other projects may change their mission after a few weeks, months, or years. Reasons for this can be related to the internal organization of the project, or external factors such as new scientific advances, new technical opportunities, change of leadership, or being acquired by another entity. When analyzing a particular project or initiative with the help of box 2.1, questions in every category should be considered separately for every stage of the project, as answers may vary.

In summary, how much influence "lay" participants have over the aim, design, and utilization of results in a project tells us something about the disruptive—in the sense of challenging dominant scientific institutions and practices—potential of a project or initiative. This disruptive potential of a project does not prejudice, however, how successful it will be in terms of the standards and metrics of traditional medical practice and science. For some projects, an assessment according to the standards of established professional practice may be ill fitting. In those participatory projects that aim at reducing treatment burden for individuals, for example, traditional metrics such as median survival rates may not be adequate. The best metrics here would be the subjectively perceived decrease of pain and burden, in a wide sense, and an improvement of happiness of the person concerned. The growing field of patient-reported outcomes research is developing excellent instruments and measurements in this respect (see Nelson et al. 2015).

## Political and Economic Dimensions of Participatory Projects in the Medical Domain

Commentators have been both enthusiastic and also concerned about the emergence of participatory projects and practices in the domain of health and medicine. There are concerns about replacing the expertise of professionally trained experts, such as clinicians and medical researchers, by that of "amateurs"–such as the participants in the lithium carbonate study organized via PatientsLikeMe. Sometimes these worries stem from a genuine concern about quality control: Because amateurs are not trained in scientific methodologies, it is feared that they cannot record or analyze data correctly and thus compromise the quality of science. Indeed, Tempini (2015; see also Kallinikos and Tempini 2014) found that data quality at the point of data entry is one of the most notorious challenges for PatientsLikeMe. But quality control is not the only concern: Riesch and colleagues (2013) found that some professional scientists also worry that the unpaid labor of citizen scientists could make some of their own, paid labor redundant.

Some participatory practices in citizen science projects bear strong resemblances with the participation required from users in Web 2.0 enterprises.[7] Google, for example, famously combined its focus on user experience with reliance on user-generated information: Google's algorithms draw on how many times users access particular websites (Auletta 2009). The assumption is often that those who contribute to participatory projects in the medical domain where they have little influence on what happens with the results, and where corporations profit from their participation, cannot knowingly and willingly be doing so; their participation must thus be driven by some kind of false consciousness. As I have argued elsewhere (Prainsack 2014a), this assumption is problematic. For many people, being part of something that they consider useful, being acknowledged publicly in publications, or learning about the scientific area in question is a strong incentive to participate. For them this is a sufficient reward. Research with early adopters of online genetic testing services has shown that at least within this group, motivations and perceived benefits included good entertainment value, playful engagement with information, unspecified curiosity, and the desire to contribute to something meaningful (McGowan, Fishman, and

Lambrix 2010; Vayena et al. 2012). But this does not mean that there is no issue here. When participatory projects, platforms, and websites—and in fact everything and everybody that collects information from patients—are not transparent, in a proactive way, about how they make money, and about who is likely to benefit from participants' contributions, then participants cannot make these decisions in an informed and meaningful manner. The need for proactive transparency in this respect cannot be emphasized enough.

## New Patterns of Exclusion? The Digital Health Divide, and the E-Health Filter Bubble

In recent years, many services similar to PatientsLikeMe or CureTogether have become available in many more languages.[8] Doctors and patients in growing economies such as China seem to be at the forefront of the early adoption of social media, despite the little attention that these developments receive in English-speaking media (see, for example, Chiu, Ip, and Silverman 2013). A common objection against predictions that web-based platforms and services will play an essential role in routine clinical care so far has been that these web-based tools attract only particularly well-educated, computer-savvy, or wealthy individuals. Therefore, the argument continues, web-based platforms are of negligible importance in today's world and will remain marginal in the foreseeable future. While this view may have held true for early phases of Internet use in the domain of health and medicine, several developments in the last few years have changed the landscape. The availability of portable devices equipped with touch screens, for one, has lowered the threshold for use: people no longer need to start up computers or use keyboards in the traditional way. This opens up the possibility of Internet use to groups who had been excluded from its use before, such as many elderly people who may never have learned how to operate a desktop computer. For many people, a large icon that can be tapped with a finger, rather than clicked upon with a cursor, is easier to operate. For all of these reasons, efforts to develop remote monitoring tools, applications to report side effects or functional changes following new medications or treatments, or other web-based devices targeted at elderly patients prefer tablet computers (for example, Fanning and

McAuley 2014; Goyal, Bhaskar, and Singh 2012; Greysen et al. 2014; K. Morrison 2012).

Similarly, the widespread use of inexpensive battery-powered devices increases the range of Internet users in countries where stable power supply is an issue. The prohibitive costs of desktop computers have been a longtime obstacle to Internet use in the developing world, and in any case they are of little use without a stable supply of electricity. Consequently, the uptake of cell phones in low-income countries has been much faster than the uptake of personal computers, due to lower cost and the use of batteries; with the emergence of smartphones, Internet use has come within reach for new groups of people. Research supported by the Rockefeller Foundation reports a growth rate of 700 percent in mobile/smartphone/PC/tablet use between 2007 and 2012 (Hatt et al. 2013; see also Kirkpatrick 2013). The World Bank (2015) reports a 433 percent growth in Internet users in low- and middle-income countries between 2005 (6.9 percent) and 2015 (36.8 percent). If calculated for low-income countries alone, the growth rate of Internet users for the same period is 956 percent (from 0.9 percent to 9.5 percent). Although exact data on the proportion of people accessing the Internet via handheld and portable devices are not available, we can assume that this proportion is considerable: The proportion of cell phone subscriptions in low-income countries has risen from 4 to 60 percent between 2005 and 2015.

This rapid growth rate in mobile smartphone use in the developing world—which is, of course, also due to the low market saturation at baseline—has led authors to refer to the phenomenon as "mobile leap-frogging" (for a critical discussion of this issue, see Napoli and Obar 2013). An additional explanation for the greater popularity of portable devices, in both high- and low-income countries, is that they can be used in the privacy of people's homes. This is relevant for many Internet users, whether they have a specific reason for keeping their searches private or not. Most of us prefer to conduct our Internet searches and check our e-mail without being monitored. In societies where public media are seen to expose people to allegedly indecent content, any Internet use, especially by women, could be discouraged (see, for example, Armfield and Holbert 2003; Crompton, Ellison, and Stevenson 2002; Hakkarainen 2012; Oudshoorn and Pinch 2003; Wheeler 2001, 2003). Portable devices such as laptops, but especially inexpensive types of smartphones and tablet computers, provide women and men in such societies with a means to use the Internet without being exposed to familial or communal scrutiny. Such devices also make Internet access available whenever people need it, not only during particular limited hours of the day. For all these reasons, for an increasing proportion of Internet users worldwide, mobile-based access is the primary form of Internet use (Napoli and Obar 2014). And this, in turn, makes it easier for people to access health information online too (Ziebland and Wyke 2012).

In high-income countries, an important reason for people using the Internet for health-related purposes has been found to be the presence of chronic health problems. In 2010, the Pew Internet national survey of three thousand U.S. residents found that a quarter reported going online to interact with others who suffered from similar health-related problems (S. Fox 2011). Four years later, a survey by the same organization found that 72 percent reported having looked for health information online in the previous year. Eighteen percent had gone online specifically to find others with similar health conditions, with chronic disease sufferers being overrepresented (Pew Research Center 2015). Although most people seem to use the Internet in addition to consulting medical professionals, and not instead of it, when it comes to managing chronic diseases, many patients seem to trust other patients more than their doctors (Schaffer, Kuczynski, and Skinner 2008; Ziebland and Wyke 2012: 221).

In low-income countries, health-related Internet use is expanding. But partly due to the unaffordability of airtime and bandwidth in many places, those who use the Internet in the health care context tend to do so to obtain information, and not to upload content.

Within the group of non-users both in high- and low-income regions, the reasons for non-use are diverse. A major factor associated with nonuse remains education; in low-income countries, poor education corresponds with lower Internet access and less possibility to contribute content (Brake 2014). But in high-income countries such as the United States, too, Internet use in general, and web use for health purposes in particular, are unevenly distributed, and education is an important factor. Women, non-Hispanic whites, younger people, and those with higher levels of education use the Internet more, and they look for health information online more frequently (Pew Research Center 2011; see also Blum 2015). Those with lower levels of formal education are less likely to use the Internet (38 percent). And they are much less likely to seek health information online; only two-thirds of people with Internet access and lower levels of education do so (note that this does not apply to people with chronic illnesses. In this group, those with lower levels of education who have Internet access are equally as likely to use it for health-related purposes as everybody else does). By comparison, 90 percent of people with college degrees had Internet access, and almost all of them (89 percent) used it to obtain health information online.

In low-income countries, women are underrepresented among Internet users (Hilbert 2011). They are also underrepresented among content producers (Schradie 2015), meaning that many women are primarily passive information consumers (Olesen and Lewin 1985: 10; Riska 2010). The reasons for this are complex; they include the aforementioned stigmatization of Internet use by women in some cultures, due to the alleged risk of compromising their moral purity. Low literacy rates among women and the higher burdens of work and caring responsibilities carried by women in some countries also contribute to this situation. When it comes to the underrepresentation of women in content creation, not only lower digital literacy skills but also difficulties in getting past male gatekeepers have been found to hinder the participation of women and girls (Stephens 2013). Moreover, the overrepresentation of women among those who access health information in the United States needs to be seen in conjunction with the fact that most respondents reported searching for health information on behalf of somebody else, not themselves. Many women are going online in their capacity as mothers, wives, and caregivers.

Media studies scholars Philip Napoli and Jonathan Obar (2015) also make an interesting argument regarding the supposed "re-passification" of online audiences by mobile web-based services. They argue that people are less likely to lean forward when using mobile devices today than had been the case during the time when social media were used mostly on desktop personal computers. One of the reasons for this process of repassification, according to Napoli and Obar, is the aforementioned problem of unequal access to bandwidth. Limited bandwidth makes it difficult to upload content. Smartphone users in rich countries experience this when trying to send files while travelling on data-roaming plans abroad; in countries and places where good broadband is not available, however, this is the default state of Internet use. Such users cannot do much more than browse sites and passively consume information; they cannot create, play, and upload (see also Haklay 2009). Another reason for the repassification of Internet use is the popularity of smartphones, which are, as argued by Internet governance expert Lisa Horner, on average much more difficult to program for a wider variety of uses than personal computers (Horner 2011: 13).

Some media studies scholars have concluded that in times when (often inexpensive) mobile devices have become the primary means of online access for many people around the world, the most meaningful means of describing the digital divide is no longer by separating people into users and nonusers. Instead, the divide is between those who use the Internet mostly in passive and basic ways, and those who engage with it in more creative and deeper ways. This distinction is independent from how much time people spend online on a daily basis (see, for example, van Deursen and van Dijk 2014; Robinson et al. 2015; Wei 2012). People with poorer education and lower socioeconomic status—among whom women and ethnic minorities are overrepresented—tend to be in the passive group, although the relationship between these factors is far from linear. The picture is complicated further by the fact that lack of Internet access is not the only reason for nonuse. Some people deliberately decide to remain offline because of what media and technology expert David Brake calls "motivational" access barriers (Brake 2014): People feel that the Internet does not have anything worthwhile to offer, or they are concerned about privacy. Is the time or effort spent worth what we get out of it? Will my data be safe? In a review conducted by information studies scholars Stacey Morrison and Ricardo Gomez, the emotional cost of Internet use was identified as the single most important factor for people to limit or even opt out of information and communication technology use (Morrison and Gomez 2014). Among those who did use the Internet and decided to stop using it, or to use it less, the observation that Internet use made them feel worse, or disconnected from what mattered most in their lives (such as spending time with their families or friends), emerged as the most frequent motivation for this decision.

## *Where Internet Nonuse Is a Problem: The E-Health Filter Bubble*

In a world where medicine is increasingly driven by digital data, and where "activated" patients are expected to play a major role in contributing such data, any barrier that prevents people from using the Internet could be seen as a problem. It could be a problem because people who cannot or will not contribute data to the personalization of their health care forego the benefits of prevention, diagnosis, and treatment being tailored to their specific characteristics and circumstances (see also Lerman 2013). It could be an issue also because, as the previous section has shown, many barriers affect people with lower socioeconomic status more severely than others. Some access barriers are particularly problematic for ethnic minorities or women. Especially in areas where more and more medical and health-related services are offered online it seems troubling that some people who would want access do not have it. In high-income countries, tasks and services that are moving from the offline to the online domain include checking symptoms, making clinical appointments, and filling prescriptions; in low-income countries, it is often access to basic health information that is at stake when people do not have access to the Internet. And there is another reason why we should be concerned about unequal access: The use of data that people upload to social media, symptom checkers, and platforms such as PatientsLikeMe and CureTogether set new standards and reference points for how we understand our own health data (Prainsack 2015a). In clinical medicine, clinical reference values are typically derived from aggregate data at population level. They often draw upon subgroup analyses, for example, between patients suffering from specific diseases and healthy controls, different age groups, or pregnant women and others (Siest et al. 2013). For a long time, the categories used for sub-group analysis have been relatively generic, such as gender and age; only in the last two decades, categories such as ethnicity and genetic variation have been considered more systematically (e.g. Horn and Pesce 2002; Shirts, Wilson and Jackson 2011).

The data collected and processed in web-based tools such as symptom checkers or participatory patient platforms are of a very different kind than information and data collected in the clinic. At first sight, the algorithms that compare our data to the data of other people in web-based health platforms do the same as "traditional" epidemiological analyses have done: They map our characteristics against those of other patients so that our health data or test results are compared with the most relevant (that is, most similar in a relevant respect) group of people. The difference between clinical reference values on the one hand, and online health services on the other, however, is that people who do not use a specific online platform are not included in the population we compare ourselves to. A patient using CureTogether, for example, to see what treatments work for other patients who are similar to her, will only see data from a very specific group: a selected subset of an already heavily biased subset of the population, namely those who use Cure-Together in the first place. Here, the "filter bubble"—the phenomenon that information from our activities is used to "personalize" what we see (Pariser 2012)—enters medicine. It reinforces existing inequalities and lines of segregation in much more silent ways than in the case of explicit stratification for socioeconomic status or race. If the only difference that we see between ourselves and others lies in the severity and combination of our migraine symptoms, or in our genetic predisposition to respond well to blood thinners, then we may fail to notice that 80 percent of the people we compare ourselves to hold a university degree.

In this way we move farther and farther away from approaches that look at the whole population. The new normal is not what is most common in our state or our entire nation, but what is most common among people who are similar to us. Here, social inequalities are made worse by moving poor people, members of minority popuations, or women out of sight: They become, quite literally, "missing bodies" (Casper and Moore 2009). Furthermore, channeling public funding into privately held biobanks (Reuters 2014), within which white and wealthy people are starkly overrepresented and which are not accountable to the public regarding this problem, exacerbates old patterns of exclusion (Aicardi et al. 2016).

Taken together, these developments increase old patterns of exclusion and give rise to new ones. Adele Clarke and colleagues' notion of "exclusionary disciplining" is helpful here: The notion captures the simultaneous exclusionary actions of biomedicine "that erect barriers to access to medical institutions and resources that target and affect particular individuals and segments of populations" (Clarke et al. 2010c: 61). Although Clarke and colleagues' analysis focuses on the United States, it applies to global patterns of exclusion as well: Especially in low-income countries, where access to clinical services can be very difficult, people are targeted as information consumers online. They become the data sources for algorithms and services put to use for the benefit of people in the rich world.

## The Blessings of Internet Abstinence? The Downsides of Being a Patient Researcher

So far I have discussed the ways in which not participating in web-based communication and data collection can disadvantage people. But can abstaining from these things also be an advantage? Is it desirable to be below the "digital radar"? To answer this question, it is again important to consider that data from activities that patients engage in—from looking up symptoms online to technologically facilitated interactions with health professionals—can be harnessed for research purposes. The two web-based platforms discussed in this chapter, PatientsLikeMe and CureTogether, are cases in point: In both cases, data curation for medical decision making and research are intertwined. Somebody who uploads data on changes in her mood and well-being when starting to take a new antidepressant, for example, could be contributing to research without even being aware of it (see also Purtova 2015).

Although some platforms, including PatientsLikeMe, place great emphasis on being transparent about how they use data and information that users share on their website (PatientsLikeMe 2014a), in the case of many other services, it is not immediately apparent to users how their data are processed and utilized by others. Not all users are conscious of the fact that by using these platforms, they are creating value for others, often for commercial enterprises. Part of the reason for this is that online platforms and services often make heavy use of language around community and sharing, leading users to believe that they are doing this for the common good when in fact they are also creating tangible financial benefits for the platform. When the latter becomes apparent to users, irritation is often the result. When the personal-genome-testing company 23andMe, which acquired CureTogether, was granted a patent for gamete donor selection in 2012, for example, many users were displeased. The patent was granted for a technology that enables prospective parents to select egg or sperm donors who would be more likely to pass on desirable traits to their offspring, developed on the basis of the DNA and phenotypic information provided to the company by their paying customers (Rimmer 2012; Sterckx and Cockbain 2014). The problem was not that the company had applied for patents; it is a commercial company after all. The issue was that it had done it behind its customers' backs. The company's self-portrayal as the spearhead of a movement that made medicine more democratic, as the driver of a revolution in disease research that wriggled power out of the hands of established experts and gave it to regular people, was at odds with the company's old school approach to intellectual property protection and their hiding of information on it in the small print of the terms of service (Prainsack 2014a; see also Sterckx et al. 2013).

## The Darker Side of Data-Driven Medicine: Three "H"s of Digital Surveillance

Digital data collection and use in our societies is characterized by what I called the three "H"s of digital surveillance (Prainsack 2015b). The first "H" stands for *hypercollection*. It refers to situations where just because institutions can collect information about customers or citizens, they do. CCTV cameras, company loyalty cards, or the retention of geolocation data by telephone companies are all based on the principle of "collect first, use later." And although many data-protection laws provide that no more data than strictly necessary for a specific purpose should be collected and processed, if people give their consent for their personal data to be collected or used for wider purposes, this is perfectly legal. Very often, this consent is given by ticking a box or clicking on "I agree" buttons online, which many people do without giving any consideration to what they are agreeing to. Such data collection takes place in the name of possible future benefits: CCTV cameras collect data that could, eventually, be useful for criminal investigation and crime control. Retail companies collect data on people's shopping patterns and behaviors because they can offer people discounts that match products of their interest—digital home assistants such as Google Home or Amazon's Echo, which switch on your heating, send your emails for you, or look for a song that you like, are but the most extreme example. Home-assistant devices are relatively cheap—because you are "paying" the company by giving them access to information about what music you listen to, what movies you watch, and when the light goes on and off in your house. Geolocation data collected by mobile phone providers ensures that they get vouchers or discount offers on their cell phones exactly at the time they are entering the shopping mall. In some cases, people can also trade personal data for cheaper drugs, or for access to other products that they would otherwise not be able to afford (Greenhalgh 2015; Robbins 2015). In other words, greater "personalization" of services is often portrayed as the boon of hypercollection. But the flip side of the benefits of personalization is that data can be used to discern patterns that can then be applied back to make probabilistic statements about individuals. As a result, as Helga Nowotny put it, people have become "more exposed to the laws of chance in the form of probabilities" (Nowotny 2016: 63).

This brings me to the second "H" of digital surveillance, which stands for *harm*. Despite the positive rhetoric about the benefits of data-driven personalization, many corporative actors do not collect data to help people, but to do other things, such as increasing revenue and profits. Although some of these goals overlap with public goods—crime control is an example—they can inflict considerable harm on individuals who, on the basis of an algorithm, have a mortgage or insurance application declined or become the subject of an investigation. This can happen to anybody, even the most upright, hardworking and law-abiding person. Taken individually, most pieces of information used for predictive analytics in this manner look entirely innocent and unable to hurt the person they pertain to. Who could do anything bad with the information that I regularly buy orange juice and like to go skiing? This is what makes today's digital surveillance so hard to see: It is not my drinking orange juice, going skiing, or accessing particular types of websites that make me suspicious, but the combination of these factors in conjunction with the insight that the same combination has been found in other people who display a particular characteristic. If predictive analytics suggests that I am a particularly "risky" or a particularly desirable customer, I may be charged less, or more, for the same service. Or I may be excluded from being offered certain services altogether.

No type of information is exempt from this dynamic. Experts suggest, for example, that hospitals and doctors should use predictive analytics to identify patients who, after a surgical intervention, have a particularly high risk of complications, and offer them extra care (King 2015; Shams, Ajorlou, and Yang 2015). It is not hard to imagine what the flip side of such extra care would look like: Risky patients are also costly patients, and costly patients are unwelcome "customers" in the health care system and elsewhere. Also, some visions of personalized medicine include the integration of wide ranges of information about people—including credit card purchases, social media activity, and even criminal records—together with their health records into the "tapestry of health data" (Weber, Mandl, and Kohane 2014). In the context of predictive analytics, it has become impossible to separate "health data" from non-health data, because any type of information can be mined and analyzed to draw conclusions for any particular trait.

The third "H" indeed stands for *humiliation*. People feel humiliated when their status or dignity is diminished. One of the archetypical examples of humiliation is when people have to participate in harming others or themselves. In the context of digital surveillance, people are regularly humiliated by having to trade their privacy for something that they cannot otherwise afford. I already mentioned patients who "agree" to pharmaceutical companies using their personal information in return for access to more affordable drugs (Hiltzik 2015). Other examples include "risky" borrowers who are pushed into consenting to having sensors installed in their cars. These sensors allow banks to know where they are, and to remotely shut down the engine if borrowers default on their repayment (Corkery and Silver-Greenberg 2014). A further example are people in low-income countries who are encouraged to download apps on their cell phones that monitor their communication patterns and online behavior in exchange for microcredits. "For example, are the majority of someone's calls longer than four minutes? Good: They may have stronger relationships and be a better credit risk" (Lidsky 2015).

The company that invented this model of asking poor people to trade information on their online and mobile communication for access to loans has been celebrated as empowering people who would otherwise not get credit to obtain one. None of these celebratory accounts considers it a possibility that the core problem to be solved is that these people live in poverty in the first place. Moreover, none of these accounts mentions the humiliation involved in a person having to agree to a company monitoring and assessing the quality of her relationships. Such practices have been normalized; they are part of what people are supposed to experience when they do not have enough resources to buy a car or get a loan. It is part of the governance regime of our societies, and it has been for a long time; with predictive analytics it is now also entering digital health.

Does this mean that the safest thing to do is to refrain from participating in health-related online activities altogether, and to limit the information about ourselves that we give consent to health care providers to use? Or is there another solution? There is a clear need for public actors here to regulate not only how personal information can be used by commercial and public entities, but also what kind of information can be collected about people in the first place. Moreover, as I will argue in the second part of this book, enhancing harm-mitigation instruments is a crucial step to start addressing the power asymmetries that exist between those whose data are used, and those who use data. But regulation is not the only answer: Laws and regulations are often toothless when it comes to large multinational companies. The latter can evade regulation, or influence the very rules that were designed to control them. Moreover, public authorities are in the seemingly paradoxical position of having the responsibility to protect its citizens from harm from digital surveillance while at the same time benefitting from it. The solution must thus also come also from us, the citizens: from citizens who resist surveillance from both "Big Brother and Company Man," as the American legal scholar Jerry Kang and colleagues (2012) called it; from citizens who demand to know what kind of information is held about them in public and private repositories (Lunshof, Church, and Prainsack 2014); and from citizens who donate data to "information commons" that use data strictly for public benefit, instead of signing them over to those who monitor us for their own profit.

## Conclusion

Although some authors and practitioners celebrate every instance of data transfer from a patient to a web-based platform as an instance of the democratization of medicine or science, others blame participatory practices and initiatives in the domain of medicine of unduly romanticizing patient "empowerment." Indeed, merely labeling an initiative as participatory or empowering does not mean that power relationships change. In order to see how power relations change, we need to take a close look at exactly how patients or others participate in certain tasks, and what they contribute. And we need to look at the wider political and economic landscape that these practices are embedded in.

Patient activist Gilles Frydman (2013) famously defined "participatory medicine" as "a movement in which networked patients shift from being mere passengers to responsible drivers of their health, and in which providers encourage and value them as full partners" (see also Hughes, Joshi, and Wareham 2008). In this view, the primary agency still lies, ironically, with health care providers, who "encourage and value" patients as "full partners"; this means that for patients to be fully "empowered," they need to be encouraged and valued by others first. Here, the metaphor of the car is useful: It is true that drivers are the ones in charge of operating the car, but they are not always the ones deciding where to go. They can also only operate the car if they have enough money to obtain a car in the first place, and to pay for fuel and maintenance costs. A more desirable picture of genuinely participatory medicine—one where the agency of people to make decisions that are meaningful to them and their significant others—would be a system of roads that allows drivers of different vehicles to go wherever they wanted in any vehicle they chose, whether it be a bike, a bus, or a high-end sports car, while allowing others to ditch these forms of transport altogether and choose to walk. People would decide what vehicle to use, if any; whether to build it themselves, rent, or share it. The fact that people's freedom to make these decisions is inevitably limited by the means and resources available to them is an issue that merits a discussion in its own right. The key point here, however, is that genuine empowerment of people in the domain of health and medicine requires (a) the provision of publicly funded infrastructures that de facto enable choice (to continue the car metaphor, this would be the provision of a road system and good public transportation), and (b) recognition that it can be the expression of a person's autonomy to decide *not* to drive a car. The opportunity to participate must not become a duty.

It is *not* a requirement for genuinely participatory medicine that medical professionals encourage and value this participation. While ethicists, clinicians, and regulatory agencies in many countries are still deliberating whether or not particular forms of patient participation are worthy of their support, and discussing how patients can be protected in areas where they are considered not to be competent enough to understand what they are doing, patients are voting with their feet—and with their computers. PatientsLikeMe and CureTogether, the two platforms discussed in this chapter, are but two examples. They illustrate how lean-forward online technologies in particular, by collecting data and information from users, turn everybody into a data source. This, as I argued, blurs the boundary between patients and research contributors. And this dynamic can turn patients into tools for cost cutting. Here, the empowerment rhetoric helps to conceal this fact. Many initiatives that call themselves "participant-led" are not actually led by participants but by the people owning and running the platforms, or by organizations that facilitate these participatory practices (see also McGowan et al. 2017). Moreover, the fact that many of these platforms and organizations are for-profit is an unintended consequence of neglect on the side of public and governmental actors: While public actors are discussing how to limit the alleged risks of online platforms for patients, they leave the creation of digital infrastructures and other health innovation to commercial actors. The acquisition of CureTogether by the personal genomics testing company 23andMe is a case in point (see also Masum 2012; Trevena 2011). Such developments contribute to an even stronger concentration of power and expertise among commercial actors, rendering—quite ironically—the very participatory practices that are often celebrated as democratizing medicine a tool to increase commercial revenue and power.

And to increase commercial revenue and power, it is necessary that patients remain engaged in participatory practices on a continuous basis. As I will argue in the next chapter, online platforms and devices turn patients into permanent contributors of data, information, time, and effort. Participatory patients need to be permanently "on."

3

# Always On

## *The Transmitting Patient*

## Introduction

In 2013, the American author Dave Eggers wrote a book titled *The Circle*. With many people it hit a nerve: The book paints a picture of a future in which people's lives take place primarily on social media. People have forgotten what it is like to live offline, and anybody who tries to reanimate their old analogous selves is cast out of society. People have *become* their social media profiles and other digital representations. And this spills over also into the political domain: In Dave Eggers' book, the social media company that provides the central setting of the story eventually takes over the role also of state authorities to run elections.

One would expect that in such dystopic visions, health care features as a *Gattaca*-like[1] enterprise where people have their genome sequenced at birth and are stratified into different groups according to their genetic predispositions. Perhaps those with problematic genetic predispositions are sorted out right away so that society saves itself the cost of investing in them. What we find in the book, however, is very different. In none of the scenes that revolve around health care—and there are quite a few of them—is DNA even mentioned. The scenarios *are* futuristic: In the first scene, Mae, the protagonist of the story, is called in for an appointment with an occupational physician upon starting her new job at The Circle. When Mae arrives, her physician knows more about Mae's health status than Mae herself, mostly on the basis of Mae's health information stored online, and through an analysis of Mae's social media activities. During Mae's visit with the doctor, a number of tests are run on Mae and she is asked to drink a smoothie containing nanosensors; these will measure a number of biomarkers from inside her body. She is also given a sensor to wear around her wrist to monitor her heart rate. Every two weeks, Mae is told, she will need to come back to see her doctor to run a battery of tests including blood work, cognitive tests, reflexes, eye exams, and occasionally also magnetic resonance imaging (MRI). When Mae inquires about the cost of the comprehensive monitoring provided to her free of charge her doctor explains: "Well, prevention is cheap. Especially compared to finding some Stage-4 lump when we could have found it at Stage 1" (Eggers 2013: 153).

How does this futuristic fictional scenario compare to the actual, nonfictional world? Even in the richest countries, most patients are not given nanosensors to swallow. Some, however, are asked to wear a rubber bangle that measures their heart rate, or tracks their sleep patterns (see also Piwek et al. 2016). Similarly, while only few patients are expected to monitor their own health information in real time such practices are becoming more common. The technologies supporting it are already available, in the form of apps such as Apple Health Kit on mobile phones and smart watches, or wearable stress sensors that feed data directly into people's health records (Schatz 2015).

Regarding the recording and use of DNA sequence information, in contrast, in most countries, DNA testing is still limited to a relatively narrow range of scenarios. These include newborn screening for specific diseases such as phenylketonuria (a heritable metabolic disorder), testing for markers of heritable genetic diseases (carrier testing), or diagnostic testing in cases where a specific genetic disease is suspected. It is unlikely that every newborn will be DNA sequenced at birth in the near future and that this information will be stored in a central registry; if only because the storage costs are too high. The cheapest way to store DNA information is still in the person herself. Whenever genetic or genomic information is needed, this can be done on an ad-hoc basis, cheaply and rapidly, and allowing health care professionals to focus on the exact markers and information that a specific diagnostic or therapeutic question requires. In this sense, *The Circle* seems a much more sober and at the same time more chilling vision of the future: There is no compulsory genetic screening and no new class of genetic cast-outs, but everybody participates in self-monitoring to improve themselves and cut costs.

In chapter 2, I focused on the changing role of the Internet in the domain of health and medicine. I explored how the role of the Internet in this domain has changed from providing information to patients to being a tool that both provides information to users and takes data from them. I also argued that patients increasingly become data providers for research and other purposes. This chapter complements this analysis by exploring how digital (self-)surveillance systems both inside and outside the medical domain include ever larger parts of our bodies and lives. This resonates with the ideal of personalized medicine bringing us closer to a situation where patients are comprehensively monitored, often in unobtrusive ways. Within this vision, any data, regardless of what they represent and where they come from, are potentially health-relevant. Any digital surveillance is potentially health surveillance. And people are becoming data transmitters by default.

## *Always On: Data Transmission as a Default State*

The proliferation of touch-screen-fitted mobile phones and portable computers not only marks changes in dominant patterns of Internet use but also serves as a powerful metaphor for how people increasingly operate in the domains of health and medicine. The simultaneity and "in-between-ness" of online and offline status symbolized by the tablet computer is paradigmatic for how people can—and are often expected to—function with regard to matters of their health. The tablet computer is always on; even when it is not being used it is continuously on standby and can be activated by a simple touch, or by opening the cover. Although tablet computers can be switched off, they are not meant to. In the words of a user of an online technology forum, "none of the electronic components in an iPad suffer from being constantly on" (Maybury 2013). The power button is mostly there to reboot when there is a problem. The long battery life of tablet computers, and increasingly also laptops, enables a state of permanent standby. Moreover, applications on most tablets can remain open without users being aware of it—because we forgot to close them, or because they are intended to be open without being visible. Cell phones transmit data even when location services have been switched off, enabling more precise geolocation. In this way, data transmission has become a default state, long before any of us have started using wearable sensors or smart glasses.

Like applications on our tablet, applications and devices used for health monitoring can be at work continuously in our homes, on our bodies, or even inside our bodies (Lucivero and Dalibert 2013), without requiring any conscious work on our part. Such sensors can monitor sleep, body temperature, or even muscle activity entirely in unobtrusive ways.[2] Information scholars Stacey Morrison and Ricardo Gomez referred to the expectation of permanent connectivity as "evertime." Like the tablet computer, we are always (at least) on standby. Telemonitoring devices, web-based tools, and data transmitting or receiving items and "the Internet of Things" (IoT) around us render this possible.

The outsourcing of clinical tasks into the homes of patients, as Brown and Webster emphasized over a decade ago, has long been a feature in the "fantasies and ambitions of medical technology" (N. Brown and Webster 2004: 86; see also Oudshoorn 2011: 6). But plans and pilots for data capture nowadays go much further: Personalized medicine, many visionaries believe, will need to capture as many data from people as possible, at any stage of health and disease. When data are collected from people throughout their entire lives, people can become their own "control group": Data at moments of disease can be compared to data during periods of health. The idea is that by establishing a baseline of normal physiological functioning of a person, irregularities become detectable by means of digital monitoring, often before people experience any symptoms (see also Massachusetts General Hospital 2016). This could, of course, be seen as another example of the phenomenon of data hypercollection (chapter 2): Data are collected just because it is possible to do so, without clear evidence on what can be achieved with this approach, and without a substantive discussion about the societal and ethical implications of this.

In addition, practices of data collection for medical purposes increasingly overlap with data collection for wider purposes, such as in the case of the Hudson Yards, an 18-million-square-foot redevelopment in New York City. Hudson Yards has been celebrated as the largest private real estate project in the United States. It will include the first so-called quantified community, where an estimated sixty-five thousand people per day—ideally everybody who lives there or passes through—will contribute data on every aspect of life, from shopping behavior to how many steps they take per day. The masterminds of the Hudson Yards project at New York University's Center for Urban Science and Progress see themselves as responding to a growing "demand" of surveillance. In their words: "This is just what residents in cities are demanding. As the urban population grows globally, if we are going to really address the most pressing problems of society—whether that is climate change or public health—it's really going to be in our cities that we do it" (Constantine Kontokosta, quoted in Leber 2014; see also Kontokosta 2016).

## The Expansion of Digital Surveillance: "Personalized" Patient Work at Home

Patient work at home, and home self-monitoring in particular, is nothing new. Some parts of people's health- and self-care have always taken place at home. For one, many patients take medicines and follow doctor's orders in their own homes. Moreover, before the establishment of hospitals, the main place for treating and coping with disease and illness and caring for the sick was the home. But in the era of digital medicine, some aspects of the collection, transmission, analysis, and use of data and information in people's homes and personal domains are being reconfigured. I have already mentioned the impact on privacy that digital surveillance technologies can have: They make patients "readable" at a distance. Patient data are read, and centrally stored, by remote actors—human or nonhuman—often without the same information being accessible by patients themselves (see also Bannan 2016).

Another concern is that for patients, the "script" provided by digital surveillance technologies in the health domain is much more detailed and much harder to deviate from than it has been the case before the digital era. As Nelly Oudshoorn (2011: 10–11) argues, there is

> an important difference between telecare technologies and devices such as the inhaler for asthma or the familiar thermometer. Whereas using a thermometer or asthma inhaler can be considered as isolated individual acts that patients can perform wherever and whenever they prefer, the use of telecare devices is materially and morally integrated into a network of care that guides and restricts the actions of patients.

Digital home surveillance technologies thus constrain patients at the same time that they give them more freedom by allowing patients to go home earlier, to move around more, etc. Digital surveillance technologies in medicine typically also enlist a wider range of actors, and sometimes even create new ones, such as the telemedicine nurse (Oudshoorn 2011: 9).

Criminologists Kevin Haggerty and Richard Ericson used the term "surveillant assemblage" to refer to systems comprising technological tools and human practices for the purpose of monitoring (Haggerty and Ericson 2000). A surveillant assemblage "operates by abstracting human bodies from their territorial settings, and separating them into a series of discrete flows. These flows are then reassembled in different locations as discrete and virtual 'data doubles'" (Haggerty and Ericson 2000: 605). When Haggerty and Ericson coined this term they had security systems in mind, such as those at airports; many of these systems have not been set up in a systematic, top-down manner but instead have grown organically to combine different tools and practices yielding different kinds of data. This focus on horizontal monitoring is different from the reality of most telemedicine and telecare systems, which typically have one center, not many. This can limit the analytic utility of the surveillant assemblage in the given context. But what the concept of the surveillant assemblage does offer is that it allows us to analyze power dynamics that work in all directions. It does not require a focus on one specific technological instrument or practice. Another advantage of the concept of a surveillant assemblage is that it enables us to see how seemingly contradictory motives and experiences, such as "desires for control, governance, security, profit and entertainment," often come together (Haggerty and Ericson 2000: 609; see also Prainsack and Toom 2010).

As the following example illustrates, the concept of the surveillant assemblage can help us understand essential aspects of contemporary digital health surveillance that may otherwise be overlooked, especially if we focus on its oppressive aspects from the outset.

## Helping Patients Get Better (People): Telemonitoring with CardioConsult HF

CardioConsult HF is a computerized decision-support system developed by Curit BV (curit.com), a Dutch company specializing in disease management and telemedicine. CardioConsult HF is not a single device, but an "ICT driven disease management system" for heart failure (HF) patients (de Vries et al. 2011: 433). It includes devices that measure blood and weight, a health monitor to be used in the patient's home, and a computerized management system based in a hospital.[3] The reason for the home device measuring patients' blood pressure and weight is that a change in blood pressure or sudden weight gain (due to fluid retention) could indicate an episode of heart failure. If a patient's biomarkers are outside a predefined range, the health monitor guides the patient through a range of questions to assess whether there is need for concern; if the patient's answers indicate that there is, the nurse on telecare duty is alerted by e-mail and text message. If the patient's systolic blood pressure, for example, is too high, the patient will be told: "Your blood pressure is higher than normal, do you have any complaints?" If the patient states that she feels fine, she is asked to monitor her blood pressure more closely in the following twenty-four hours. If the patient feels unwell in any way, the nurse is alerted and supposed to contact the patient within two hours. She will also check and adjust the medication if necessary (see de Vries et al. 2011: 435).

In 2011, the Dutch health care professional Arjen de Vries and colleagues published a detailed case description of a fifty-year-old patient with a high number of hospital readmissions due to heart failure over a number of years. The patient had already had a cardioverter defibrillator, a device to detect and treat life-threatening arrhythmias with electrical pulses, implanted. When the patient was admitted to hospital five times within only six months with symptoms such as dehydration or decreased blood flow in the brain, his medical team decided it was time to sign him up to a telemonitoring program (de Vries et al. 2011: 433).

CardioConsult HF was the system of choice. The specific patient in this case study is reported to have been very happy with the system. In the words of the authors, the "presence of the telemonitoring devices at home, as well as the reassurance that deviating or missing data generate an alarm, gave him a sense of safety and had a positive effect on his compliance" (de Vries et al. 2011: 436). The patient also said that he could integrate the activities that the system required him to do "into his life without any problems" (de Vries et al. 2011: 436). Despite this positive account of the patient, and the authors' conclusion that "we were probably able to prevent at least two readmissions for heart failure in a period of 10 months" (de Vries et al. 2011: 432), the authors remained skeptical of the benefit of telemonitoring overall. They noted that evidence on the effectiveness of telemonitoring was inconclusive and that it was currently not possible to determine in advance what types of patients will benefit (de Vries et al. 2011: 433).

Why is it so difficult to determine in advance what types of patients will benefit from telemonitoring? One reason is that telemonitoring—which, according to de Vries (2013), is used in about 35 percent of all heart failure patients in the Netherlands[4]—cannot normally monitor all relevant parameters (see also Dierckx et al. 2015). It could thus be the case that relevant information is not recorded. Moreover, for some patients, the constant presence of the disease in their homes, as well as the need to inform the hospital when leaving the home, is burdensome (de Vries et al. 2011: 437). Ethics experts Tom Sorell and Heather Draper also argue that because the devices enable people to spend more time at home rather than in the hospital or in the doctor's office, telecare technologies in particular bear the risk of increasing social isolation (Sorell and Draper 2012). This is even more dangerous for people who are already marginalized. Finally, telemonitoring systems could also give patients and those caring for them a false sense of security, suggesting that the system will "think for them" (de Vries et al. 2011: 437; see also Ridderikhoff and van Herk 1999).

It is neither desirable nor possible to conclude in general terms whether the use of digital surveillance tools is a good development within the personalization of medicine. Practices of digital surveillance empower some people in specific contexts and disempower others in other contexts, and it requires an analysis of concrete cases to say when they do what. What the concept of the surveillant assemblage helps us do is not to look at individual surveillance technologies in isolation but to see them as driven by the desire "to combine practices and technologies and integrate them into a larger whole" (Haggerty and Ericson 2000: 610). This "whole" is not merely a technological supersystem but is, as the term suggests, an assemblage of technologies, practices, and discourses. If we looked only at the CardioConsult HF system in isolation, as a technical system to address a specific medical problem, we would miss the larger story outside of clinical and medical parameters;

we would be missing the societal expectations and practices that are key enablers of the system.

In the case of the patient discussed by de Vries and colleagues, what exactly is the problem that the telemonitoring system was supposed to solve? According to the authors, it was meant to reduce the hospitalization risk for a person with heart problems. But there is an interesting dimension in de Vries and colleagues' case description that the authors do not elaborate on. In the beginning of their paper, they introduce their patient as a "50-year-old, unemployed, man, who was living alone" (de Vries et al. 2011: 433). As the likely cause for the man's frequent hospitalizations they identify "a combination of factors, including a lack of compliance with dietary and fluid restrictions, symptoms of depression, and a delay in seeking care when symptoms of deterioration occurred" (de Vries et al. 2011: 433). This tells us a totally different story from the main narrative in their paper: The reason for including the patient in a telemonitoring system seems to have been that the patient lived alone. It is standard procedure in high- and middle-income countries to advise patients with heart failure to weigh themselves regularly and keep track of any relevant changes. If the patient in this study had done this, telemonitoring would not have been necessary. We can only speculate about the reasons for this specific patient's inability to be "compliant enough" to manage without telemonitoring. Had it to do with his depression? Or with the absence of significant others in his home environment who could have helped him keep track of his weight or blood pressure, or motivated him to try to get better? The paper remains quiet about these factors. But it is clear that the purpose of telemonitoring, in the case of this patient, was not only to detect early signs of heart problems and avoid the need for rehospitalization but also to compensate for some perceived deficiencies in his social and home environment. The system did not only seek to help him get better, but also sought to compensate for the lack of his social networks—in a medically relevant way. The help offered to the patient in the CardioConsult HF case does not address the problem by its social roots, such as having somebody visit him on a daily basis. Instead the patient is offered a technological solution that captures data. What is then analyzed is thus not the patient himself but an inevitably incomplete and skewed digital representation of him.

This digital data-driven approach resonates with a vision of personalized medicine that sees the future of health care as treating the digital data doubles of people (ESF 2012; Hood and Auffray 2013; National Research Council of the Academies 2011; Topol 2015). What is noteworthy, however, is that these visions do not plan for patients to have any say in what *types* of data from and about them will be used for this purpose. Their only way of influencing what data will be used about them is by refusing to participate in telemonitoring in the first place. Doing this, however, could have serious repercussions for patients.

The de facto absence of a feasible opt-out scenario is also noteworthy because efforts to integrate health data are not limited to data in the medical domain. The neuroscientist and self-tracker Rachel Kalmar draws a particularly vivid picture of what a future of comprehensive data capture and data integration could look like: the "possibilities, and the fun," says Kalmar, "increase dramatically when [ . . . ] devices talk to each other: when the refrigerator door won't open until your health monitor registers a minimum number of steps" (quoted in Denison 2013). Whether or not we agree that such a scenario would be fun, Kalmar's vision shows us how closely medical and moral aims can be intertwined in seemingly value neutral disease management plans, and how fluid the boundary between lifestyle and health care have become (Lucivero and Prainsack 2015). All of these points are also apparent in the next example, which is one where data are, quite literally, taken out of thin air: It concerns an activity tracking metric offered by the sportswear company Nike.

### Just Do It? Nike's Fuel

In 2012, Nike launched an activity tracker in the form of a bracelet called FuelBand. The wearable components of the FuelBand consisted of a black plastic bracelet with a rubber surface and an illuminated digital display. The bracelet contained an accelerometer and a USB connector to be used for synchronization with the computer, or with Apple portable devices. It also gave the time.

FuelBand received its name from the company's operating metric, so-called fuel units. The creation of this generic activity metric meant that FuelBand users could compare their activity levels across different times and dates irrespective of the kind of activity they were engaged in—playing tennis, cleaning the house, or running after a bus. It also enabled users to compete with each other for activity ("fuel") ratings. Users who entered their height, weight, and age could also see the average number of Fuel points that people with similar characteristics obtained in a single day. Since 2014, Nike FuelBand users have also been able to analyze and visualize user data longitudinally (see Nike 2014). In the fall of the same year, Apple launched its Health Kit, an integrated platform for fitness and health data; soon thereafter it was announced that the iPhone could do the activity tracking directly so that FuelBand users would no longer need to wear the bracelet. Fuel tracking was integrated in iPhones or other Apple devices via a Nike+ app, which in the meantime has also become available for other types of smartphones. (Shortly after launching this app, Nike stopped selling FuelBand bracelets, although it retained the name for its activity-tracking software and app working via smartphones.)

In order to explain how Nike's Fuel and other very popular fitness and activity-tracking devices—such as Fitbit or Jawbone—operate, I will use the example of Jesper, a student in his early twenties living in Copenhagen.[5] Jesper liked many types of sports, ranging from sailing and cycling to golf. During a visit to the United States in the summer of 2013, he bought a FuelBand wristband, and by the time I spoke to him a year later, the two had become inseparable: Jesper said that he took it off only to take a shower ("it's 'water resistant,' but not really waterproof. I don't want to take the risk"), but then wore it for the entire day. About twice an hour, Jesper told me, he looked at his wrist to see how many Fuel points he had received; in the evening he usually also looked at the data on his iPhone or at his desktop computer: "I look at my Fuel points and when I see I have not yet reached my goal, I may take a walk to get my Fuel points for the day. [ . . . ] You get this little satisfactory feeling just because you've reached your goal." When I asked him whether it would be correct to say that FuelBand made him work out more, Jesper corrected me: "I wouldn't say 'work out more,' but 'move more.'" For Jesper, the FuelBand was clearly not only a sports tool but something that was integrated into his day-to-day routines. Jesper had no problem treating the FuelBand as something that was part of his life and yet something "foreign" at the same time. Although it was a piece of technology that was conceivably his, it also entailed elements that are the intellectual property of somebody else. For example, Jesper was well aware that Nike kept the algorithm used to translate raw activity data into Fuel secret, but he did not mind. He had his own ideas about it ("it must have something to do with steps and how fast you go"), but he had never tried to find out exactly how it works.[6]

At the end of our conversation I asked Jesper whether he viewed FuelBand as something that could be relevant to his health. He said he could envisage that it could be used to compare people with a very active lifestyle on the one hand, and people who lead a very sedentary lifestyle on the other:

It's not completely accurate, because a bodybuilder gets Fuel points for going to the gym, but he doesn't get as many Fuel points as somebody who runs 20km every day. And with regard to diet, you could go [out] on a limb and say that people who lead more active lifestyles also eat more healthily. And maybe for myself, if I use it for a couple of years and if I [then] look at my app, where you can look back at several years, and I can see that two years ago I was more active than I am now, I could want to do something about it.

By wearing his FuelBand, Jesper collected and transmitted data by default, even when he was not actively and consciously involved in it, and even when he was asleep; he was both online and offline at the same time. Here we encounter a surveillant assemblage that does not stop with the specific monitoring system that the hard- and software of FuelBand represents; it links together virtually all aspects of a person's life. In Nike's own narrative, the Fuel system makes people formulate goals and try to reach them, encouraging them not only to compare their own performance longitudinally over days, weeks, and a year but also competing with others. The company actively encourages users to include virtually every activity that they are involved in, work and play, in their competition for best performance; to "turn every day into a game" (Nike 2015). The only parts of the day that do not count are those when people are unproductive; when they rest, relax, or sleep, and when not even their wrists move over a keyboard. FuelBand thereby also serves a particular kind of governmentality: It aims to make people want to be more productive, while feeling they are playing a "game." Corporate wellness programs where employees get rewarded for being physically active use the exact same rationale (see also P. Moore and Robinson 2016; Till 2014).

This connection between digitally measurable activity and productivity also solidifies the association between stereotypically masculine forms of physical activity, such as vigorous sports, and productivity. Physical labor done mostly by women remains, literally, pointless. Nursing and other caring activities, for example, do not often entail rapid movement, which scores the most points. Activity trackers thus perpetuate the traction of mainstream theories of production and value, which have, throughout history, had a bias toward what was seen as typically men's work. In David Graeber's words, "burly men hammering away at glowing iron, sparks flying everywhere—the term 'production' brings most readily to mind" (Graeber 2001: 68; see also M. Stacey 1984). This applies also to the production of Fuel points.

## *Activity Tracking in the Name of Personalized Health Surveillance*

Activity trackers such as FuelBand do not just play a role in fitness tracking for leisure; they are also relevant for health-related uses. They have the potential to bring information about a patient's activity levels, muscle power, and other relevant information to the table—the kind of information in between doctor's visits that gets us closer to comprehensive personalized patient surveillance. For Dennis Ausiello and Stanley Shaw at Massachusetts General Hospital, the next big challenge in medicine is to "quantify wellness and disease in a more continuous manner, and as our patients lead their daily lives" (2014: 221). They propose that smartphones, wearable devices, and other sensing devices should be used to "make the gathering of measurements more unobtrusive to the individual" (222). Another advantage that they see is that data from such devices can be sent directly to medical teams and caregivers to make data capture more "complete." But such visions, as well-meaning as they may be, also construct anyone not willing or able to participate in such passive data capture as incomplete.

Incomplete Patients: Technological Challenges and the Pleasures of Self-Surveillance

One challenge that visionaries such as Dennis Ausiello and Stanley Shaw still need to solve on the way to continuous and unobtrusive patient monitoring is the integration of data from different devices. Making different devices and systems of digital health surveillance "speak" to one another is a difficult challenge. The Google Maps metaphor put forward by the National Research Council of the U.S. National Academies of Sciences (chapter 1) proposes a health data system comprising multiple kinds of layered and integrated data sets to underpin personalized medicine (National Research Council of the Academies 2011). It could be seen to suggest that the challenge of integrating different kinds of data into a meaningful whole has already been solved. But this is not the case: It is a vision, and not a depiction of what is currently possible.[7] Although approaches such as the "semantic web"—a collaborative quest to enable the sharing of content beyond the boundaries of applications and websites[8]—are making big advances in addressing data integration issues, we still lack solutions that could make the Google map of health or similar integrated personal health repositories a reality. Medical practitioners and patients complain about the lack of portability of data between electronic health records of different institutions, not to mention between different countries (see, for example, B. Smith et al. 2007; Taweel et al. 2011). Moreover, there are no universal standards for how data should be structured, or what metadata (such as annotation) should be provided with them (see also Özdemir et al. 2014).

Another currently unresolved issue is the trustworthiness of data collected outside of the clinic. We briefly encountered this issue when discussing the lithium study that patients on the PatientsLikeMe platform had organized (chapter 2). Problems of data quality also pertain to data collected in the clinic, but this does not normally affect the willingness of clinicians to work with them because these data have been collected by their colleagues, or by other academically trained professionals. Some clinicians and other professionals, however, are hesitant to work with data collected by patients. This concern must be taken seriously, especially in contexts where measurements are difficult to standardize. Where measurements concern parameters that are in themselves subjective, such as mood, or pain, many experts agree that patients are better placed to collect and record these data than others (for example, Dawson et al. 2011). In the words of Ethan Basch (2009), an oncologist at Harvard Medical School, in the area of evaluating drug safety, patients have a key role to play: When data on drug safety are collected by clinicians, certain types of information are often left out. This can be the case because doctors or nurses are not used to asking about certain topics, or patients do not feel comfortable volunteering certain types of information. And if symptoms are not recorded it is usually impossible to say whether they were left out because the patient did not have them, or because they were not discussed (Basch 2009: 1905). These problems can be mitigated if patients themselves record symptoms. Comparing clinician-collected and patient-reported assessments in a study with lung cancer patients, for example, Basch and colleagues (2009) found that while data collected by clinicians did better in predicting unfavorable clinical events, data recorded by patients reflected their daily health status better.

These findings highlight that data collection by patients and by clinicians should be treated as complementary, and not as mutually exclusive strategies. Guidelines and policies from regulatory bodies increasingly require that patients report these outcomes to authorities *directly,* rather than via their clinicians (Food and Drug Administration 2009; see also Ahmed et al. 2012; Basch 2013). As a result, a lot of work is currently put into developing so-called patient-reported outcomes measures (PROM) and other metrics to assess the quality and effectiveness of interventions from patients' perspectives (Nelson et al. 2015).

As pointed out earlier in this chapter, the concept of the surveillant assemblage focuses on the human body being taken apart and put together again by various systems of surveillance at different levels. Because it does not require a focus on only one specific technological instrument, mechanism, or practice, but on how different systems come together, it lends itself to analysing power dynamics that work horizontally, and from the bottom up, such as the self-monitoring of individuals—and not only power that is exercised from the top down. It draws attention to the voluntary and even pleasurable practices that keep these systems going and helps us to see the extent to which contemporary forms of surveillance capitalize on the active and enthusiastic participation of those being surveilled—often because this participation is "fun," or even "liberating" (see also Haggerty 2006: 28). This clearly also applies to our example of Nike FuelBand, where self-tracking not only serves a motivational purpose—such as for Jesper, to "move more"—but also entertains, and for many people is fun to engage with.

It has often been argued that there is an inverse relationship between the practical utility of a technology—such as experience of pleasure, or any kind of other personal, social, work-related, or financial utility—and people's willingness to act upon their concerns about privacy or confidentiality (see, for example, Martin 2014; Wellcome Trust 2016). In other words, the greater the benefit of a technology to users, the more they are willing to accept that their privacy is compromised. Others have argued that there are no such trade-offs; instead, people are resigned and have given up even trying to prevent corporations from using their data (Turow, Hennessy, and Draper 2015). As we have seen in the case of Jesper, who is well aware that by wearing FuelBand he is handing over his personal data to Nike, the utility of being able to track changes in his movement and performance outweighs any potential concerns. And even if Jesper were to refuse to wear a digital activity tracker, he would be very unlikely to suffer negative consequences. The situation of patients being signed up for telemonitoring is different. Even if patients are uncomfortable with some of the surveillance-related aspects of it, the pressure to use telemonitoring technologies is often so high that they decide to use them anyhow. If they refuse to participate, they risk being labeled as noncompliant, difficult patients.

And there are other obvious differences between telemonitoring systems such as CardioConsult HF and lifestyle devices such as Fitbit or FuelBand. The former are medical devices that are used to monitor vital functions of ill people, while the latter are fitness gadgets targeted primarily at healthy, wealthy, and young cohorts. The costs of the former are covered, or subsidized, by health insurers, whereas the latter are marketed to people whose pockets are deep enough to shell out one hundred dollars or more for the "sports bangle," or several hundred for a trendy smartphone. Moreover, while data produced or received by health care providers is protected by special laws in most countries—such as by the Health Insurance Portability and Accountability Act (HIPAA) in the United States—the data that Jesper collects on his activity tracker are not covered by special privacy laws, other than generic data-protection laws such as the European General Data Protection Regulation. There are also striking similarities between activity tracking and medical telemonitoring. First of all, both systems leave the monitored person little leeway in how to use the device (see Bratteteig and Wagner 2013; Oudshoorn 2011). Both require a certain level of self-discipline from their users and motivate them to become even more disciplined. Indeed, both devices aim to change the person wearing or using them, either by changing their behavior, or by compensating for "deficiencies" in their living circumstances. With patients, the digital surveillance system may do this in very immediate and explicit ways, for example by trying to enhance a person's mobility. The digitally surveilled patient is supposed to be healthier, happier, and often also "cheaper" for the health care system. Fitbits or FuelBands also try to change their wearers: They are not built merely to quantify their owners' every moves, but also to change their behavior, and to make them healthier and more active (see also Albrechtslund and Lauritsen 2013; Gilleade and Fairclough 2010; Peppet 2012: 80).

Another feature that both CardioConsult HF and activity trackers have in common is that they both represent instances of datafication (Mayer-Schönberger and Cukier 2013); they render visible and quantifiable something that used to be exempt from quantification. They thus mark the end of "structural privacy" in their fields, namely the end of the protection of privacy due to technological or physical barriers (Surden 2007). Certain types of data that are captured today used not to be collected because there were no technological means to do.

## Privacy in the Era of Datafication: The Search for New Concepts and Instruments

I argued in the previous chapter that looking at how much influence people have in what and how data and information about and from them will be used is helpful in classifying participatory practices in health and medicine. I also pointed out that the indiscriminate use of the terms "participation" and "empowerment" conceals differences in formats of participation that are politically, ethically, and morally meaningful (see also Del Savio, Buyx, and Prainsack 2016; Harris, Kelly, and Wyatt 2016). In the remainder of this chapter I will foreground another crucial aspect of digital data use in the domain of medicine, namely data protection and privacy.

It is very difficult to summarize what privacy is; it is easier to say what privacy *concerns*. The English data-protection expert Mark Taylor defines privacy as "a relevant stage of separation [ . . . ] established by norms regulating access to individuals or groups" (M. Taylor 2013: 25, here following Laurie 2002). What exactly the norms are that determine what and who is excluded from access to information needs to be determined in a context-specific manner (M. Taylor 2013: 56). Taylor uses the example of a private conversation on a crowded train to illustrate this: Although the people involved in the conversation are not physically set apart from other passengers, social norms still expect that other passengers will refrain from intruding in the conversation (or, one could add, recording it). Thus, although the conversation between the people on the train is observable, it is still private in important respects. In his emphasis on the contextual nature of social norms determining the who and how of exclusion, Taylor's understanding of privacy is strongly influenced by New York–based media studies scholar Helen Nissenbaum's notion of "privacy as contextual integrity" (Nissenbaum 2004).

Digital surveillance systems pose complex challenges for data protection and privacy. Some of them are related to the scale and breadth of data collection. They emerged due to novel ways to link, integrate, and mine datasets, and to the power structures that digital data collection and use is embedded in. Large corporations collect, analyze, and concentrate data much more easily than is the case for individual citizens or citizen groups (see A. Taylor 2014; Wellcome Trust 2016). One of the reasons for the difficulty in addressing these challenges is that traditional concepts and instruments do not get us very far. If we continued to focus on informed individual consent, for example, the digital surveillance systems discussed in this chapter would be unproblematic. Both in the case of FuelBand and of CardioConsult HF, users give consent to their data being collected and used, technically speaking: In the former case they do so by accepting the terms of service of the activity tracking software, and in the latter by giving consent to participate in the disease management plan. Both systems are thus based on data that are supposedly voluntarily disclosed by participants because they have given individual consent. The problem is, however, that the idea of voluntary disclosure assumes not only that people knowingly and willingly share data or information about themselves, but also that they know how the data will be used. With many digital health surveillance systems, this is regularly not the case: Only rarely are users told in a meaningful and intelligible way how their data will be used (see also Pasquale 2015). In the words of legal scholar Scott Peppet: "We may be stuck with an architecture in which firms collect self-surveillance data for consumers and use the data in various ways, including in marketing or other transactions that may or may not always be in the consumer's best interest" (Peppet 2012: 78).

This means that companies who charge for storage and processing services may be a "safer" option for users in many instances. Users pay the service provider for storage or processing and have a say in what the provider can and cannot do with the data, instead of enjoying a sup-posedly free service when the business model of the company actually lies in exploiting the data. In the words of an article in *The Economist* in September 2013, citizens worried about their privacy in the era of ubiq-uitous data collection have two choices: "Pay up or shut up."[9] Anything that users share online, so the argument goes, "will inevitably be bought and sold and, sooner or later, used against them in some way. That is the price people tacitly accept for the convenience of using popular web ser-vices free of charge" (N.V. 2013). Calling any part of this self-surveillance voluntary would be ironic.

When I spoke to Jesper about this, he seemed aware but unfazed by this situation. He was well aware that Nike owned the data coming from his activity tracker, but he did not mind. He explained:

> I can't really be bothered to care. My data is everywhere nowadays, and if I needed to think about all the places my data can go, then I would need to become a zombie: I would need to give up Facebook, my smartphone, my Gmail address, basically my entire existence on the Internet. We are in a transition period right now, when people who are not used to it, they find it very weird that people know everything about you, while people in my generation don't care. We need to learn to live with the fact that everything is public.

It is interesting to note also that in our conversations Jesper did not distinguish between privacy and ownership: for him, Nike's ability to analyze his data was the same as Nike owning the data. This resonates with Nike's own conflation of privacy and ownership in their communication with customers. When I wrote to the company as a potential customer asking about their data *ownership* policy related to FuelBand,[10] I received a response with a link to their *privacy* policy, telling me that "it covers everything that you would need to know."[11] The information itself was written in jargon-free, easily understandable language. I was also told that were I to use any of their "website, mobile application or NIKE product or service on any computer, mobile phone, tablet, console or other device," I would consent, by default, to the company's use of my data for a range of activities, including "analyzing user behavior and trends." I would thereby also grant permission to Nike to pass my information on to other companies and to law enforcement authorities. Moreover, if I were to share data publicly via any of their platforms, I would automatically consent to Nike's use of these data for promotional purposes. Finally, I learned that "like other companies, NIKE cannot guarantee 100% the security or confidentiality of the information you provide to us" (Nike 2012).

Jesper told me that if companies provide a "free" service, it was only fair that they should profit from people's activity and personal data. And although not everybody may be as sanguine about companies owning their data as Jesper is, this does not seem to prevent people from using activity trackers: In 2015 one in five people in the United States reported using a wearable activity tracker, with Fitbit being the market leader (Fleming 2015). While I could not find corresponding information on Europe, where Jesper was based, sales data for health and fitness trackers indicate that the European and North American market shares at the time of writing this book were roughly equal (Statista 2016).

There are currently no satisfactory solutions to the problem of data ownership by companies, or to the issue that some people hand over data that they never meant to transfer. The instrument of consent cannot address this problem, because it considers voluntary self-disclosure as presenting no privacy issues if the consent is valid (Peppet 2012: 83). Some scholars argue that effectively tackling the challenges posed by data collection and use in the digital area requires that we move away from a control-based view of privacy. I will explain this further in the next section.

## Control, Flow, or Travel? Conceptualizing Data Privacy

Legal scholar Jerry Kang and colleagues' concept of data "flow" offers an alternative to a control-based understanding of privacy. For any type of data, Kang and colleagues argue, we should ask where, how quickly, and with what bandwidth they move through the system. It would then become apparent that some types of data flow faster than others, and that sensitive data in particular often move more slowly (Kang et al. 2012: 821). The question of the adequate pace of data flow should not be answered solely on the basis of a principle-based ethical assessment; it should also consider changes in societal understandings of what sensitive data are, Kang and colleagues argue. The flow metric is, in their view, unique in that it remains sensitive to the privacy implications of such changing social practices and values:

> If we as a society become sufficiently exhibitionist such that most of us regularly and voluntarily broadcast naked pictures of ourselves on the Internet, our privacy may not have decreased under a control metric. By contrast, the flow of such information will have increased and, conversely, privacy (in the flow sense) will have decreased under the flow metric (Kang et al. 2012: 821–822).

Although the flow metaphor abolishes the implicit assumption that it is possible to effectively control who can access and use data, its disadvantage is that it suggests that data are constantly in flux, like a river, the blood in our body, or electricity.[12] Although the flow of data can be temporarily interrupted, the assumption is that flux is the normal state. This assumption is problematic in the context of privacy protection, as the point of the latter is often specifically to prevent or restrict the movement of data, and not only to slow it down, as suggested by Kang and colleagues. For this reason, philosopher of science Sabina Leonelli (2016) uses the term "data journeys" to refer to the movement of data through systems. Like travelers, data should not be expected to be constantly moving; sometimes they remain in one place for prolonged periods of time.

Internet and Society scholar Sara Watson (2013) suggests a radical approach to thinking about data protection in the digital era: She proposes to give up concepts such as privacy and ownership altogether. The reason is that these concepts stem from the paper age, when data sets could be locked in a cabinet or burned or hidden from somebody. Notions such as privacy or ownership, so Watson argues, are unsuitable for capturing the realities and concerns of data subjects in an era when we, ourselves, "are becoming data." Watson suggests that instead of talking about ownership, we should talk about the "right to use" personal data (Watson 2013; see also Purtova 2015).

## Toward a New Understanding of Data Use

I agree with Sabina Leonelli's critique of the data flow concept as implying the problematic idea that the default state of data is to be *in flux*. Moreover, the idea that data are more valuable when they "flow" suggests that in a healthy economy data are a commodity that should be in circulation. This is closely related to the equally problematic assumption that people who do not want others to use their data are considered selfish "data hoarders." At the same time, the term preferred by Sabina Leonelli, "journeys," could be seen to ascribe agency to data, instead of to the people who collect and use them and make them move. My own approach is to refer to the "storage" or "movement" of data and be as specific as possible about how data move if they move, who makes them move, and for what purpose. Spelling out who makes data available to whom and for what purpose is a good way to describe what is happening without resorting to morally laden or otherwise problematic terms such as data "sharing" or "flow." The following schematic typology of practices pertaining to data collection and use can help us demarcate areas that are particularly problematic and thus deserve particular awareness and public scrutiny. What sets this approach apart from other work on this topic (for example, Dyke, Dove and Knoppers 2016) is that I do not consider particular *types* of data as particularly sensitive, but instead I focus on the conditions of collecting data and on how they are *used*. In chapter 6 I will go into more detail about how regulation should treat different types of data use differently. Building upon the argument that privacy is both a personal and a collective interest (Casilli 2014), I will also lay out ways to enhance collective control and oversight over data use.

## Conscious and/or Active Participation in Data Collection

The first aspect to consider is whether people are conscious of, or even actively participating in, their data being collected. It is not a given that people are aware that data from and about them are collected. This is often not the case when data are recorded passively by remote sensors and when people actively use online services without being aware that data about them will be retained and analyzed. In the context of medicine specifically, people contributing information to the personalization of their health care can do this by different means: they can let their bodies speak for them, as in the case of a patient undergoing clinical genetic testing to determine her breast cancer risk, a woman undergoing a gynecological exam, or a person taking a blood test. Alternatively, they can collect and disclose information *about* their bodies, lives, or symptoms. A person taking a genetic test with a commercial provider in order to learn which drugs she is able to metabolize more efficiently and who, in turn, shares this information with her doctor, is an example of the latter.

These various forms of creating and providing information can be conscious and deliberate on the part of the patient. In some situations patients are aware that the information from and about them is being collected, stored, and analyzed. In many instances the information is collected without the person knowing that their information will be used for any other purposes than the one they provide it for (for example, for diagnosis). As pointed out earlier in this chapter, the existence of the person's consent is not an appropriate criterion to distinguish between deliberate and unwitting contributions; patient data can be collected with the person having given consent—such as by accepting the terms of service of an online service, or signing papers when entering a hospital—even if the patient has not read the materials or has not made a voluntary and deliberate decision to accept the conditions.

## Data Collection or Use for Health-Related Purposes

Many people consider the use of their data for individual-level health-related purposes as particularly sensitive or important. For this reason, regulation and policy making should not only consider whether people are aware of their data being used by others but also whether their data are used for health-related purposes for specific individuals. In a clinical setting, this will be straightforward: People will normally be aware that their information will be used for health-related purposes. But in the case of somebody's credit card purchases being used by a commercial company to calculate their health risk score—that is, their risk of suffering from a chronic condition or needing emergency care in the next months, or otherwise being or becoming a costly patient—their data are used for health-related purposes at the individual level without their knowledge and consent (see Dixon and Gellman 2014). Unless data are kept in a place where they are legally and technically insulated from access by any outsider, such as is the case with police databases in many countries, we need to assume that all data can be used to make health-related inferences about individuals at least in principle.

When we bring the dimension of conscious versus unwitting participation together with whether or not data are used for individual-level health-related purposes, table 3.1 is the result.

| TABLE 3.1. Types of patient involvement in the creating, collecting, or providing of data and information in the health domain | | |
|---|---|---|
| Activities in the dark gray box (in the upper right corner) are the most problematic; those in the white box (in the lower left corner) are the least problematic. | | |
| | *Data and information cannot be used for individual-level health-related purposes* | *Data and information can be used for individual-level health-related purposes* |
| *People were not conscious of, nor actively voluntarily involved in, the production of these data* | Data that people are not aware of being collected but that are legally and/or technically insulated from use for individual-level health-related purposes; for example, surveillance video footage collected by the police in many countries | Data that are not insulated from use for health-related purposes and that people were not aware of being collected, such as metadata from users of symptom checker websites being used for consumer scoring |
| *People were conscious of, or actively and voluntarily involved in the production of these data* | Data that people are aware of being collected and that are legally and/or technically insulated from use for individual-level health-related purposes; for example, people's votes in an election | For example, information on side effects of drugs collected and reported directly by patients |

Activities in the dark gray box in table 3.1 are the most contentious in terms of their possible negative effects on the agency and interests of people. They are most likely to contribute to three particularly problematic practices of digital surveillance, namely hypercollection, harm, and humiliation (chapter 2). Activities in the white box are the least problematic in this respect. In an ideal world, the dark gray area in the table would not exist; at the very least, the practice of giving away information for one purpose without being aware that it will be used for another should not be called "participatory," even if people have formally given consent.

### Addressing Data Privacy Challenges: Privacy-by-Design, Privacy-by-Default, Personal Data Guardians, and Making Your Own Devices

I already mentioned that many of the most pressing societal and ethical challenges related to digital data use cannot be adequately described, not to mention addressed, with the conceptual and legal tools of the paper age. A reason for this is that traditional distinctions between sensitive and nonsensitive data, between identified and nonidentified data, and between health- and nonhealth-related data cannot be maintained. Any data set, regardless of what it signifies and where it was collected or produced, can be used for potentially any purpose. Even the most trivial, nonhealth-related piece of information, such as whether somebody buys sports goods online, can be used to make probabilistic inferences regarding their health status (in the case of sports goods, that they are more likely to overuse hospital emergency rooms; Dixon and Gellman 2014).

Just as it is impossible to maintain the distinction between medical and nonmedical, and health-related and nonhealth-related data, it is impossible to uphold the dividing line between sensitive and nonsensitive, and identified and deidentified data. In the last few decades, the label "sensitive" has been applied to information that is particularly likely to cause harm if used in an unauthorized manner. Medical information, names, and addresses, as well as information on trade union memberships, political affiliations, and sexual orientation, have typically been subsumed under this term. Today it is possible to link almost any type of data to make probabilistic predictions about people that can harm them. Thus, virtually any type of information and data is potentially sensitive. And as we know very well from genomic and other studies, any type of information can potentially lead to reidentification (Gymrek et al. 2013; Prainsack 2015b; Slavkovic and Yu 2015).

Scholars, practitioners, and policy makers have been working toward solutions for this problem, but these solutions do not go far enough. The European Union's (EU) new general Data Protection Regulation, for example, which will come into effect in 2018, explicitly refers to the need to rethink data protection in the digital age (European Commission 2016). The new Regulation has been hailed as a milestone "fit for the digital era" (European Parliament 2016; Trevor 2016) because it will place stronger burdens on organizations processing personal data and give citizens more control over how their data will be used. The term "personal data" here is defined very broadly as data pertaining to identified or identifiable natural persons. They include names, addresses, ZIP codes, and IP addresses. The burden is now on data processors to inform citizens of privacy and confidentiality breaches. EU citizens will have a right for decisions of their data-protection authority to be reviewed by courts in their own country, even if the organization using the data is based in a different country. Last but not least, EU citizens will also be able to move personal data from one service provider to another. This is not currently possible because data are seen to belong to the service provider, not to the person they came from (European Council 2015).

The new Regulation also codifies two principles that have featured prominently within discussions on data protection everywhere in the world, Privacy-by-Design, and Privacy-by-Default. The first principle, Privacy-by-Design, obliges businesses or services that utilize personal data to integrate data-protection requirements into the design of their services. The second principle, Privacy-by-Default, prescribes that only the minimum set of personal data necessary for a purpose should be processed. This also means that whenever a user acquires a new product or service, the strictest privacy settings must be offered "by default." It also prescribes that service providers can collect and use only the data that they absolutely need to provide the service. This rule seeks to avoid that companies collect data just because they can—in other words, that they engage in hypercollection (chapter 2). Similarly, other than in exceptional circumstances organizations or businesses can retain personal information only as long as they need it to provide a service.

Although at first sight these changes look as if they were changing things for the better, it remains to be seen how effective the new Regulation will be when implemented. I already pointed out that its use of outdated dichotomies such as sensitive versus nonsensitive data will limit its effectiveness. Moreover, its success in mitigating the current power asymmetry between organizations using data and the people the data come from will also depend on whether fines levied by authorities will be painful enough for big companies to make them comply with the law.[13] And it is important to note that the EU's new data-protection framework will be binding only for organizations and companies operating in the EU; it will thus not be a remedy for data-protection problems in other parts of the world.

But besides legal solutions there are also technical and practical approaches to addressing privacy issues. Computer scientist Daniel Le Métayer and legal scholar Shara Monteleone (2009), for example, believe that privacy preferences of users could be "learned" by an automated agent who then, for example, could alert users when a website they want to visit does not correspond with their personal privacy preferences. Other solutions suggest the introduction of state-funded human "Personal Data Guardians" negotiating adequate data protection on behalf of the citizens, and securing it in so-called "Personal Data Vaults" (Kang et al. 2012: 828).[14] Users would upload their personal data into the Personal Data Vault, which is maintained by the Personal Data Guardian, "instead of into some amorphous cloud owned and operated by some faceless third party" (Kang et al. 2012: 828).

Yet another approach is taken by people who argue that, in order to avoid a situation where others can access, process, and profit from our data, we should use devices that we built ourselves: "[I]f you can't open it, you don't own it" (Mister Jalopy n.d.). The so-called maker community (Hatch 2013; Tocchetti 2014) set out to build their own tools. This is indeed a very good way to avoid issues regarding data ownership and data protection for tools that do not need to be interoperable with other personal or health care devices because they "merely'" track different aspects of our own lives. It would be more difficult to use this approach for digital health surveillance more broadly. But it would not be impossible:

Instead of every patient having to build her own devices, prototypes of nonproprietary "open" devices could be developed and scaled for use by hospitals and other health care providers.

## Conclusion

Patients, in any capacity, are rarely ever entirely passive: health care systems rely on their participation and compliance (see also Strauss et al. 1982; 1997). Across different times and places, patient participation has manifested itself in a myriad of ways, from self-care to actively seeking a doctor's advice to filling in a prescription, measuring one's blood pressure, or even filing a complaint. The more health care aims to be tailored to individual characteristics of patients, however, the wider and deeper the participation of patients needs to be. Similarly, the more a health care system needs to know about people in order to tailor services to their characteristics and needs, the more information people are expected to provide in the first place. And the information provided needs to be more detailed: a characteristic or need that is not known or only poorly characterized cannot be adequately responded to.

This rationale has led some people—clinicians, researchers, and also policy makers—to assume that comprehensive data capture from patients is the best way to realize personalized medicine (see also Vogt, Hofmann, and Getz 2016). In this scenario, which is sometimes referred to as "continuous health," every aspect of a person's life would be monitored, and the data would be added to a personal health data repository that can support prevention, diagnosis and treatment decision making. Although unlike in Dave Eggers book *The Circle,* most patients are not yet swallowing nanosensors that monitor them from inside their own bodies, researchers are working toward this scenario, and the use of wearable and remote sensors for health-related purposes is expanding fast (see, for example, Hicks 2016). As digital surveillance becomes less invasive and less intrusive (Ausiello and Shaw 2014; see also Schatz 2015), the ways in which people contribute to the personalization of their health care becomes more passive. Patients become data transmitters who typically have very little influence over what data are collected from them and how they are used. This situation undermines assumptions that digital self-monitoring and telemedicine empowers patients, or makes medicine more democratic. On the contrary, in many contexts, it entails rigid scripts of how instruments and systems are to be used by patients and other actors. At the same time, because the tools, instruments, and software used for digital health surveillance are typically produced and owned by companies, power asymmetries between citizens and corporations are increasing (see also Zuboff 2015). One of the essential lessons of the digital revolution is that formally equal access to digital technologies does not mean that power and expertise are distributed more equally. In the clinical domain, power remains concentrated in the hands of professionally trained experts such as doctors and other medical professionals. And power is increasingly also in the hands of corporate actors who develop tools and instruments and thus become de facto decision makers in some domains of medicine (Sharon 2016).

I argued in this chapter that the most problematic types of data use are those for which people are not aware that their data are collected and used, and where the data are used for individual-level health-related purposes. This informational asymmetry between people and the corporations using their data is accompanied by widening power gaps between them also in other ways. In the next chapter, I will take a closer look at how technological practices in the context of personalized medicine in particular contribute to shifting power between different actors.

4

# Beyond Empowerment

## Introduction: How Do We See Power?

*Milena's Story*

Milena is a medical student in Vienna, Austria.[1] In her genetics class a lecturer mentioned a test sold online that enables people to learn about their genetic disease risk and some traits such as reading ability or response to exercise. Milena cannot quite imagine that such a test would find anything that could be useful to her. But she is curious and wants to see it for herself. She goes for a test by the Californian company 23andMe, if only because it seems to be a very popular service.

When Milena logs on to the website she finds that although the "spit kit" and the DNA analysis itself is relatively affordable at $99, the shipping costs to her country are very high; she would have to add another $48 to have the test kit shipped to her home and then on to the laboratory in California. She is annoyed about the hidden costs. After thinking about it for a few days, however, she decides to pay the shipping costs anyhow, as there is no other way for her to get her hands on such a test (Milena is not aware of bio.logis, a personal genome testing service based in Frankfurt, Germany, that offers genome-wide testing for a more limited range of diseases than 23andMe. Milena is not aware of this because bio.logis does not market its services as widely as other companies). Milena also decides to keep a diary of her experience of taking the test and write one of her term papers about it. She considers the money spent on the test a good investment in this sense.

The spit kit arrives within a week. It is very easy to use. Every step is clearly explained. Nevertheless, in order to make sure that she gets it exactly right, Milena watches a few short clips on YouTube of people who videotaped themselves taking the same test. She fills her tube with saliva and mails the kit back to California, where the company selling the test is located.

About eight weeks later Milena receives an e-mail informing her that her test results are available online. She receives this e-mail while in class; she can't help but log on immediately to see her results. There is nothing surprising. The test got her eye color wrong: it predicts blue eyes with 72 percent probability, while Milena's eyes are brown. Other physical traits, however, are described correctly. Hearing that she has a higher genetic risk of heart disease—20.5 percent instead of the population average of 15.9 percent in people with European ancestry—is not nice, but it does not come as a shock either; many of her relatives have had heart problems, and some have died from them. The website tells Milena that the heritability of atrial fibrillation is over 60 percent; this means that genetic factors are more influential than lifestyle. This worries Milena; she had assumed that by living very healthily she could reduce her heart disease risk to a minimum. Momentarily she feels trapped by her DNA—but then she sees that the testing company recommends a range of lifestyle changes to reduce risk, including eating a "heart-healthy" diet, and exercising. So there is hope that she will escape heart disease after all. Milena reminds herself that in her father's family, where some relatives have died of heart attacks, there are at least as many who have reached old age in very good health.

The other news that initially worries Milena is that her genetic risk of suffering from Parkinson's disease is also elevated. It is calculated at 2.4 percent compared to the population average of 1.6 per cent. Milena's aunt died of the disease; nobody else in her extended family suffers from it, though. By reading additional information available on her test result pages Milena learns that the heritability of Parkinson's disease is estimated at 27 percent, which she does not consider very high. And her math skills are good enough to know that the increase in relative risk is too low to tell her anything useful. She dismisses her concern about Parkinson's disease and clicks on the breast cancer risk tab, which is something that she has worried about all her life; besides heart disease, breast cancer is very common in her extended family. Milena carries out very regular breast exams, and once a year her gynecologist examines her breasts as well. She is relieved to see that her genetic risk of breast cancer is lower than the population average, namely 10 percent instead of 13.5 percent. The website warns her, though, that if she has a family history of breast cancer, she should consider clinical genetic testing, because the test that she took does not sequence the genes that carry the most impactful genetic mutations. Milena knows about these mutations; she discussed it with her physician because of her family history but decided not to do a BRCA1 and BRCA2 test at that time. Instead she opted for regular breast exams and mammographies. She still feels it was the right decision.

Milena then moves on to her carrier status results, only to find that there seems to be nothing to worry about. Her genetic ancestry results are unexciting; she learns that she is 39 percent "Eastern European," which corresponds roughly with what she knows about where her ancestors came from. The company tells her she has some fourth and fifth cousins who apparently all live in the United States—she plays with the thought of contacting them but dismisses it; she is not aware of any of her family moving to North America in recent generations and assumes that these "cousins" are not really related to her. Also, the idea of speaking to somebody just because she shares a stretch of DNA with them is not appealing to her.

Next Milena clicks on the tab with "Drug Response" information. Her response is predicted as "typical" in most cases, except for two instances: She is told that she is a slow caffeine metabolizer and that drinking coffee would increase her heart attack risk. Milena feels vindicated when she reads this, as she has often said to her friends that having too much coffee made her feel that she was poisoning herself. Some of her friends had dismissed this as a neurotic fad. At the same time, Milena does not like the idea of being a slow caffeine metabolizer because caffeine has been found to protect against Parkinson's disease, for which she has an increased genetic risk. What should she do? Drinking coffee increases her risk of heart disease even further, not drinking it might put her at higher risk to develop Parkinson's . . . . But given how low her absolute genetic risk to develop Parkinson's is, compared to her much more serious risk of suffering from heart disease, Milena decides to restrict her coffee consumption. She does not believe in radical solutions, so she does not plan to give it up entirely, but just to drink less.

The other thing she learns here is that she is likely to metabolize a certain kind of blood thinner very poorly, and that existing guidelines already recommend that people with her genotype should be given a different drug when needed. Milena writes this down in her diary; she will tell her parents and her sister about this. She might even suggest to her family to also take this test to see whether they have the same predicted poor response to clopidogrel (that's the name of the drug). As heart disease runs in her family, knowing what drug not to use in case of a heart attack is very useful information. Milena thinks of suggesting taking the test to her boyfriend, Mike, too, whose father died of a brain aneurism at a young age; Mike has always been worried about suffering the same fate. But when Milena clicks on her own genetic risk information for brain aneurism, she realizes that all scientific studies on brain aneurism that the company bases their risk calculations upon included only Europeans. Mike is Eritrean; Milena has no idea whether any of the test results would even apply to him. She will discuss this with Mike; perhaps he knows the answer.

*How Do We See Power?*

Has the test changed Milena's life? Has it helped her to become more engaged with her own health? Has it empowered her? And what are the effects of her taking the test on her partner, who just found out that most of Milena's test results are applicable only to "European ethnicities," as the website puts it? Large parts of the literature on patient participation in medicine (Agus 2016; Meskó 2014; Topol 2015) portray digital tools as the major drivers for change in medicine and health care. That medicine is supposedly becoming more personal, more precise, and more participatory is seen as an effect of "disruptive technologies," such as the genetic test that Milena took, which in turn had become possible via the advancement of DNA analysis tools. But technologies by themselves do not disrupt, reinvent, or empower anything or anybody. Some information and communication technologies have been used to create the opposite effect. They have been used to conserve and reinforce traditional hierarchies, values, and practices. They have helped institutions that are already rich and powerful to become richer and even more powerful as they became gatekeepers to tools or data sets, for example. Moreover, it has been argued that the way electronic health records and digital decision aids are being used often leads to poorer quality of health care. This is the case when doctors look at screens instead of their patients (Lown and Rodriguez 2012; see also Wachter 2015b). And when health care professionals rely on electronic alerts instead of their own judgment when checking drug doses, for example, health care also becomes less safe (Wachter 2015a).

These undesirable effects of technology use take up relatively little space in the scientific literature, compared to the promises that technologies are seen to make. Similarly, while problems such as the widening of health disparities in our societies remain unsolved, large sums of public and private money are invested in creating digital infrastructures for medical practice and research. The U.S. Precision Medicine Initiative, which received $215 million during its first year in 2016, and the National Institute of Health's (NIH) Big Data to Knowledge (BD2K) funding initiative are but two examples (Huang, Mulyasasmita, and Rajagopal 2016). The problem is not that these are badly designed initiatives; on the contrary, they have been set up in a very thoughtful manner. The issue is that taken together these initiatives place technology in the center of how we think and act "precision" and personalization into being. They underscore the idea that personalized medicine will make medicine more precise, more effective, and thus also cheaper. And here the circle closes: Because personalized medicine is seen to require new technological infrastructure and more data, prioritizing investments in these areas seems the logical thing to do.

Are patients empowered or disempowered by this development? In the previous chapter I argued that the digital and operational infrastructures that foster personalization turn patients into permanent data transmitters. At the same time, despite the rhetoric of empowerment, patients typically have very little say about what data about them are collected and how these data are used. Thus, it is tempting to conclude personalized medicine as such will disempower, rather than empower, patients.

But the story does not end here. In this chapter I will argue that personalized medicine does indeed change the distribution of power between different actors in medicine, but not merely by taking power away from some actors and giving it to others. Power is not a zero sum game where one entity has less power if another one gets more. Some types of patients, namely those who can afford to decide what self-monitoring, data collecting, or conversations with clinicians they participate in, will benefit from more personalized medicine and health care. The scope of agency for those unable to do these things, in contrast, will typically become smaller. At the same time, technological practices in the service of personalization, such as the calculation of personalized genetic risk scores on the basis of genetic testing, or personalized prognosis on the basis of imaging, also change what patients and others expect from medical professionals. They bring new actors to the scene: the telemedicine nurse, the commercial genetic testing provider, or the long-distance radiologist.

Like many other scholars in the social studies of medicine, my understanding of power is influenced by Michel Foucault's work. As is well known, for Foucault, power does not "sit" within powerful people or authorities, but is exercised whenever people act. Power is concentrated in some places rather than in others, but there is no space in life that is entirely devoid of it.[2] Moreover, people are hardly ever merely passive objects upon whom power is exercised. Instead they actively exercise power—on others, on their environments, and regularly also upon themselves.

With regard to *how* we exercise power upon others and on ourselves, different conceptions can be found, even within the scope of Foucault's own work. What distinguishes them is the extent to which actions of individuals are seen as determined by external factors, such as sovereign rulers, teachers, or authoritative discourses, rather than by forces that come from within the person herself.

In systems of sovereign power, power is highly visible and tangible: the monocratic ruler is the master over life and death. In such systems, power often expresses itself in physical ways: people are killed or penalized by means of corporal punishment. In Europe, the mechanisms of power became subtler and increasingly complemented by mechanisms of *discipline* during the course of the eighteenth century (Foucault 1991 [1975]). In disciplinary societies, power does not take the form of repression and coercion as much as it unfolds in less visible ways. People discipline themselves because they know they are being monitored. In situations where there is no open conflict, power tends to be less visible—it has all but disappeared.

In his later work Foucault placed ever more emphasis on the self-regulation of individuals through non-direct ways of intervention. These "technologies of the self,"[3] as he called them, move another step farther away from the traditional understanding of coercive and centralized power (see also Lemke 2001; 2011). People act in particular ways not only because of outside pressures, whether they are visible or not, but also because they have internalized the values and commitments underpinning these pressures. For example, in genetic counseling, people are not threatened with punishment if they do not choose what seems the most rational option, such as undergoing yet another test, or opting for abortion. Instead, they are "helped" to behave rationally (see also Markens, Browner, and Press, 1999). Here, power is the least visible, yet is perhaps the most effective, and the most sustainable: "[P]ower is tolerable only on the condition it masks a substantial part of itself. Its success is proportional to its ability to hide its own mechanisms" (Foucault 1980 [1978]: 168; see also Rose 1999).

Although Foucault linked these different archetypes of power to particular forms of government throughout history, he did not claim that they neatly succeeded each other, or even that they ever existed in a pure form. Instead, he assumed that authorities and people use different modes of power and (self-)governance simultaneously.

*Risk*

The notion of risk is intimately linked to power. Risk is not an entity that is just "out there" and can be measured objectively. It is a conceptual instrument that helps some people in interacting with the world around them, and it also helps authorities discipline and regulate people and populations (Beck 1992; Clarke et al. 2003; Ericson and Doyle 2003; Rhodes 1997; Rose 1999, 2007). The political scientist Giandomenico Majone famously spoke of the emergence of the "regulatory state," where decentralized and private actors—including individual citizens—increasingly participate in rulemaking and administration. This does not mean that governmental control is waning: What has changed is how such control is exercised (Majone 1997; Moran 2001). Other scholars have observed that governments increasingly outsource the task of ensuring that populations are healthy and productive (Gottweis 1998). Many aspects of this task fall upon private actors, or upon citizens themselves. This is one of the reasons for the current emphasis on prevention in public health: Prevention is something that individuals can be held responsible for. They are told their individual risk and expected to reduce it. At the same time, measures to tackle the social determinants of ill health, for example, by reducing air pollution or providing affordable housing, have been neglected due to budget constraints or ideological commitments. The less governments do to enable everybody to lead a healthy and happy life, the more they need to rely on citizens to police their own behaviors, and to take the blame if things go wrong. Risk is the fuel that is hoped to keep the machinery of people's self-governance running (Clarke et al. 2010b; Kerr and Cunningham-Burley 2000; Petersen and Lupton 1996).

## Four Faces of Power

But how do people govern themselves—and how do authorities get them to do it? The field of political science and international relations is particularly rich in conceptualizations of power (see for example, Gallarotti 2011; Haugaard 2012). Especially after the end of the Cold War, when analysts had to explain the emergence of a new world order that was no longer determined by the size of armies and nuclear threats, their attention shifted from "hard" to softer manifestations of power. While "hard" power is expressed with material force, coercion, and by opposing parties directly interacting with each other, "soft" power manifests itself in the ability to shape what others want. Political theorist Joseph Nye referred to hard power as "command power" and to soft power as "co-optive power" (Nye 1990, 2004). In a remarkable move for a field whose mainstream has been, and still is, staunchly positivist, this has led to an embrace of interpretive approaches to understanding power among some political scientists. In 1992, political philosopher Peter Digeser wrote a seminal article titled "The Fourth Face of Power" in which he endorsed Foucault's understanding of power as particularly helpful for political analyses (Digeser 1992). He distinguished between four different "faces" of power: The first two faces are easiest to see, as they are characterized by open conflict or disagreement. The first face materializes when an actor makes another actor do something that the latter does not want to do, either by use of force or direct pressure (Dahl 1957: 202–203). It is the oldest form of power that political scientists have learned to analyze and for a long time it had been the only form that they were able to see.

The second face of power refers to situations in which an actor prevents somebody from doing what they want to. The recognition of this less openly visible dimension of power is largely owed to the work of Peter Bachrach and Morton S. Baratz who, in a landmark article in the early 1960s, drew the attention of political analysts to "instances of power where actors are not constituted as parties to a conflict and/or issues are not defined as contentious" (c.f. Bilgin and Elis 2008: 9; see also Bachrach and Baratz 1962, 1963). Analyses of the second face of power often consist of explorations of decisions that were not made, or processes that resulted in certain items never making it onto policy agendas.

The third face of power that Digeser added to his list drew upon the work of NYU political theorist Steven Lukes (1974). As a mechanism of soft power the third face captures something that the first two faces do not encapsulate, namely scenarios in which an actor or institution willingly—without the use of brute force or open pressure—does something that another actor wants him or her to, yet is against the interests of the person or institution doing it. This expansion of the remit of power to situations where there is neither an open conflict between the parties nor an apparent *disagreement* represents a significant conceptual advance beyond the first two faces. In the words of Digeser, "the first two faces are blind to a form of power in which the very desires and wants of [an actor] are manipulated" (Digeser 1992: 979; see also Lukes 1974: 23).

Digeser's fourth face of power is influenced by the Foucauldian notion of power. Within this fourth face of power, there are no open conflicts or clearly defined interests, and neither are people's subjectivities predetermined (or manipulated). Instead, within such a Foucauldian understanding of power, it is assumed that people's subjectivities are created through their actions and their interactions with others (such as humans or technological devices). In other words, actors "make themselves" in and through interactions with others, and always against the backdrop of societal "truths" (discourses). A person's identity as a good patient or as a good doctor is not established according to stable and objective criteria but is shaped by societal understandings of good conduct in a specific situation, by other political, economic, and cultural values, or by interactions between patients and doctors with their human, natural, and artefactual environments.

Such a nuanced understanding of power sheds a very different light on participation in medicine than celebratory accounts of patients being "empowered" through technologies. Employing an understanding of power as something that is present in all social systems, and something that can be invisible and even nonintentional makes us ask different questions than we would if we treated power as shaped by the material capabilities that an actor has at her disposition and assumed that actors exercised their power rationally. This is not to say that material capabilities or rationalities do not matter; a patient being forced to undergo a treatment against her will and against her interest by enforceable law is a very stark example of the exercise of power. But instances of this first face of power have become relatively rare in medicine and health care in contemporary Western liberal democracies. This is because physical force and other forms of access to people's bodies against their will are seen as unacceptable unless there is a strong justification, such as the containment of an infectious disease, or the prevention of self-harm or harm to others.

It is also because of the relative scarcity of brute force and open conflict that scholarship investigating Western biomedicine has focused on softer expressions of power. Soft power is often expressed in the decisions that people make, and those that they do not make. The elderly man who does not ask for better palliative care because he does not want to make a fuss, or the parents who feel they have to agree to a sex-assignment surgery after the birth of their infant born with "ambiguous" genitalia, all act upon social norms and contribute to establishing what is normal and responsible (see also Casper and Moore 2009; Lemke 2011). As Nikolas Rose (2007) pointed out, in advanced liberal democracies it is usually no longer state authorities that "improve" people by introducing measures at the population level, such as by operating forced sterilization or detaining the morally and mentally "abnormal" (see also C. Mills 2011). Today, individuals are increasingly being called upon—and are calling upon themselves—to enhance themselves, by eating the right food, by keeping fit, or by taking genetic tests to determine disease susceptibilities or potential genetic issues of their unborn (see also Cetina 2005; Clarke et al. 2010b). They do this not because they are coerced to do so, but because they *want* to be healthy, fit, and responsible. These values are in turn closely aligned with norms of production and reproduction, including norms about sexuality, as Natalie Boero's study of the American obesity "epidemic" masterfully shows (Boero 2012). Many of the societal truths that we translate into our preferences and commitments in this manner are indeed highly gendered: a female healthy body is seen to need different things than a male healthy body, and different types of behaviors and environmental factors are seen to make women and men sick (S. Moore 2010; see also Casper and Moore 2009: chapter 5). Moreover, because women are seen as responsible for feeding and caring for their families, many health, lifestyle, and obesity prevention campaigns are targeted at them. This places not only the work of managing the health of the family on the shoulders of women but also a large part of the responsibility for failing to do so effectively. And such societal truths are highly racialized too: Explicit and implicit bias leads to black patients being considered "tougher" and able to put up with more pain, or less able to understand complex medical information (Matthew 2015).

## A Powerful Opposition: Social Determinants versus Individual Behavior Change

The stigmatization of obesity is an instructive example of the relationship between medical evidence, societal truth, and personal practices. It would be tempting to explain the significant role that the "fight against obesity" plays on public health agendas by referring to the considerable medical problems that are associated with higher body mass. They include diseases such as diabetes, coronary heart disease, and respiratory problems. But this is not the whole story. In his book *Fat Politics* (2006), political scientist Eric Oliver challenges the assumption that overeating *causes* diseases. Instead, he argues, obesity is mostly *correlated* with health problems because in America, poor and ill people are likely to have higher body mass. Moreover, that people eat a lot and exercise little, argues Oliver, is a manifestation of America's consumer culture. As long as politics and culture will not change, overeating will not go away.

With his analysis that obesity is a political and cultural practice, Oliver is a lone voice amidst the large choir of those who see overeating as an individual choice that places significant burdens on society. The literature on the costs of obesity is vast.[4] As a result, authorities channel funds and efforts into prevention, increasingly also by "nudging"[5] people into leading healthier lives (see G. Cohen, Fernandez Lynch, and Robertson 2016; Marteau et al. 2011; Michie and West 2013; Quigley 2012; Thaler and Sunstein 2008).

The idea that the obesity "epidemic" is best addressed at the level of individual behavior change makes intuitive sense to many people, but it should not. Social and economic factors have been found to play a key role in shaping the health or illness of people (Marmot 2015; Institute of Medicine 2014). In the United States, the gap in life expectancy between the richest and the poorest 1 percent of the population is almost fifteen years (Chetty et al. 2016). The reasons for this are unequal insurance, unequal access to health care, and unequal access to healthy food, clean air, and education. Epidemiologist Michael Marmot called these factors "the causes of causes" (Marmot 2005: 1101) because they make certain healthy behaviors harder or even impossible to achieve for some people, such as those who live in unsafe neighborhoods, who have no access to fresh produce, or those whose financial worries prevent them from sleeping.

Another critical factor that influences health outcomes is the experience of discrimination and shame. African Americans have worse health outcomes than Caucasians and other groups even when the data have been controlled for access to health care and socioeconomic factors. Stress resulting from structural discrimination plays a big role here, but so does lower quality of health care received, not least due to the conscious or unconscious bias of health care professionals who treat members of different ethnic groups unequally (Duster 2015; Matthew 2015; Roberts 2011).

That formal access to health care is not the only factor that matters in terms of health inequalities is also illustrated by data from England. The United Kingdom has tax-funded universally accessible health care that is free at the point of use; people with little means even get their travel to the hospital reimbursed, and their drugs paid for. But the difference in life expectancy between the poorest and the richest 10 percent within the same inner-London district, the Borough of Westminster, is almost nine years, and similar discrepancies are found between the wealthier regions of the south and the more deprived regions in the north of England, just to name two examples (Buck and Maguire 2015). The reasons for this lie, again, in social and economic determinants that represent the "causes of causes" for lives led in greater stress and distress, with more humiliation, and fewer opportunities to take time off work or take a rest when needed, and in a greater need for escape or coping mechanisms such as alcohol, tobacco, or "comfort food."

Despite the fact that inequalities by income and race are increasing, public funding for population and public health goals in the United States has been declining (Khoury and Galea 2016). A similar trend can be observed in Europe, which has been swept by a wave of austerity politics since the financial crisis in 2008. At the same time, attention to so-called Omics research—the study of data representing different types of molecules in a cell, such as genomics—has been increasing. Besides such data-driven science, also research on how individuals can be "nudged" to adopt healthier lifestyles has seen a surge in funding and in public attention. This prioritization of data-driven science and "new public health" (Petersen and Lupton 1996) strategies aiming at behavior change, at the cost of more investment into improving the social determinants of health, is a reflection of a political economy where the failures and losses of corporate actors are collectivized—think bank bailouts with public money—while the supposed failures and mistakes of citizens are individualized. Citizens are advised to behave well, and sometimes given some support to do so, but if they do not succeed, they are increasingly left alone.

## The Powers of Patient Participation

Against this backdrop, it seems important that people manage themselves and their health effectively. And if people do get sick, they have the duty to do what they can to get better. This duty is not enforced by the use of brute force, or even by legal means. It is enforced by making people *want* to get better. I already referred to Foucault's understanding of how people internalize the norms and values of authorities to govern themselves in accordance with these norms, a mechanism that Peter Digeser called the fourth face of power. But other scholars have also drawn links between illness and deviance that are relevant for our understanding of people's self-governance. A prominent example is the

American sociologist Talcott Parsons, who developed the notion of the "sick role" in the early 1950s (Parsons 1951). Parsons argued that sick people assume a role of "sanctioned deviance." Sick people are perceived as dysfunctional as they cannot be fully productive members of society. But for the effective functioning of society it would be dangerous to leave sick people to their own devices. To do so would mean that sick people would be outside the remit of societal control. This is why, according to Parsons, societies have always given sick people certain privileges: They are exempt from many of the duties of healthy people, including work or caring for others. In many societies they have been entitled to receive help in the form of social care or financial support. In return for such assistance, however, they are also assigned specific duties: they need to do their best to get better, and try to become fully functioning members of society as quickly as they can. If they refuse to work toward this expectation, they lose the privileges that come with the sick role and become fully deviant.

Albeit writing from very different perspectives, Michel Foucault and Talcott Parsons both concluded that sick people can never merely be passive; they are expected to be active members of society at least in the sense that they actively seek to get better. This simultaneity of passivity and activity also lies at the core of the notion of participatory medicine. On the one hand, patients are, by definition, in need of help and care; in this sense they are at least structurally in a more passive place than those who help them. At the same time, the strong emphasis on empowerment and participation in current public health and medical discourse emphasizes the need for patients to be proactive in pursuing what is good for them, *and* for society. The inevitable tensions between these two goals are obscured, but not removed, by the empowerment rhetoric. This is also reflected in definitions of participatory medicine that describe patients as "responsible drivers of their health," while "providers encourage and value them as full partners" (Frydman 2013). In this vision people should be active decision makers and managers of their own health ("in the driving seat"), while they are also expected to fit into existing structures and institutions at the same time. They should innovate, but not at the cost of changing the system too much. Most importantly, they must not hurt the vested interests of Big Brother and Company Man (Kang et al. 2012).

In the next section I will use two case studies to explore how practices and technologies associated with personalized medicine are involved in articulating and redistributing power. In the first case I return to the type of personal genome tests taken by Milena, whose story opened this chapter. The introduction of such tests to the online market at the end of the 2000s received a lot of attention from public media, clinicians, and scholars alike (for an overview, see Harris, Kelly and Wyatt 2016). Although there was little agreement on the risks and benefits of these tests, most commentators did agree that new testing technology having become available to the public was the cause of the problem. The tests looked at variations at the level of single nucleotides in people's DNA and then calculated the genetic risk for a broad variety of conditions and characteristics. Clinicians, ethicists, and regulatory agencies alike saw these tests as insufficiently robust and predictive to be released for public access.

But what happens if we stop seeing the test technology itself as a key agent of disruption and innovation, but instead treat the social meaning of the technological practice as the key agent? Disagreement on the reliability and ethical use of a new type of test then becomes a controversy over the personal and societal meaning of genetic information, and over the acceptable contexts of its production and use. If we do this we also see, as I will show in the case description below, a struggle over the authority to make predictions about the future (see also Prainsack 2011a). The question of who can make legitimate claims about the future is crucial to how we envisage and implement personalized medicine. If we consider evidence produced by technical devices and algorithms as the highest form of evidence within personalized medicine, we will end up with a very different kind of personalization than if we put shared decision making, dialogue, and "subjective" values of patients in the center of personalization (see also NHS Scotland 2016).

## Empowering Companies by Empowering Users? The Case of Personal Genome Testing

Employing a broad understanding of power comprising all four faces discussed by Digeser (see table 3.1) begs the question of how structural aspects of power and practices of self-governance come together to shape practices of participation in medicine. The example of DTC genomics illustrates how the introduction of a technological practice to personalize health-related information can affect the distribution of power between different actors in partly unexpected ways.

Although online genetic tests had been available for almost two decades, a particular variant of them sparked a particularly heated controversy in the late 2000s. In 2007, to be exact, a small number of companies started to market genome-wide tests looking at genetic markers that corresponded with risk for diseases or traits.[6] Initially costing about one thousand U.S. dollars, these tests deviated from previous forms of clinical genetic testing in several ways. First of all, they were offered online and DTC and thus cut out health professionals. Anybody with Internet access, a credit card, and the necessary economic resources could order the test and receive results online without going to see a health professional. A handful of companies offered tests for genetic predispositions to diseases; some included drug metabolism status and genetic carrier information, and some gave information on genetic ancestry. The California company 23andMe also gave information about a person's genetic predisposition to traits that were not related to health, such as freckling or bitter-taste perception.

These tests also differed from previous DTC online genetic tests in their genome-wide approach; they were not limited to a particular region in the genome but scanned for markers across the entire genome. Results were thus highly speculative and often inconsistent across different test providers and across time. Different companies used different markers and algorithms, and new markers became available as new scientific studies were published. As testing technologies and methodologies changed, so did people's test results.

Not surprisingly, the tests drew strong criticism from ethicists, health authorities, social scientists, and clinicians. Much of their criticism focused on classical bioethical concerns such as data protection, the right not to know (see also Chadwick, Levitt, and Shickle 1997, 2014), and on the analytic validity and clinical utility of test results.[7] Many of these concerns were related to the fact that testing algorithms were based on research findings that had not been replicated or validated. Many also addressed the problem that DTC genetic testing bypassed medical professionals. Later on, concerns about the systemic effects of the provision of personalized genetic information by commercial companies became more prominent. Specifically, it was feared that test takers would turn to the publicly funded or supported health care system for help with interpreting their results and thus drain collective resources (see, for example, Caulfield et al. 2010; Selkirk et al. 2013).

But was the problematic accuracy and predictive value of the new test the root cause of this controversy? I believe that the core issues lay much deeper. If we treat DTC genomic testing as a technology-in-practice (Timmermans and Berg 2003a), and if we look at the discursive and institutional landscape that it has been embedded in, it appears that the controversy around DTC genetics stemmed also from the challenge that DTC personal genomics posed to some core categories and assumptions of clinical medicine (Lucivero and Prainsack 2015). First and foremost, the idea that people should have unmediated access to their genetic information runs against preconceived divisions between science, health care professionals, patients and publics.[8] Not only did DTC companies bypass health care professionals, but many DTC testing companies also openly challenged the idea that clinicians *should* be gatekeepers to genetic information. Many users of DTC companies were (and are) highly educated people who—if only via their engagement with genetic factors influencing health—understood genetic risk data better than many medical professionals. Most medical professionals, after all, have not been trained to interpret such data (see, for example, Szoka 2013). Second, as mentioned earlier, DTC genomics services did not sequence genes to test for specific mutations but instead created large datasets that could be reanalyzed in light of new findings. These new findings could lead to changes in individual genetic risk scores. DTC genomics thus also challenged the idea that genetic information was something stable and reliable (see also Turrini and Prainsack 2016). Third, by disclosing personalized genetic risk information regarding nonhealth-related traits such as alcohol-flush reaction or genetic ancestry alongside health-relevant information, some companies portrayed genetic testing as a recreational activity, or even as something pleasurable. This unsettled traditional understandings of genetic testing as a serious and often painful process that responds to health concerns.

In short, DTC genomics services challenged several assumptions underpinning clinical medicine: that medical experts are legitimate gatekeepers to genetic information; that genetic information given to individuals should always be validated and clinically useful; and that genetic testing is inevitably robust and health related. They also unsettled the delineation of different roles and functions within clinical practice: patients who seek advice, treatment, and care; doctors who provide expert knowledge and who practice medicine on the basis of that knowledge; and genetic counselors and other specialists who each contribute what they have been specifically professionally trained to do. DTC disturbs the way clinical medicine is set up.

My argument here is not that DTC genetics turned patients into market consumers. Although such an observation is accurate, it is incomplete. It misses that what changed here were not only the relationships and power dynamics between different actors, but also the configuration and nature of some of the very actors themselves (see also Harris, Kelly, and Wyatt 2016). DTC genomics has been controversial not simply because it rests upon a novel technological approach but because the people who run the testing services set out to challenge the gatekeeping position of certified health professionals to genetic information. DTC genomics companies promote the idea that users can make sense of their personalized genetic risk information on their own, without the help of health professionals. If they do need help, they can get it from the data-visualization tools and background information provided by the company—and perhaps from online communities and free software tools such as OpenSNP (opensnp. org). In addition, at least some DTC genomics companies give their users access to their raw SNP data. By doing so, they challenge the idea that scientific information should flow in one direction, namely from the biomedical realm to the realm of patients and publics, and that the concentration of knowledge should follow a gradient from its source (science) via medical professionals on to lay people.

So how does this affect the distribution of power? In the case of DTC genomics, we see very little of the first face of power. There is no open pressure or coercion, apart from the power exerted by regulatory authorities such as the U.S. Food and Drug Administration (FDA), which first stopped personal genomics companies from disclosing health-related information in 2013 (Wagner 2013). Instances of the second face of power—actors preventing others from doing something that the latter want to do—are discernable. For example, the price and language of the

DTC genetics testing service creates socioeconomic barriers: Almost ten years and several price drops after their launch, an SNP-based genome-wide analysis still costs at least one hundred U.S. dollars. This means that many people are excluded from even considering taking a DTC genomics test because they lack the money, the necessary technological tools, or language or computer skills.

Determining instances of the third face of power is the most difficult: Have people been manipulated into doing something that is against their interests? Some critics of DTC genetics would argue that people who have their genome analyzed without the involvement of a physician must have been manipulated into it, because it is a dangerous thing to do. It is dangerous because genetic test results, once seen, cannot be unseen. If we agree with this stance, then the entire field of DTC genetics becomes an example of the third face of power. If we do not accept that getting one's personal genetic risk profile without the involvement of a medical professional is dangerous as such, however, it is much harder to discern any instances of the third face. The term "interest" is difficult to operationalize in this respect: Who determines what somebody's interests are? If the person herself determines what her interests are, then we need to take what she says at face value. In that case the third face of power is irrelevant in the context of DTC genetic testing: if I had been manipulated into *willingly* doing something, then I would, by definition, not consider this to be against my interests. Interpretive approaches would suggest that it is impossible to determine interests objectively (Wagenaar 2011); it is not possible to assume the position of an objective observer with a "God's eyes" perspective.

Luckily, the problem of having to decide what people's objective interests are does not emerge regarding the fourth face of power. The fourth face assumes that interests and subject positions are shaped in social interactions and are not stable or objective. Analyzing the fourth face of power requires us to look at the dominant discourse prevailing in a given field, and then determine the position and role of actors and practices vis-à-vis the dominant discourse. In the context of DTC genetics, the dominant discourse is constituted by certain ideas about how power, authority, and expertise should be distributed in the medical domain, and by how the medical field is organized—and who is in charge of making these decisions.

If we stick with the concrete example of 23andMe, we can say that the company clearly positioned itself in opposition to the assumption that doctors should be gatekeepers to medical information. According to Anne Wojcicki, 23andMe's founder, the desire to overturn this assumption had been one of the driving forces behind setting up the company. "People should have access to their own genetic information," she told a reporter for the *New York Times:* "It belongs to them.[9] Get rid of the paternalism" (quoted in Miller 2014). This rhetoric labels the clinicians, ethicists, and regulatory authorities who have criticized 23andMe for bypassing medical professionals, or for disclosing information that is not clinically useful, as anachronistic defenders of the established discourse. They deserve to be "disrupted" by DTC companies and their users who grant and obtain direct access to genetic information under the guise of making biomedical research more democratic. The emphasis on "opening up" science conceals the strategic commercial interests of the company, who now own a unique biomedical resource. This is not just happenstance: As Astra Taylor argued, "open" access to digital technologies often has the consequence of amplifying domination (Taylor 2014: 214). Similarly, social theorist Kean Birch and colleagues pointed out that open science can be "another attempt to create a 'knowledge commons' that can be enclosed through new property rights or technical arrangements" (Birch et al., 2016: 39; see also Tyfield 2012).

Besides keeping their proprietary interests covered by a varnish of openness and community, the democratization rhetoric has also enabled the company to enter a discursive alliance with "regular" citizens that conceals the profound power asymmetries between the two. The language of patient empowerment bears a strong connotation of individual autonomy, choice, and freedom from paternalism, especially in the North American context. By adopting this rhetoric, 23andMe managed to position itself alongside citizen activists in opposition to supposedly oppressive state authorities seeking to restrict their natural rights. This discursive alliance between antiestablishment activism and libertarian consumerism has made also other commercial companies in the field even more powerful.

Today, very few of the DTC genomics companies that made headlines in 2007 are still operational. After the first push-back from regulatory authorities in the late 2000s, and following relatively low consumer demand, one company after another changed its business model or gave up entirely. Some started to involve physicians in their activities: doctors now order tests for patients, or disclose results to them (Prainsack and Vayena 2013). One of the last remaining "pure" DTC companies on the health market is 23andMe, which notably has been backed by Google. The FDA ordered 23andMe to cease disclosing health-related genetic risk information to new customers late in 2013. But the company started offering its health-related tests to consumers in the United Kingdom and Canada in 2014, and relaunched its services in the United States a year later—only to stop showing health-related results to customers in some countries early in 2017. As a holder of one of the world's largest DNA databases it is now stronger than ever. It attracts considerable amounts of public funding for its research arm and leads impactful research collaborations with public and private entities.

Two main groups of actors have been empowered by the emergence of DTC genomics. The first are people who are interested in their genetic and genomic information and who have the necessary means and resources to get it. They are now able to obtain this information directly, without needing a clinical indication, or going through health professionals. The second group of actors that has been empowered by this development are companies that were already very powerful, such as 23andMe and Google; 23andMe, besides owning one of the world's largest DNA databases, has also obtained crucial influence in policy making and regulation. By creating facts on the ground, namely by building a cohort of more than a million people who have direct access to information about their genome, the company forces regulatory agencies to deal with this situation.

That empowerment is not a zero sum game becomes clear when we look at who has lost power through these developments. It would be easy to assume that health care professionals lost the most, specifically their position as gatekeepers to health-related genetic and genomic information. But for some health professionals this is not an issue at all; many genetic counselors and doctors have told me that they would not want to discuss DTC genetics results with patients. They did not want to become health information managers for the worried well: They would rather help people with "real" problems. Most of the people who voiced this view to me were employed within publicly funded health care systems.

The situation may be different for self-employed health care profession-als for whom DTC customers seeking help in interpreting their results may be a vital source of income. But it is clearly not straightforward to conclude that health professionals as a group have been disempowered by the introduction of DTC genetics in the health domain.

One group of actors that has clearly been disempowered by these de-velopments are public organizations and civil society more broadly. The fact that one of the largest DNA databases is owned by a privately owned company does not help advance public interests—not only because public funding now goes to support commercial companies instead of going to publicly owned research institutions, but also because privately owned companies are not accountable to the public for key decisions they make (Aicardi et al. 2016). Moreover, in public perception, the link between Google and 23andMe—despite all the criticism that this alli-ance has received—seems to have helped Google to establish itself as a player in the health domain. When Google financially backed 23andMe in the late 2000s, it still raised eyebrows: Do we want a giant, multi-national corporation to hold our DNA information? When it became known, less than ten years later, that Google was the company of choice to help the British National Health Service with the analysis of clinical data, very few eyebrows moved anywhere anymore (Google DeepMind 2016). Google has solidified its position as a legitimate service provider, data collector, and de facto regulator in the health care field.

In sum, in the case of DTC, one of the most profound instantiations of the fourth face of power is that large commercial companies have entered the scene and are seen as posing legitimate challenges to regu-latory authorities. They are seen as the harbingers of innovation and creative "disruption" while public authorities are associated with inertia and paternalism. If public actors want to change this situation, they need to take a much more active role in formulating and realizing their own visions of medicine and health care, and to invest in publicly owned infrastructures and innovation. Their own role must not be limited to having to take the edges off the worst consequences of the visions that privately owned corporations create and realize.

What Biomarkers Do

As a second example of shifts in the distribution of power in the domain of medicine is the increasing focus on biomarkers in medical imaging. In contrast to the previous example, there is no public controversy here, and no open challenge to traditional categories or knowledge flows in the domain of health care. Nor does this case, as the previous one did, openly challenge anybody's professional expertise or gatekeeping position. What we do find in this case, however, is that shifts in technological practices in the name of personalization have had wide-ranging effects on the duties, responsibilities, and options of different actors. And, as I will argue at the end of this section, they also contribute to the reshaping of some fundamental categories in our societies.

The increasing use of biomarkers in medicine has been a key component of personalized medicine. Defining the term "biomarker" is not straightforward, and the use of the term in literature is not consistent. Some authors understand biomarkers as objective indications of stages of pathology that can be measured reproducibly (for example, Strimbu and Tavel 2010; see also Biomarker Definitions Working Group 2001). In this understanding, if biomarkers reflect characteristics that are expected to change as a result of therapeutic interventions, such as tumor size, for example, they also make good clinical endpoints: They enable comparisons between two time points, such as before and after chemotherapy.

A smaller group of authors use the term "biomarker" to refer to any marker that correlates with the working of the body more broadly. In the latter understanding, weight and sex may also be seen as biomarkers. Regardless of what definition is used, it is clear that biomarkers play an increasingly important role in medicine, especially if they are quantifiable and digital. In many instances, biomarkers have replaced other clinical parameters, especially nonquantified, narrative, or palpable characteristics and variables that reflect a patient's functioning and wellbeing. In stroke diagnosis, for example, images—for example, from computed tomography (CT) or MRI—are increasingly complementing or replacing traditional means of diagnosis based on clinical symptoms.

Medical imaging is a field that has undergone a particularly rapid process of "biomarkerization" (Metzler 2010). A key reason for this is that the use of imaging devices and software has made medical images digital and computable, and they (semi-)automatically quantify what can be seen. It would be wrong to speak of a *quantification* of imaging, of course; in the early days of nuclear medicine in particular, results were numerical and had to be visualized for medical practitioners to understand them. MRI, for example, started out as a numeric measuring technique; numeric representations had to be translated into visual images as MRI was becoming more widely used also by radiologists, who were seen as less comfortable interpreting numeric measurements than nuclear medicine specialists were (see, for example, Joyce 2008; Beaulieu 2002). In this sense imaging has had a long history of quantification. Throughout this history, however, the goal has been to visualize the numerical, whereas we are now seeing the re-quantification of the visible. For many decades, medical imaging had relied mostly on trained and experienced experts looking at the image with their bare eyes ("eyeballing"). Today, imaging software quantifies certain parameters such as the diameter of a tumor.

An example for how this plays out in practice is the diagnosis of heart disease. For a long time, the diagnostic standard was to determine the degree of stenosis on the basis of eyeballing an image. This means that trained experts rated the degree of narrowing of a vessel by looking at the image. The result was neither digitally recorded nor necessarily quantified in discrete figures and numbers. Today, guidelines prescribe that certain interventions, such as the widening of the coronary artery with the help of a balloon catheter, should be done only after an analysis of the blood flow through the heart muscle (perfusion scan) and a quantitative stenosis assessment have been carried out. The latter is done with the help of a specific heart-imaging technique called quantitative coronary angiography. The images that are produced are digital, and they are accompanied by quantified evaluation. Triangulating the diagnosis in such a manner, it is argued, helps to avoid the treatment of nonsignificant arterial alterations.

Initially, quantifications based on digital data were produced as a by-product of the primary function of the instrument. They made something visible that could not otherwise be seen. Later, because such quantified data were available, their collection and analysis became established as a new standard. They replaced the embodied expertise of the human expert. And here is where the analysis of the different dimensions of power becomes relevant again: Human radiologists are disempowered by these developments in that they need to follow more extensive and detailed protocols, while a growing proportion of the evidence that shapes decision making comes not from them but from machines. In principle, radiologists could decide to dismiss the machine-produced digital evidence if they believed it was wrong. But if they did so, they would open themselves up to challenge and perhaps even litigation. This is a clear case of the second face of power; and an example of the third or fourth faces as well if radiologists themselves believed that machines produce better evidence than their own experience.

Another instance of disempowerment of human actors becomes visible when we consider, as Lisanne Bainbridge did in her seminal piece on the "ironies of automation," that "the more advanced a control system is, so the more crucial may be the contribution of the human operator" (Bainbridge 1983: 775). In other words, the key question is not whether machines will replace humans in making diagnostic and treatment decisions, but how humans and machines can work together. The more machines there will be, the more human input will be required. Automated systems can inevitably only be designed for some, and not all possible scenarios, and they typically rely on human operators to "do the tasks that the designer cannot think how to automate" (ibid.). In medical imaging, humans are needed to detect and correct the errors of machines, and to help the machines see: Human experts need to tell the software where the tumor or the artery is that is being measured (brain imaging is an exception). To illustrate this, figure 4.1 shows the measurement of plaque thickness in a carotid artery carried out by the imaging device, but only after the human operator has marked the outer contours of the artery. The imaging device cannot reliably find the artery by itself.[10] Artificial intelligence and learning algorithms are making strides toward automating the analysis of images, but full automation may never be achieved. As a result, the radiologists using the imaging device that produces quantified digital data are responsible not only for following the script or protocol but also for giving the machine accurate information about what to see. Once this is done, they need to be alert to possible errors of automation. The quantification of images also has systemic impacts on the organization of health care. As Robert Wachter (2015b)

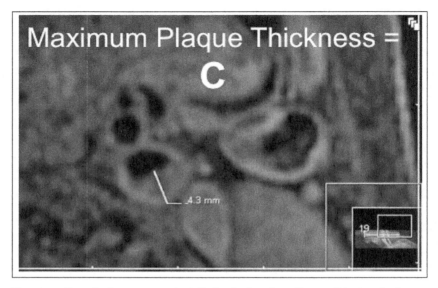

Figure 4.1. Once the human operator tells the device where the carotid artery is, the imaging device quantifies the maximum plaque thickness. Image courtesy of Gabriel Krestin, Erasmus University Medical Center Rotterdam, The Netherlands.

argued, the digitization of radiology had already abolished the need for radiologists to physically meet with the clinicians who requested their expertise. The ability to transmit and read images remotely led to what Richard Gunderman and Allison Tillack called "the loneliness of the long distance radiologist" (Gunderman and Tillack 2012). What is even more concerning than the psychological well-being of radiologists, however, is that without physical meetings, much of the "thick" information about patients that used to be exchanged informally is now lost from the interpretation of the image. While followers of Daniel Kahneman may be inclined to celebrate this as the removal of priming bias, it can also be considered the loss of contextual information.

That radiologists have become data managers spending a lot of time on data validation and treatment monitoring also has implications for their training: With imaging software getting better at "knowing" what the image shows, and measuring key parameters, the interpretation of images requires a different type of expertise than before. Because visual evidence in radiology does not depict something that most other people can easily recognize, a crucial part of radiological training has so far been to teach radiologists how to see: Radiologists learn how to obtain information from a place where others see only noise, and they develop an ability to distinguish physiological variation from pathology. The increasing use of quantitative biomarkers that appear automatically on a screen contributes to a de-skilling. In addition, radiologists face increasing competition from colleagues in other countries: Advances in computing power and the speed of data transmission make it possible for images to be interpreted far away from where they were produced. Experts in India or China can interpret medical imaging materials from clinics in England or Australia in "real time" (Venco 2012). This also gives patients greater independence from their treating physicians. They could (and some do already) submit their imaging data to experts of their choice for interpretation. Their ability to do so is, of course, dependent on whether they can get their hands on their own imaging data, whether they can pay for secondary or independent analyses, and whether they are even aware of having this option. This situation illuminates how contingent on "external" socioeconomic and political factors empowerment and disempowerment attributed to technological practices can be.

At the same time, the increasing reliance on digital, (semi-)automatically quantified biomarkers opens up a new range of possibilities and business opportunities for different actors. The most obvious one is that it improves diagnosis and treatment: In the context of cancer treatment, molecular imaging is already used for disease staging, which is the determination of the severity of a disease, such as lung cancer. Imaging has also been used more widely to guide drug delivery, and image-based treatment monitoring, such as monitoring the change of blood vessels or the size of a tumor. This allows early identification of treatment responders and nonresponders, which could prevent unnecessary side effects for those who do not benefit from a given treatment, and save unnecessary costs. The term "theranostics," a composite of the term "therapy" and "diagnostics," further signifies a growing area of tools and practices representing an "image and treat" approach (Bouchelouche and Capala 2010). The combination of targeted imaging and targeted therapy also aids the identification of localized responses to treatment (European Society of Radiology 2011). And in the domain of prevention, imaging biomarkers can guide the stratification of patients according to their risk of developing a disease: For example, relatively small sizes of particular parts of the brain have been associated with an increased risk of developing dementia (Lupton et al. 2016; Yang et al. 2012). If these findings are confirmed, patients with a smaller hippocampus or amygdala could be singled out for special measures to prevent, or at least push back, the onset of dementia while they are still young.

Similarly, the quantified visualization of cellular and molecular processes also means that some symptoms can be diagnosed much earlier than before. And imaging can replace *ex vivo* tissue analysis, enabling less invasive diagnosis. It allows the identification of localized pathophysiology of diseased tissue as well. All of this not only means more work for those providing imaging services but also much higher revenue for service providers, and for the companies producing imaging devices and software. And typically higher costs for patients.

## Changing Age

Moving from imaging biomarkers specifically to somatic biomarkers more broadly, another thing that biomarkers do is contribute to an increasing quantification not only of disease but of life (see also Rose 2007; Vogt, Hofmann, and Getz 2016). This challenges, at least conceptually, Georges Canguilhem's famous argument that the normal and the pathological are not merely different ends on a quantitative scale, but that they are qualitatively different: Canguilhem considered health to be a state of flexibility defined by the ability to adapt to different environmental impacts. Although there can be "normal" ranges of illness, it is the absence of the ability to tolerate and adapt to external impacts that characterizes illness. This sets illness categorically apart from health (Canguilhem 1989).

But what about biomarkers that measure an oscillating yet overall gradual decline in health that is part of physiological aging? Canguilhem developed his argument in the 1940s, when the average life expectancy was lower than today. With growing life expectancy in many parts of the world, more people now live long enough to experience chronic health issues in old age. The growing proportion of people who need health and social care is seen as posing an additional strain on health care budgets, pensions, social care, and training. Personalized medicine has been hailed as a way to address this challenge. The use of biomarkers to support the diagnosis and treatment of problems associated with old age has been part of the personalized medicine agenda all along. What has not been an explicit part of the personalized medicine agenda, however, is the quantification of age based on biological instead of chronological information.

The use of biomarkers to establish the age of a person is of course not new per se. Forensic scientists have used biological markers of aging to learn more about unidentified human remains. Biological markers for age have also been used in the context of immigration, such as when people claimed to be minors but looked older. A common way of estimating a person's age so far has been the analysis of proteins in teeth or bones (Gibbs 2014: 269). A disadvantage has been that these methods could only be used on a limited range of tissues. When such tissue types were not available, age could not be determined.

Recent science has led to a better understanding of the dynamics of aging at the cellular level, with epigenetics having been a particularly active area of study. In general, epigenetics looks at changes to the genome that do not alter the DNA sequence as such. It focuses on the way in which environmental impacts modify the regulation of genes. Research in another field of study, microbiomics, has found that changes in the composition of human gut bacteria can reflect age-related inflammation (so-called "inflamm-aging"; Zapata and Quagliarello 2015). With the help of such biomarkers, the biological quantification of age is now entering the domain of living beings. One method, developed by UCLA biostatistician Steve Horvath, utilizes the fact that the activity of genes changes over a human life course. Horvath and his team developed an algorithm, a kind of epigenetic "clock" that determines cell age. One of the benefits of this method is that it works in different kinds of tissue, and the accuracy of the algorithm seems to be high (Horvath 2013).

The potential applications of methods to determine biological age are numerous. We already know that people age at a different pace, and being able to assess the biological age of relevant tissues can inform medical decision making in more meaningful ways than chronological age. In the domain of assisted reproduction, for example, age cutoff points—typically between the ages of forty and forty-five—are used to determine the eligibility of women for in vitro fertilization or insurance coverage of fertility-related procedures. Reasons for the age limit include the negative effect of higher maternal age on egg quantity and quality that has been found in population-level data, as well as typical hormonal changes over the lifecourse. It is possible that in the domain of assisted reproduction, chronological age cutoffs will be abolished entirely and give way to the exclusive use of relevant biomarkers.

Personalized medicine, by making increased use of biomarkers and quantified digital parameters, is expanding this approach to wider areas. The availability of biomarkers that correspond with "somatic performance" by ascertaining how young or "functional" somebody's body is compared to a variety of standards is particularly relevant in the context of a backlash against age discrimination in many countries. In many societies, mandatory retirement age provisions have come under fire. The more scientifically robust and clinically useful age-related biomarkers become, the more likely it is that such biomarkers will replace chronological age as a criterion for access to certain benefits or services. For example, could somebody's ability to remain in paid employment until a higher (chronological) age be justified by age-related biomarkers? Do social justice–related arguments support such an approach? It could be argued that those of us who experience more stress, which is, in turn, correlated with social and economic hardship, tend to age faster (Cherkas et al. 2006; Robertson et al. 2013). Do those of us to whom this applies deserve to retire earlier? Those of us whose living circumstances, jobs, or genetic predisposition let us age more slowly, in contrast, could be seen as having the duty to work longer, or to contribute more to society in another way. In sum, medicine's increasing reliance on biomarkers can spill out of the medical field and affect categories that legal and regulatory frameworks have traditionally operated with.

## Conclusion

This chapter started out by discussing different ways of seeing and analyzing power. Inspired by Peter Digeser's (1992) distinction between four "faces" of power, I have looked at shifts in the distribution of power within two areas: The first was DTC personal genome testing, and the second the increasing use of biomarkers in the field of medical imaging.

I deliberately used two examples that display critical differences: While personal genome testing has received a lot of attention from public media and in scientific communities alike, the quantification of medical imaging has received relatively little. Personal genome testing is a "loud" technological practice that is seen to raise controversial ethical issues, and it openly challenges traditional categories that clinical medicine has operated with. The requantification of medical imaging, in contrast, is a much more silent development, but when it comes to the changes in power that they contribute to, the latter one is perhaps even more impactful.

What we can see in both cases is that technology cannot be analyzed in an isolated manner; as scholars in STS and related fields have argued, the agency of technology is always technology-in-practice (for example, Timmermans and Berg 2003a). The concrete uses of a technology determine their involvement in changing power relationships. A smartphone that is used for stalking a person is very different from one that provides a light source during a power cut, or one that is used to monitor somebody's pulse. And if most people used their phone for one purpose rather than the other, this would in turn shape the evolution of mobile phone technology.

Both cases discussed in this chapter illustrate practices of "personalizing" medicine in the sense of making probabilistic predictions on the basis of a person's genome information or medical images respectively. In both cases, even those aspects of the technological practice that are framed as diagnostic or predictive, such as calculating somebody's genetic disease risk, or the degree of the stenosis of her artery, are future-directed; the process of diagnosis does not only have implications for the selection of the treatment regime but also for prognosis. The stratification of people into different groups, according to what genetic markers they carry, or according to the pace with which their tumor shrinks during treatment, also puts them into different therapeutic and prognostic groups. In this sense, controversies over legitimate expertise in the field of diagnostic and therapeutic knowledge, technology, and practice are also always struggles over the authority to act upon the future.

Last but not least, the cases discussed in this chapter also highlight the need to think carefully about how we can avoid a scenario in which personalized medicine will increase social inequalities. The example of aging biomarkers has shown how plausibly medical "evidence" could spill out of the medical domain and redefine criteria for legal duties or entitlements—such as, in our example, in the case of retirement. This is not necessarily a bad thing, but it requires careful consideration of the potential political and social consequences. With improved, data-rich characterization of people and their diseases, the choice between different diagnostic and treatment options will be guided more strongly by probabilistic outcome predictions (see also Hood 2014; Hood and Flores 2012), shifting power from health care professionals to digital datasets and algorithms. People whose chance to benefit from a certain intervention is algorithmically determined to be worse than another group of people could be excluded from this intervention in the name of "fair rationing," without the algorithm being open to examination.

There is also the concern that treatment choices will increasingly also be determined by what patients can afford (see also McGowan et al. 2014). The rhetoric of personalization emphasizes that medical decisions are based on seemingly objectively measured personal characteristics. It thereby conceals that some of these characteristics are directly related to financial resources—and most of them are connected to socioeconomic factors. Thus, there is indeed a risk that personalized medicine will further empower those who have the means and resources to pay for expensive care and treatments and disempower those who cannot. Such a scenario would disadvantage those people who cannot, or do not want to, contribute to the personalization of their own care in the ways that systems expect or prescribe.

The next chapter will be devoted to making explicit the economic and political context in which personalized medicine is currently taking shape. I will discuss the extent to which profit-driven commercial goals are intertwined with philanthropic and activist initiatives, especially in the realm of digital health. I will argue that this entanglement has made it more difficult than ever for people to decide who to entrust with their data and information, and, ironically, how to plan for the future.

# 5

## Just Profit?

### Introduction: "If You Were a Company . . ."

The making of financial profits is often contrasted with rationales that foreground social value or societal benefit. The way that current health entrepreneurism is organized, however, does not fit this distinction. Today's health entrepreneurism is situated within a political economy whose dominant discourse considers it possible to combine social benefit and capitalism. This means that personalized medicine unfolds in a situation where it is assumed that "commons and commerce" can be symbiotically aligned (Van Dijck and Nieborg 2009: 863; A. Taylor 2014).

A number of social scientists have discussed the marriage of profit orientation and idealist activism in the domain of health (for example, Cooper and Waldby 2014; Hayden 2003, 2007; Pálsson 2009; Parry 2004; Tutton and Prainsack 2011). Most of these analyses, however, treat profit orientation and nonprofit health activism as distinct types of practices that only come to converge in some specific instances. But today, their convergence is no longer a rare occurrence; it is becoming the norm. This is particularly apparent in the digital health sector, where data can travel very quickly between the public and private realms[1] and where entrepreneurial forms and practices can change rapidly.

And the digital health sector is growing. The global market for electronic health records alone was estimated to be worth over $22 billion by 2015 (Price 2014), and predicted to exceed $33 billion in 2025 (Grand View Research 2016). In 2014, almost half (47 percent) of all venture capital–backed health care companies were launched into the stock market ("Healthcare Startup Boom" 2015). While it is true that strict data-protection standards for clinical data, as well as low levels of data interoperability, remain obstacles for digital companies to enter the health care field, recent regulatory developments provide strong incentives. In the United States, the Affordable Care Act (ACA) has mandated that insurers invest between 80 and 85 percent of the premiums they collect in measures to enhance the quality and efficiency of providing health care. Although it is not clear whether this provision will be retained in Republican plans to replace the ACA, digital health enterprises have already benefitted from this (Griffith 2014). Another example for the increasingly important role that digital companies play in the health care sector is the collaboration between Google—or technically speaking, Alphabet, the multinational conglomerate that owns Google—and NHS England. Early in 2016, and without any prior public or political debate, the NHS gave Google access to about 1.6 million patient records (Hodson 2016; Powles and Hodson 2017). The official story is that Google helped the NHS support patients with acute kidney injury. But Google also had access to much wider data sets that it could use to improve its artificial intelligence systems.

What these examples show is that we need new ways of conceptualizing entrepreneurism in the health domain. Many powerful players in the health domain today are consumer tech companies that have no prior or specific health focus—Apple and Alphabet (Google) are the two best-known examples (Sharon 2016). And there are also start-up companies that started as nonprofit initiatives and were later acquired by commercial players that decided to retain the emphasis on social value creation—only that it now also serves to increase revenue.[2] For patients and citizens more broadly, this situation means that the distinction between for-profit and nonprofit is less useful than ever to inform decisions about whom to support, whom to engage with, or whom to trust with their health information. In terms of protecting the confidentiality of patient data, for example, we can no longer assume that data are safer in public hospitals than in the commercial domain. One reason for this is, as examples in the following sections will show, that the mission to create public benefits has been perforated by commercial stakes almost everywhere in medicine and health care—and vice versa.

## The Marriage of Commercial Interests and Health Idealism

In chapter 2 I discussed the online platform PatientsLikeMe to show how services that provide information to patients also take information from them. But PatientsLikeMe is paradigmatic in yet another respect: It exemplifies the many ways in which for-profit and nonprofit goals overlap. Founded by family and friends of a patient suffering from motor neuron disease, the platform had initially set out to facilitate the sharing of information about the diseases that its members or their loved ones were afflicted with. It also facilitated the sharing of information on new research, clinical trials, personal experiences, and the provision of mutual support. With the growth of its user base, PatientsLikeMe has become an influential commercial player, making money from selling patient information to commercial companies. But the site has also remained faithful to its initial mission: It joins forces with nonprofit organizations carrying out research on a range of diseases and it is particularly active also in the development of new patient-centric methodologies (PatientsLikeMe 2014b). The platform also emphasizes that it only works with companies that develop products to improve the lives of patients, and it is very transparent about who they work with specifically, and how. And it is open about how patient data are used to create profits (PatientsLikeMe 2014a).

The story of PatientsLikeMe is thus not simply one of a patient initiative being hijacked or bought up by commercial interests. Instead it is a multilayered cluster of financial, political, and societal interests that do not merely coexist but that mutually enforce each other. At the same time, and despite the patient-centered rhetoric and nomenclature used by the platform, patients have little say in what PatientsLikeMe does: They can suggest new conditions for the platform to include, but apart from that, they are mostly data contributors. It is the owners of the platform who call the shots and reap the financial profits. Patients benefit by obtaining information and support from other users.

This symbiotic relationship between for-profit and nonprofit goals is characteristic of contemporary health entrepreneurism more broadly. The case of data entrepreneur Nathan Eagle is another example. Eagle started out as an epidemiology researcher at the Harvard School of Public Health. He used geolocation data from cell phones and other sources to link with longitudinal data about access to health care or education to find new correlations and patterns. In 2009 he funded a company named Jana, which helped enterprises to reach people in poor world regions for political or market surveys and campaigns. Initially, Jana mostly enabled companies to contact "emerging market consumers," as the company called them, via their mobile phones and get them to watch specific content. People targeted in this manner were typically too poor to pay for mobile airtime. The company turned this obstacle into a business opportunity: Instead of paying for it, people received free mobile airtime as a reward for watching content created by Jana's clients. Later Jana started helping companies get people in low-income countries to download their apps in return for free mobile data.

At first sight, Nathan Eagle's story may look just like any other story of a person creating a for-profit spinout from university-based publicly funded research. Such spinouts have been a common phenomenon since the second half of the twentieth century. At the same time, Eagle's oscillation between publicly funded academic research and the private sector is emblematic of current health data entrepreneurism. Since founding Jana, Eagle has remained involved also in nonprofit research projects. In his book *Reality Mining: Using Big Data to Engineer a Better World*, coauthored with technology journalist Kate Greene in 2014, he emphasizes his unbroken commitment to good causes at the same time as he is trying to make money.

There are many other stories like Nathan Eagle's. Today's health-data entrepreneurism is part of a political-economic system whose dominant discourse assumes not only that nonprofit and for-profit activities are compatible but that they create valuable synergies. Public-private partnerships are high on the agenda of funding bodies and politics, couched in a discourse that sees market mechanisms as distributing resources effectively and prudently, while public ownership and management are seen as ineffective and wasteful. This discourse is hegemonic in the sense that even many of those working for public bodies are part of it. The DTC genomics company 23andMe, for example, prides itself with a quote from a research scientist at the New York State Department of Health: "What 23andMe did in a matter of years would have taken several decades and tens of millions of dollars if done conventionally" (23andMe 2017). Even public officials praise the private sector as dynamic, unconventional, and effective, while the public sector is associated with red tape and paternalism. For many academics working in publicly funded institutions and universities, collaborations with commercial companies provide a way to score points for having impact on the "real world," for stepping out of the ivory tower, and for valorizing research.

At the same time that the pressure on publicly funded researchers to create financial value is mounting, so is the expectation that commercial companies "give back to society." The practice of data philanthropy is an expression of this. Data philanthropy works as follows: Companies or for-profit organizations that routinely collect large amounts of data as part of their core business "donate" these data, with personal identifiers removed, to researchers who use them for common benefit. Geolocation data and call logs held by telephone companies, for example, can be mined in order to learn about likely disease outbreaks, based on the idea that disease outbreaks correlate with changes in patterns of movement of people in a particular area (Wesolowski et al. 2012). Such data can also be used to monitor the movements of people after a natural disaster in order to aid the distribution of emergency relief (Bengtsson et al. 2011), or to improve the understanding of the spatial distribution of diseases (for example, Stresman et al. 2014). Data philanthropists donate data not only to researchers in academic or public institutions but also to commercial start-up companies.

Despite data philanthropy often being portrayed as a sacrifice that companies make for the sake of public good, for most companies, it is an inherent part of their business strategy (see also McGoey 2012; 2014; 2015). For Robert Kirkpatrick (2011), one of the key promoters of the idea of data philanthropy, it seems obvious that it is driven by the same commercial considerations as companies' core business activities. Speaking about his work at the Global Pulse,[3] a United Nations initiative to facilitate and catalyze data-driven research into the "impacts of global and socio-economic crises" (United Nations Global Pulse 2014), Kirkpatrick explains:

> The companies that engage with us, however, don't regard this work as an act of charity. They recognize that population well-being is key to the growth and continuity of business. For example, what if you were a company that invested in a promising emerging market that is now being threatened by a food crisis and that could leave your customers unable to afford your products and services? And what if it turned out that expert analysis of patterns in your own data could have revealed all along that people were in trouble, while there was still time to act? (Kirkpatrick 2011)

Altruism, we are told here, is in business's own best interest. Why let an opportunity to do good and be seen doing it go to waste?

## Don't Be Evil: The Bubble of Idealistic Capitalism

The combination of for-profit strategies bound up with health idealism is a variant of the kind of fluffy capitalism that the Slovenian intellectual Slavoj Žižek considers characteristic of the early twenty-first century. In the mid 2000s, Žižek observed that global capitalism was adopting the ethos of some of its most fervent critics. It is worth quoting the key part of his argument in full:

> Since 2001, Davos and Porto Alegre have been the twin cities of globalization: Davos, the exclusive Swiss resort where the global elite of managers, statesmen and media personalities meets for the World Economic Forum under heavy police protection [ . . . ]; Porto Alegre, the subtropical Brazilian city where the counter-elite of the anti-globalization movement meets [ . . . ] It seems, however, that the Porto Alegre reunions have somehow lost their impetus—we have heard less and less about them over the past couple of years. Where did the bright stars of Porto Alegre go? Some of them, at least, moved to Davos. The tone of the Davos meetings is now predominantly set by the group of entrepreneurs who ironically refer to themselves as "liberal communists" and who no longer accept the opposition between Davos and Porto Alegre: their claim is that we can have the global capitalist cake (thrive as entrepreneurs) and eat it (endorse the anti-capitalist cause of social responsibility, ecological concern, etc). [ . . . ] *Liberal communists do not want to be mere for-profit machines: They want their lives to have deeper meaning.* (Žižek 2006: 10; emphasis added)

Žižek is conscious, of course, that the concept of the good capitalist is not an invention of our time. Indeed, the idea that "the ruthless pursuit of profit is counteracted by charity" (ibid.) is as old as capitalism itself; it has featured in the creation of the welfare state, and been part of the spirit of many family-owned small and medium-size enterprises (Fraser 2015; see also McGoey 2015). Moreover, even the father of laissez-faire capitalism, Adam Smith, was convinced that humans have a natural propensity for "sympathy," as he called it, towards other people. Smith's book on this topic, the *Theory of Moral Sentiments* (1759), preceded his much more famous *The Wealth of Nations* (1776), in which he laid out his main vision of a capitalist economy. Smith assumed that egoism and welfare were compatible; he thought that selfish motivations had the potential to lead to modes of production and exchange that could increase welfare. In other words, welfare, for Smith, was a by-product of capitalist systems, and in fact any system, due to the intrinsic features of human nature. Even Smith's own vision of capitalism thus presupposed that a society where the cruelest edge of capitalism could be purged by people's innate urge to help those in need.

The suggestion that the harshest aspects of capitalism could be mitigated by the charitable actions of capitalists also has a prominent place in popular culture. Some of the most popular TV series in the United Kingdom and in the United States feature capitalism with a human face. The highly popular British drama *Downton Abbey,* for example, launched in 2010, follows the lives of the noble and affluent Crawley family living on a country estate. The family and their servants are separated from each other not only by their distant living quarters on the estate but also by their clothing, their habits, and their language. They live in different worlds, and when they meet, it is always in their roles as masters and servants. This setting bears clear resemblances to class divisions in British society today (Byrne 2014), which are more deeply engrained and more visible than anywhere else in Europe. In *Downton Abbey,* however, these harsh differences are eased by the protective attitude of the aristocratic masters. The Crawley family is portrayed to care for the well-being of its servants. Although it is unclear how much of this is done out of habit and how much out of genuine concern, they ensure that nobody is left alone in their hour of need. This fictitious symbol of a good-hearted upper class prepared to compromise its own comforts for the benefit of those in need stands in stark contrast to the war on the poor that is currently taking place in contemporary Britain. In the United States, the NBC television series *West Wing* (1999–2006), a fantasy of a truly progressive and humane presidency committed to decreasing social inequalities, did a similar service to viewers. And it could be argued that Donald Trump's election as president of the United States embodies a perversion of this phenomenon: A property tycoon who pretends that he deeply cares about the "common man" (arguably a bit less so about the common woman).

Another contemporary articulation of ethical capitalism in the actual world is the concept of corporate social responsibility.[4] It is so popular that it has its own acronym, CSR. It is based on the idea that entrepreneurs and managers have a responsibility not only to shareholders but also to stakeholders (Spreckley 1981). CSR gained currency in the 1970s and obtained additional momentum in the 1980s and 1990s, when global players such as Nestlé and Nike faced mounting criticism following their involvement in the baby milk scandal and their exploitation of child labor respectively. (For summaries of these affairs see Boggan 2001; Muller 2013). The core idea of CSR is often described as "organizations hav[ing] to meet the expectations of society" (Beurden and Gössling 2008: 407). Its growing popularity, however, is linked to the idea that profits can be increased when a company displays its socially responsible and "ethical" awareness (see also McGoey 2015). Unsurprisingly, there is also a sizable literature assessing the extent to which the embrace of CSR improves market performance (for example, Beurden and Gössling 2008). Doing good should not mean that one loses money.

The traditional big players in the domain of health and medicine, such as pharmaceutical companies, have run CSR programs for decades. Since the HIV/AIDS crisis in the 1980s and 1990s, when the pressure on pharmaceutical enterprises to lower costs and ease intellectual property protection to improve access to drugs increased, investments in CSR have increased further (see, for example, Horrigan 2010; Knowledge@Wharton 2012; Weeden 1998). The sincerity and positive effects of these efforts have been the subject of doubt. If large corporations take social responsibility seriously, many wonder, why is access to essential medicines, for example, still such a big problem in many countries (see, for example, Hogerzeil 2013; Leisinger 2005; see also Access to Medicine Index 2014, McGoey 2015)?

For global pharmaceutical enterprises and other large commercial players, an investment in CSR is often a necessary investment in reputation management. For smaller and younger companies in the health domain, the stakes are different. Many newer companies in the health field weave CSR into their organizational fabric from the very start. Role models and infrastructures to help them do so are available: The Salesforce Foundation, for example, headquartered in San Francisco, promotes the so-called 1/1/1/ model, encouraging for-profit companies to devote one percent of their employee time, product resources, and profits to charitable causes (Salesforce 2014; see also Beato 2014; Parrott 2014). The Effective Altruism movement takes the idea of ethical capitalism a step further by applying business metrics to philanthropy. Its goal is to help the global elite "combine the heart and the head" when making investments in society (Centre for Effective Altruism). Effective altruists, we are told on the website, do not merely want to make a difference, but the *most* difference; they look at the evidence and then decide to invest their money in a cause where the marginal benefit of their investment is the highest. The movement believes that the effectiveness of all charities should be assessed objectively, and that "it generally doesn't make sense for individuals to donate to disaster relief" (MacAskill 2015). In this way, philanthropy becomes part of business, and business becomes part of philanthropy. Data philanthropists have already realized this, of course: "We're trying to track unemployment and disease as if it were a brand," says Robert Kirkpatrick, the chair of the UN Pulse Initiative (cited from Lohr 2013).[5]

At least in this sense, Slavoj Žižek was right: More and more actors manage to be in Davos and in Porto Alegre at the same time. Many organizations in the health domain, and particularly those whose activities revolve around health information and digital health, do not fit into traditional binary categories such as public versus private, ethical versus unethical, or bottom-up versus top-down. Despite this, in large parts of the scholarly literature and mass media, publicly funded academic research is still portrayed as striving for public benefits, while commercial research and development is taken to aim solely at maximizing profits. The pharmaceutical industry in particular has certainly done much to deserve the current decline in public trust (see for example, Angell 2005; Goldacre 2012), and critique of ruthless profit making is of essential importance. Because of its focus on large corporate enterprises, such as global pharmaceutical players, device manufacturers, and health management organizations, however, the value of this critique for an analysis of participatory and personalized medicine is limited. Today's health landscape is characterized by a much greater fragmentation of tasks, providers, and locations. And the pace with which new start-ups can become influential players is greater than ever (see also Clarke et al. 2010a). As noted earlier, although the health field has been known for its high entrance barriers, these barriers are much lower in the context of digital health. In 2014, new start-ups focusing on personalizing health data emerged on an almost weekly basis.[6] Companies were built around personalized advice on the basis of pictures of people's lunches and activity-tracking data, or on the basis of an analysis of microbiomes inhabiting our bodies, to name just a few examples.

## Reasons for the Increasing Convergence of Financial Profits and Social Responsibility

What developments have made it easier for new players to enter the health(care) domain? First, web-based tools have reduced the cost and difficulty of communication and marketing. A wider range of people can be approached to become potential investors and at a faster pace. Crowd-sourcing has become an option to complement and in some cases replace other funding strategies. Web-based tools have also made it much easier for people without a preexisting interest in health to find projects or organizations to support. Many of the new initiatives and companies focus on activities that are not clinical, or even medical, in the strict sense of the word, but that have a tangible impact on the lives of patients in other ways. They can improve lab report delivery, increase the effectiveness of patient scheduling (Chu 2014), or enhance the communication between patients and medical professionals. Such initiatives can launch, grow, or disappear very quickly, or change their legal status and organizational form. They are sometimes led by patients or doctors, such as in the case of the British creators of the anti-insomnia smartphone app Sleepio (www.sleepio.com). Some of these initiatives have both a for-profit and a nonprofit arm.

Second, there is more specialization in the health care field today than there has been in the last decades. Many big pharmaceutical and medical technology companies no longer try to keep everything in-house and instead prefer to collaborate with smaller, often younger companies (Chu 2014). Moreover, due to the increasing amount of digital data produced and used in the health domain, health information management and health care IT are growing (see, for example, Gold 2014). As Niccolo Tempini points out, new business opportunities are often created around collecting, processing, or repackaging data from various sources (Tempini 2015; see also Kallinikos 2006; Weber, Mandl, and Kohane 2014).

Third, public actors and private insurers have new incentives to invest in preventive measures. This contributes to a kind of "function creep" of health care into new domains. The increasing convergence of lifestyle and health care (Lucivero and Dalibert 2013) in turn widens the scope of organizations and enterprises that play a role in the health domain.

These developments have contributed to the interlocking of nonprofit and for-profit goals and practices. This applies not only to high-income countries: People in low-income countries have become valuable customers for digital enterprises that often also promote global health, such as mobile phone companies who use text messaging services for data collection or monitoring. All around the globe, the distinction between for-profit and nonprofit can no longer serve as a moral compass for people when deciding whom to support, engage, or entrust their data with. To ensure that people's contributions go and do what they want them to, new approaches are necessary.

In chapter 3, I have argued that practices where people are not actively involved in, or even aware of, data collection ("passive" data collection), and where data can be used for individual-level health-related purposes, are most in need of public scrutiny. In the next section, I will add to this analysis by unpacking the notion of participation further. I will argue that it is virtually impossible to avoid "prosumption," namely the value-cocreation for corporations on the side of patients and citizens. All of us who upload seemingly trivial or innocuous information to online platforms, who use online services, or who have medical records in health care systems that share them with commercial companies for research purposes, have become prosumers.

## What Does the Marriage of Nonprofit and For-Profit Mean for Participation?

For digital humanities scholar Antonio A. Casilli, one of the most original thinkers on the topic of data governance, the notion of participation can serve to connect societal and commercial value. Participation bears the connotation of user-centeredness and individual choice, while at the same time enlisting participants in causes that support the commercial and political interests of powerful actors. This is why participatory design is also a core feature of contemporary digital surveillance systems:

> By "participatory," we mean a mutual, horizontal surveillance based on the intentional, agonistic disclosure of personal informations [sic] by users of digital services, mobile applications and online platforms. It is accompanied by a loss of control over the terms of service of the infra-

structure where personal data are stored and circulated. *This surveillance is participatory insofar as it is mutual and involves a generalization of bottom-up moderation mechanisms and of the way online communities enforce norms within social platforms.* (Casilli 2014; emphasis added)

Casilli argues that in such an understanding, participation has no intrinsic value. It merely denotes contributions that people make, either in terms of time and effort—for example, when they post content online—or in terms of personal information to which they give commercial companies access. Such a thin understanding of participation also resonates with how the term is often used in the context of empowerment-based reforms in medicine (Chiapperino 2014). It has made it possible for participatory initiatives to be enlisted in the quest to personalize medicine in a way that makes it, first and foremost, more cost-effective. But if we want to broaden the understanding of what personalized medicine is about, we need to repoliticize the notion of participation. The debate on prosumption—a composite of production and consumption—is a good place to start.

## Is Prosumption Always Bad? Three Types of Health Information Prosumers

Those with whom people share personal health-relevant information can be clinicians, medical professionals, friends, family members, or companies. In every instance, our contributions—in terms of data, time, or effort—create value: either value for ourselves, for our families and friends, for entire communities, for researchers, or for companies and their shareholders. The notion of prosumption has been used to describe the latter scenario of consumers creating value for companies (Tapscott 1997; Toffler 1980; Ritzer, Dean and Jurgenson 2012). The paradigmatic case of prosumption is a consumer who helps produce what the company makes money with: consumers uploading music files to file sharing platforms, or using loyalty cards to provide information that companies can use for marketing.

Many people have pointed out that health data and information are becoming essential assets in the production of value and capital in the medical domain. Prosumption is arguably most pronounced where people are actively involved in collecting or providing data or information that create value for commercial companies or other organizations. When people are not actively engaged with—or even not aware of—data collection, the term "value creation" is more fitting than the label of "prosumption." This leads to the seemingly ironic conclusion that situations where people are aware of what they are doing (which is good) are the most clear-cut cases of prosumption (which is supposedly problematic). How do we solve this conundrum?

The answer is twofold. The first part of the answer is that cases where people are aware that they are creating value for commercial actors are simply the lesser evil compared to people not being aware that they are doing it. In other words, active data contributions are less problematic than passive data contributions. The second part of the answer is that not all practices of prosumption pose the same challenges. In the domain of health information specifically, we can identify three different types of prosumption (table 5.1). The first is hedonistic prosumption. A hedonistic prosumer is a person who engages in this practice primarily because she is seeking entertainment or pleasure. If somebody plays an online game and in this process "shares" data about herself with the game provider, or shares health information in social networks mainly because it is pleasurable, then she is a hedonistic prosumer in this situation. The second type of prosumption, which I call idealistic prosumption, refers to activities undertaken in the pursuit of a greater good. If my main motive for playing a computer game is to help to improve algorithms for the automation of malaria diagnosis in resource-poor countries, or if I participate in a crowdfunding campaign because I want to support a particular area of research, then I act as an idealistic prosumer. People who participate because they want to reach a concrete goal to satisfy an immediate need are the third type: utilitaristic prosumers. If I enter personal data on CureTogether, for example, because I want to find out what treatment may be most effective for my particular type of migraine, then I am an utilitaristic prosumer in this situation.

I deliberately left the distinction between prosumption for for-profit and nonprofit enterprises out of this typology. Especially in connection with online platforms where users (co)create content, the line between for-profit and nonprofit can be difficult to draw. The confusion over whether Wikimedia, for example—the organization supporting Wikipedia and other "open knowledge" projects—is truly a nonprofit organization, given the high proportion of its donation income that it pays out to the organization's leadership, is a telling example of this difficulty (see, for example, Sawers 2012; Tkacz 2015).

| TABLE 5.1. Three types of health information prosumption | | |
|---|---|---|
| Type of prosumption | Description | Exemplary reference |
| Hedonistic prosumption | Prosumption for entertainment or other "hedonistic" purposes; sharing personal information with others because it is an enjoyable social activity, such as chatting online or playing a computer game. Also playing "serious games" (computer games for science) is hedonistic prosumption if done for entertainment purposes. | Boyle et al. (2012) |
| Idealistic prosumption | Participation due to commitment to the goals or values underpinning an initiative or activity. (Note that this does not preclude that people benefit themselves from participating.) Also playing "serious games" can be idealistic prosumption if executed out of idealistic motives. | Nov (2007) |
| Utilitaristic prosumption | Prosumption for strategic reasons that are more specific than advancing the well-being of society, such as helping disease research. Prosumption of this type typically serves to reach a clearly defined goal. | S. Fox (2013) |

## Prosumption and Personalized Medicine

What is the relationship between prosumption and participation in personalized medicine? I have argued that every person who contributes data, time, or effort to the personalization of her health care can be called a prosumer if her contributions create value for actors with commercial interests. This means that most patients are prosumers in some respects, and that prosumption is a ubiquitous feature of data-rich personalized medicine.

I believe that not all instances of prosumption are equally troubling. Rather than assuming that prosumption is always bad, it is possible to separate the problematic from the less problematic cases by asking two questions: Who benefits from the prosumption? And what influence do prosumers have in the type of value that is being created? Box 2.1 in chapter 2, which helps assess the types of participation that specific initiatives or projects invite or promote, can also be helpful here. Not everybody who knowingly and deliberately prosumes has fallen victim to some kind of false consciousness (Comor 2011). As noted, prosumption can be a conscious and considered decision of people and may be pleasurable (hedonistic prosumption), do good (idealistic prosumption), or help reach a specific goal (utilitaristic prosumption). In all these forms prosumption can also increases the agency of patients in a meaningful way.

In the domain of medicine, prosumption is problematic if it is the only way for a patient to get a service or treatment that they need and that they could not otherwise access or afford. Much has been written about the emergence of personal data as a new currency in our societies: Customers give away personal information to obtain discounts via loyalty cards, or even to obtain access to affordable prescription drugs. This phenomenon is not limited to wealthy customers in high-income countries. "Bottom of Pyramid" (BOP) consumers—the poorest people in the world—are especially targeted by companies. The poorer people are, the more willing they are to trade personal information for discounts or benefits. In fall 2015, the California-based company Amgen offered patients a cholesterol-reducing drug for a significantly discounted price if they allowed the company to access and use their personal data (Hiltzik 2015). Similarly, target marketing in any sector, not only the health domain, benefits people who cannot afford to care more about privacy than about the convenience of a "free" online service or a discount for which they pay with their data. The value that these people create for companies by handing over their personal data is not only a troublesome instance of prosumption, but it is an unfortunate extension of "patient work" (Strauss et al. 1982; see also Comor 2011; Lupton 2014; Stewart 2016). In the words of a British patient, commercial companies are putting up a one-way mirror toward the people whose data they use: "They know everything about you, but we don't know what they are doing with that" (quoted in Wellcome Trust 2016: 5).

Prosumption in the field of personalized medicine could be seen as posing specific ethical problems. Health has very high value for us, not only our own health, but also the health of our friends and families. Due to the lengths that most people are prepared to go to in order to protect, regain, or improve their health and the health of their family or friends, special measures need to be taken to protect them from exploitation.

Desperately ill people who pay large sums of money for unproven treatments and remedies can be a troubling example of such exploitation. In comparison to a family losing their house to pay for a stem cell treatment with unproven efficacy, the fate of a prosumer whose data could be used to her disadvantage does not seem particularly harsh. The threshold for doing the latter, however, is much lower, and the number of people who engage in prosuming is much higher. A survey carried out by the Health Data Exploration Project (University of California 2014) found that the majority (57 percent) of the 465 U.S.-based individuals surveyed were happy to make their personal health data available for research.[7] What these people wanted in return was the assurance that their data would remain "anonymous," and that they would not be deceived about the commercial interests of the companies. But if we consider the failure of organizations to disclose commercial interests a form of deception, then research contributors are routinely deceived.

## Prosumption, Do-It-Yourself (DIY) Biology, and Open Science

Knowing that many people are willing to make health data available to others for a good cause (see, for example, Geppert et al. 2014; Sikweyiya and Jewkes 2013; Wellcome Trust 2016), some commercial companies deliberately use the rhetoric of community and solidarity to increase people's willingness to "share" data on their site. Writing about web-based businesses that rely on prosumption for content generation (such as file sharing sites or social media) or for dissemination (such as viral marketing), media studies scholars Van Dijck and Nieborg consider "We-Think" to exemplify

> a currently popular way of business and management books that favor terms such as collectivism, participation and creativity to argue their economic benefits for Web 2.0 business models. A decade of experimenting with e-business models appears to have resulted in a smooth integration of communal models of production into the largely commoditized infrastructure of the internet (Van Dijck and Nieborg 2009: 856).

It is indeed important to treat the present emphasis on community and "sharing" in the rhetoric of web-based platforms and enterprises as part of a deliberate business model (see also John 2012). It is a business model that capitalizes on practices that the web is particularly good at, namely facilitating horizontal sharing and value cocreation by users. As Van Dijck and Nieborg (2009: 865) note, "every user who contributes content—and for that matter, every passive spectator who clicks on user-generated content sites (such as YouTube) or social networking sites (such as Facebook)—provides valuable information about themselves and their preferred interests, yet they have no control whatsoever over what information is extracted from their clicking behaviour and how this information is processed and disseminated."

At the same time, we need to avoid drawing an overly simplistic picture. Initiatives and organizations vary greatly in how they facilitate data collection and the exchange of information. This variation is also reflected in different levels of transparency about issues such as commercial interests, different decision-making procedures, and accountability. Moreover, for the various reasons discussed in this chapter, it is becoming increasingly difficult to separate socially valuable initiatives (that is, transparent ones that also pursue a positive political or societal goal) from bad apples. The nonprofit versus for-profit distinction is no longer very helpful in this respect. Organizations such as PatientsLikeMe, for example, are hybrids; they are for-profit, but they often also host or convene nonprofit research for communal benefit. Likewise, the British care.data initiative, announced early in 2014 with the aim of enabling the "sharing" of patient data held by the English National Health Service (NHS) with researchers and corporate actors in the UK and abroad, plays into the hands of corporate gains despite being a public initiative.

The ethos of sharing also plays a central role within the Open Science movement. This movement seeks to make all elements of research, from lab books and research notes to raw data and research findings, accessible to the public with as few barriers as possible. Barriers could be cost-related, technical, or they could consist of license requirements. Some authors also subsume IT and other technical tools used for this purpose, such as social media, infrastructures, and software, under the one label of Open Science. However narrowly or broadly defined, Open Science is fused with the promise of making science more transparent and democratic. And this has not remained without effects: The growing pressure to remove access barriers to research findings, for example, has made it much easier for people outside of the ivory tower to obtain medical information. But Open Science can cut both ways. It can increase the power of those who are already in the privileged position of having the skills and resources to do research that can be shared openly, and to pay for article-processing charges to see their findings published via open access. Open-access mandates from research institutions have been criticized for increasing the gap between well-resourced researchers whose grants pay open access publishing fees on the one hand, and those who do their research without external funding on the other (Caball et al. 2013; Leonelli, Spichtinger, and Prainsack 2015). It is thus premature to celebrate Open Science as a way to make science more democratic and equal—similar to "the Internet," which was initially imbued with the hope that it would democratize the world but was later found to serve the purposes of the powerful at least as much as those people had hoped it would empower (Turner 2010; Morozov 2011; 2013; A. Taylor 2014). As Julie Cohen argues, increasing access to information is not an emancipatory activity in itself. It depends on whether this activity serves to enhance the wellbeing of people in that society ("information-as-freedom") or to enhance domination and control ("information-as-control") (J. Cohen 2012: 6; see also Taylor 2014).

The "biohacking" and "DIY biology" movements, which are underpinned by some of the same values as the proponents of Open Science, try to address the problem of commercial interests and power asymmetries head-on. In mainstream public media, "biohacking" has so far featured mostly as an arena for maverick hobby scientists manufacturing potentially dangerous organisms (see, for example, Charisius, Friebe, and Karberg 2014). In academic scholarship, the political context of biohacking has only recently started to be explored (see, for example, Tocchetti 2012, Delfanti 2013). As Sara Tocchetti and Sara Aguiton summarize, a large part of the DIY biology movement is driven by the commitment to overcome the dependency on corporate money that established research institutions suffers from (Tocchetti and Aguiton 2015). The leaders of the DIY biology movement include professional scientists who seek to free biology from its links with commercial and strategic interests and turn it into a shared civic practice serving the common good (see, for example, Loukides 2014).[8] One of the characteristics that unites the otherwise very heterogeneous movement is the commitment to produce knowledge that is not locked under intellectual property regimes. This latter aspect also sets the DIY movement apart from most practices of prosumption: while prosumption affirms and partakes in the commodification and commercialization of science and medicine, many DIY biologists emphatically oppose commercialization (Delfanti 2013; Ratto and Boler 2014). Although it can be the case, of course, that the same person engages both in prosumption and DIY, the practices can be distinguished in terms of their normative thrust. DIY posits itself as an alternative to established power structures, not as part of it.

Another thing that most DIY biology groups share is the central role that ethical practice plays. This is partly related to the great concern with which DIY biology has been viewed by those who worry about biohazards created in the garage next door (see also Marris 2015). The focus on ethics in the DIY biology community is partly a reaction to this, but it is not merely instrumental. Many DIY biologists want to act in more responsible and ethical ways than professional scientists working in established institutions. In the words of Jason Bobe, one of the founders of the DIYbio movement:

> The DIYbio community is positioned better than any other organization to develop a positive culture around citizen science and to "set the pattern" for best practices worldwide by establishing a code of ethics, developing norms for safety, and creating shared resources for amateur biologists. (quoted in PR Newswire 2010)

As Kathleen Eggleson, in her comparative analysis of DIYbio ethics codes summarizes, "Open Access is number one on the North American list" (Eggleson 2014: 188). Good access to information and availability of tools to a wide group of people are indeed preconditions for participation in DIY biology and thus of practical importance. Openness is also symbolically important because of its discursive proximity to transparency, which, in turn, is often associated with accountability and democracy. The conflation of openness and transparency with accountability and democracy, however, runs the risk of glossing over a range of critical nuances, for example, different types of transparency (see, for example, Koops 2013) and the role of inclusiveness in democratic decision making. That more people see or know something does not always make processes or institutions more democratic, or even more "open," in the sense of inclusiveness. For example, how "open" is a highly technical paper on DNA methylation in an open-access journal if it takes specialized knowledge to read, or even to find it? How democratic is a funding decision if it was motivated by the fear of bad press, even if virtually every aspect of the decision making process were recorded and made public (Gurwitz, Milanesi, and Koenig 2014)? How desirable is a majority decision that undercuts minority interests? The latter concern is particularly relevant in the context of participatory practices and forums that are used mostly, or even exclusively, by elite groups—which has been held also against the biohacking and DIYbio communities (Delfanti 2013). Openness and "sharing" are thus not intrinsically positive and democratic (Stalder and Sützl 2011). Whether they are or not depends on what is shared with whom, on what terms, and at whose costs. Costs, here, are not limited to monetary expenses, but include the social, ethical and technological-organizational costs of "sharing." Openness and sharing can have unintended consequences: "Open" data are as accessible to insurance companies, right wing parties, and religious fanatics as they are to charities, patients, and teachers. Last but not least, the "opening" of data sometimes also includes data that people shared unwittingly, or that they would have preferred not to share if that were an option.

## When Opt Out Is Not an Option

As media and privacy scholars Finn Brunton and Helen Nissenbaum (2011) remind us, there is nothing inherently problematic in collecting and processing data. What renders these practices contentious in some contexts are the profound power asymmetries that they are embedded in (see also Stalder 2009). When Big Brother and Company Man (Kang et al. 2012) collect data in order to increase financial profits, from people who have no realistic way of opting out, this is what makes them politically and ethically contentious. As Brunton and Nissenbaum argue, only rarely

> do we get to choose whether or not we are monitored, what happens to information about us and what happens to us because of this information. We have little or no say when monitoring takes place in inappropriate contexts, and is shared inappropriately with inappropriate others.

[. . . Equally important] is an epistemic asymmetry: we are often not fully aware of the monitoring, and do not know what will become of the information produced by that monitoring, nor where it will go and what can be done to it [ . . . ] (Brunton and Nissenbaum 2011).

Governments and major commercial enterprises—with Alphabet/Google being but the most prominent example—have the power and potential to use data in ways that people may consider intrusive or outright damaging. Notably, in the case of commercial companies, the issue is exacerbated by their not being subject to mechanisms of democratic control and public accountability in the same manner as public actors are. Even when people are conscious of this situation, it is often difficult or even impossible for them to opt out of "sharing" data with these organizations and companies.

Having no realistic way of opting out does not only mean that it is legally or technically impossible to refuse to participate—like refusing to pay tax, for example—but it also applies to scenarios where people would suffer considerable negative consequences if they did. It is similar to the "request" to be searched before traveling on a plane: Compliance is voluntary, but if we refused, we would be denied boarding. In the health domain, there are many situations where patients would need to invest significant time and effort, or suffer negative consequences, if they opted out. A recent example is the aforementioned English care.data initiative, a government-imposed scheme to share patient data with other health care organizations and commercial companies (Weaver 2014). The scheme presumed people's consent, meaning that patients needed to actively opt out if they were not happy to participate. Moreover, information on the opt-out process was difficult to find, and many people had to go to pick up forms from their doctors. In some cases, such as my own, they even had to convince their doctor to hand them a form in the first place. The form itself was written in such a way that it made potential opt-outers feel that they were obstructing efforts to improve health care (see figures 5.1a and 5.1b). To top things off, it turned out that some family physicians had failed to pass opt-out information on to the Health and Social Care Information Centre. This meant information about seven hundred thousand patients who had in fact opted out were shared with third parties nevertheless (U.K. Government 2015). Because of all these problems, care.data was aborted in 2014.

Figures 5.1a (above) and 5.1b (facing page). Patient information sheet on the English care.data initiative, which renders patient data accessible for research outside of the NHS. The information provided to patients implied that opting out could compromise the quality of their health care, despite stating otherwise [source: information sheet handed to the author by her family doctor].

## Summary Care Record: Opt in / Opt out Form

Please tick one of the options below:

☐ Yes, I would like to have a Summary Care Record

☐ No, I do not want a Summary Care Record

☐ I don't know whether I want a Summary Care Record, I will decide later

| Forename(s) | |
|---|---|
| Surname | |
| Phone number | |
| Date of birth | |
| NHS number (if known) | |

Representative's details (if signing for someone else):

| Your name | |
|---|---|
| Relationship to patient | |

Signature ................................................ Date ...............................

| For GP practice use only | |
|---|---|
| 9Ndm added – consent | Y / N |
| 9Ndo added – dissent/don't know | Y / N |
| Initials + date | |

---

## Care.data: Opt-Out Form

Please tick one or both options below:

☐ I do NOT want my personal confidential data from my GP surgery to be released for the care.data programme.

☐ I do NOT want my personal confidential data from hospitals and other care providers to be released by the Health & Social Care Information Centre (HSCIC) for the care.data programme.

| Forename(s) | |
|---|---|
| Surname | |
| Phone number | |
| Date of birth | |
| NHS number (if known) | |

Representative's details (if signing for someone else):

| Your name | |
|---|---|
| Relationship to patient | |

Signature ................................................ Date ...............................

| For GP practice use only | |
|---|---|
| 9Nu0 added – GP data | Y / N |
| 9Nu4 added – hosp data | Y / N |
| Initials + date | |

Feb 2014

## Resistance, Obfuscation, and the Commodification of Privacy

The difficulty of opting out is not the only problem related to technology-mediated personalization in medicine. Scholars have argued that digital health technologies in particular leave very little room for alternative, insurgent, and alternative uses (see also Oudshoorn 2011). In a recent book edited by Matt Ratto and Megan Boler (2014), authors discuss creative and innovative ways for citizens to resist or divert data collection. For example, people swap loyalty cards (Brunton and Nissenbaum 2011), or they use web browsers that produce decoy queries to drown people's genuine queries in a cloud of noise (Brunton and Nissenbaum 2011; Howe and Nissenbaum 2009; Milberry 2014).

The aims of data obfuscators can be manifold: to resist commodification, raise awareness of public surveillance, or bypass monopolies. Almost always they seek to enhance privacy. But also the relationship between privacy and corporate power has become increasingly complex. Computer science scholars Constantinos Patsakis and Agusti Solanas argue that privacy has transitioned from being "a *need* that people struggled to cover" to "a *right* recognized by the Universal Declaration of Human Rights" to its most recent iteration as a *service* (Patsakis and Solanas 2013: 1; original emphasis). Privacy is no longer merely a negative state, namely the state of excluding others from access to something: It has become a product (ibid.). It is something that people are willing to pay for, directly or indirectly. This is also reflected in the new European General Data Protection Regulation, which requires that some types of organizations carry out privacy impact assessments (see, for example, Wright 2011). It also requires that organizations engineer privacy-enhancing features into their processes and technologies (Privacy-by-Design). Despite their good intentions these requirements contribute to the commodification of privacy: it is not only a value in the process of innovation, but also a financially and economically *valuable* feature of a product.

Does this make data obfuscators, whose aim is also to increase privacy, unwitting accomplices in the process of data protection and commodification? It does not, if we assume that there is a key difference between privacy as a product, and privacy as a personal, social and political value. Data obfuscators do not ask for money in return for their "services"; they are motivated by the desire to protect a social good. To paraphrase Julie Cohen, they are working toward a society where information is in the service of freedom and the flourishing of people (J. Cohen 2012: 6), and not in the service of corporate interests. Data obfuscation in the service of privacy enhancement is thus a very different animal from privacy as a product. The value of privacy services can be assessed in financial terms; they have a market value. Data obfuscation for the sake of information-as-freedom, in contrast, explicitly resists being priced and commercialized. It resists the commodification of privacy also by enacting it as a "collective effort" (Casilli 2014).

## Health Data and Participatory Medicine: How Not to Sell Out

In an ideal world, health data would be generated, collected, and used in such a way that people have a say in what others collect, know, or "predict" about them, and they could trust that their data would be used sensibly and carefully. In theory, this should already be the case: The U.S. Federal Trade Commission (FTC) "fair information practice" principles are but one example of a framework aimed at improving self-regulation of the industry (Federal Trade Commission 2000). But they are not enforceable by law, and the level of compliance is, put euphemistically, a bit patchy. Within the European Union, the aforementioned General Data Protection Regulation (European Council 2015) will give people more rights to control over how their personal data are collected and used. It remains to be seen, however, whether the new regulation will be an effective tool to fight practices that can be more easily hidden, such as consumer scoring or health scoring—that is, the use of big data analytics to stratify people into different groups according to characteristics that have been found to correlate with particularly risky or costly behaviors. The legal requirement that data processors need to notify data subjects of the fact that their data are being processed does not solve this problem: As Julie Cohen argues, "even highly granular, dynamically updated purpose and recipient disclosures would not necessarily shed light on the operational significance of collected information" (J. Cohen 2012: 236). In other words, the type of notification required by law would not convey the utility and value that the processing of data has for those who process them.

These examples show clearly that data protection is not just a matter of protecting individual privacy; it is also a collective and societal concern. If we do not treat it as such the imbalance between citizens and organizations using their data will increase further. But if we are serious about treating data protection as a collective concern we need to ask a painful question: Is *individual* control over data really always the best way to counterbalance the power of corporate data use? Or should we focus instead on giving collective actors more control over enforcing good governance of data use?

Collective responsibility also requires increasing the trustworthiness of institutions. Much of the literature on health data emphasizes how important it is that people trust institutions that collect and use their data and information. But this way of phrasing the challenge puts the onus on the people, who ought to trust institutions. Instead, it should be the responsibility of the institutions to be worthy of people's trust. Recent discussions about data collection practices of the U.S. National Security Agency (NSA) or the aforementioned English care.data project have done great harm to the trustworthiness of public institutions in this respect. As noted earlier, public actors are often in the seemingly paradoxical position of having to protect citizens from harm from digital and "big data" surveillance, while at the same time benefiting from it by receiving tax revenue from companies that headquarter on their territory in exchange for industry-friendly laws. This makes public authorities both regulators and facilitators of digital surveillance.

One step in the right direction would be to stop using the term "sharing" when we speak of data (Prainsack 2015c). At present, a wide range of diverse activities—from research institutions making interpreted results of genomic research available to participants, to individual patients posting information about their illness online, to customers of online companies allowing the latter to use information on how they use their services—are all lumped together under "data sharing." If, instead, we talked about making data or information accessible to somebody for a specific purpose, this would serve two purposes at once. First, we would avoid the moralistic undertone of the term "sharing" and thus the implication that those who oppose certain ways of exchanging, collecting, or using data have dubious motives. Second, we would need to be very specific about who is given access to what data and for what purpose:

Are we talking about individual people making health-related or other information about themselves available to organizations? Or are we talking about organizations exchanging data about individuals? What information is it that is being exchanged or made available, and for what purpose is this done? Is it done for biomedical research, for criminal investigation, or to increase profit margins? This would be a start to enabling us to differentiate between "good" ways of data sharing driven by solidarity and the aim to create public benefits, and calls for data sharing that see people as little more than data sources that hand over their information for the benefit of shareholders. It would ensure that our well-meant efforts to support knowledge creation for common benefit do not end up being used for purposes that are not in the public interest.

## Conclusion

In this chapter I have argued that it is increasingly difficult to disentangle for-profit and nonprofit motives and organizations, and that taking the distinction between public and private enterprises as a guide for whom to trust with our data is no longer a feasible approach. For users of health-related websites, it is often impossible to tell, without engaging in detailed background research, who funds a particular project or platform and whether it is for profit or not. Moreover, it is not always apparent to outsiders who the "real" customers of a service are—advertisers, users, or other companies who buy user data?

Some people have started to create their own platforms or citizen cooperatives. Openhumans (openhumans.org) or DNAland (dna.land), for example, are nonprofit online platforms that allow people to upload health-related data and make them available for anybody to access and use. These data include results from DNA tests, but also, in the case of Openhumans, data from other tests or fitness trackers.

In the past, some nonprofit platforms—such as CureTogether.com (see chapter 2)—have been acquired by commercial companies. They often retain at least part of their initial public mission at the same time as pursuing for-profit strategies. Such entanglements between health idealism and commercial stakes are paradigmatic for entrepreneurism in the health domain. In the context of data-rich medicine specifically, the roles of Big Brother and Company Man (Kang et al. 2012) are no longer played only by governments and big pharma, but also by Google, Apple, and other consumer technology companies that have had no prior interest in health specifically (see also Sharon 2016).

But even here, the picture is not black and white: At the same time that big global players are gaining more power, the "digital revolution" has also made it easier for innovative and socially responsible, solidaristic health initiatives to find support from across the globe. In the next chapter, which opens the solution-oriented part of the book, I will discuss how a change in the way we understand the person in personalized medicine can suggest tangible ways to change medical research and practice.

# 6

## Beyond Individualism

### Atomistic Individualism in Medicine and Health Care

While dichotomies such as online versus offline, health-related versus not health-related, and for-profit versus not-for-profit have all been challenged by the turn toward data-rich personalized medicine, a dichotomy that is still surprisingly intact in the medical domain is that between self-interest and care for others. It shapes many ethical and legal frameworks that underpin Western medicine. The concept of altruistic organ donation is an example: This notion assumes that donation is motivated either by self- or other-serving interests, and that they are mutually exclusive.

Whether we assume people to be self-interested, gain-maximizing rational actors, or people whose identities, needs and interests are also shaped by their relations to and concern for others, has profound consequences for how we envisage and realize personalized medicine (see also Widdows 2013; Prainsack 2014c). Although many have criticized dominant visions of personalized medicine as not being truly "personal," few studies have started to scrutinize the notion of person in this context (for an exception see Reardon 2011). By leaving the meaning of the word "person" in personalized medicine unexplored, however, we risk taking on board two impactful yet problematic assumptions of Western thinking: first, that social practice and social institutions can be reduced to the actions of individuals, and second, that individuals are normally clearly separable from one another. In the field of medicine, both of these assumptions have caused tangible problems.

The idea that we can distinguish clearly between self-serving and other-oriented practice is closely related to the central position that the autonomous individual has had as the bearer of agency in Western thought (see, for example, Battersby 2007; Douzinas 2000; C. Epstein 2013; Richardson 2007; C. Taylor 1985a). The assumption that individual human action is the core unit of social life and that societies and political institutions are reducible to the actions of individuals is known as methodological individualism (see also Scott 2000). In many other parts of the world, and in other times throughout human history, self-hood and human practice have been conceived in a more communal sense (see, for example, Bird-David 2004; De Craemer 1983; D. Tsai 2001). For example, a person's actions could be considered as determined by the role that the acting person fulfills as part of her family or her community, instead of being seen as the result of reasoned individual decision making (see also Strathern 1988; Siedentop 2014). But in the field of medicine, the Western distinction between self-interested and other-oriented action has been influential across the globe, not least due to the influence of North American and European bioethical norms and standards in other world regions (see, for example, Chadwick and Schüklenk 2004).

In this chapter I will discuss some of the implications that such an understanding of personhood in the tradition of Western dualism and the rational actor paradigm has had for the practice of medicine. In the second part of the chapter I will suggest ways to overcome an unproductive focus on atomistic individualism, and explore how this could contribute to a personalized medicine that does not force us to choose, as Donna Dickenson called it, between We medicine and Me medicine (Dickenson 2013). I will argue that personalized medicine has the potential to bring personal and collective needs and interests closer together.

## The Person as a Rational, Bounded Entity

In the Western world, the idea of a clear separation between self- and other-serving motivations has important roots in the strong foothold that a particular conception of rational action has had.[1] The early beginnings of the rational actor paradigm, in turn, are often traced back to John Locke's work on self-ownership (1988 [1689]). The nuances within the existing scholarship on self-ownership are too manifold to do justice to in a short overview. The following characteristics, however, are central to self-ownership: self-awareness, free will (independent from, and unmanipulated by, others), and the capacity to formulate life plans (see also Christman 2015). Some understandings of self-ownership are strongly influenced by Immanuel Kant's idea that human beings—as rational agents in the way just described—have an inherent dignity and must not be treated merely as a means to an end (see also G. A. Cohen 1995). Other understandings of autonomy qua self-ownership draw upon a more *strategic,* instrumental understanding of rationality whose early beginnings are often traced back to John Locke's work on property (1988 [1689]) as well as to his, and Thomas Hobbes's (1651), conception of the "state of nature." As is well known, the "state of nature" is short-hand for the (fictitious) circumstances under which humans lived before politically organized societies emerged. Hobbes saw social institutions in the state of nature as reducible to individual choices; an idea that the Australian political scientist Charlotte Epstein called the "traditional founding myth for the rational actor" (C. Epstein 2013: 289; see also I. Murdoch 1992; Neal 1988). The rational-actor paradigm entails that social and political space is shaped by the effects of the choices of people and other entities—collective actors such as corporations, organizations, or states—who can be assumed to behave rationally. Two assumptions are of crucial importance here: that individual action is the "elementary unit of social life" (Elster 1989: 13; see also Macpherson 1962), and that individuals are presumed to aim to increase their individual gain. A rational actor is one that is guided by self-interest.

While the idea of rational choice has been influential within many academic disciplines, its penetrance across different fields has been uneven. Economics, political science, and law have been strongly influenced by it. Within sociology and social theory, in contrast, many strands of scholarship have treated rational action as only one among several elements of human practice. Scholarship in these fields has considered other, nonrational elements, such as habits and emotions, as at least equally important (see also Scott 2000). In philosophy, a more relational understanding of personhood has been prevalent. Martin Heidegger (1996 [1927]) is but one well-known example of a philosopher who rejected the idea of a subject as a fixed, bounded, self-aware entity, which he argued did not capture the meaning of human existence. Heidegger used the German term *Dasein,* an untranslatable notion of being in, of, and with the world, to refer to "a complex and open-ended interconnection with the world" (Sharon 2014: 140). Other important influences on current scholarship employing nonlinear and relational understandings of personhood were Durkheim's critique of "the cult of the individual" (1969 [1898]), Friedrich Nietzsche's deconstruction of the self as a social construction and moral illusion (Nietzsche 2011 [1886]), the important role that Ludwig Wittgenstein gave to language in making the world (Pitkin 1993; see also Rorty 1989), and Jacques Lacan's deconstruction of ego identity (Lacan and Fink 2002; Lacan 1977 [1966]). A deeply relational understanding of how individual subjectivity comes into being can also be found in Hannah Arendt's work (for example, Arendt 1978 [1973]).

The increasing popularity of postmodern philosophy in the 1960s and 1970s, with its emphatic rejection of a dualist worldview, meant an irreversible departure from the idea of the self as a fixed and bounded entity for those associated with this thinking. Particularly influential on the conceptualization of subjectivity and agency was Michel Foucault's early work, in which he questioned the very concept of the modern individual. Instead, he saw individuals as the product of power configurations that he referred to as discourse (Foucault 1991 [1975]; see also Paras 2006). The work of the French philosopher Gilles Deleuze and the psychiatrist Félix Guattari (Deleuze and Guattari 1977 [1972]) has also informed nondualist understandings of subjectivity in wider areas of theory and practice. Based on an analysis of how psychoanalytical understandings of consciousness are related to modern subject positions, these authors support an understanding of subjectivity that is fluid and decentered, which resonates very strongly also with feminist scholarship (see Butler 1990; Chodorow 1980; Haraway 1991; Kristeva 1980; Meyers 1994; K. Oliver 1998).

Feminist scholars, including proponents of the care ethics approach, explicitly emphasized that the human ability to reason is developed through relationships with others (see, for example, Gilligan 1982; Strathern 1988; Butler 1990; Meyers 1994). For authors in these traditions, such human relationality is a precondition for subjectivity, not the other way around (C. Taylor 1985b: Chapter 7; C. Taylor 1989; Mackenzie and Stoljar 2000). We are who we are because we relate to others.

Feminist scholarship has also challenged the rational-choice paradigm in its home discipline, economics. The ideal of the self-interested, rational, and competitive *homo oeconomicus* has a clear masculine bias (see, for example, Nelson and Ferber 1993). Moreover, already in the 1970s, vocal critique came from experiments in "behavioral economics" (Kahneman, Knetsch, and Thaler 1986). These experiments seemed to consistently contradict one of the core assumptions of rational choice, namely that actors can be assumed to behave rationally. The only thing that was predictable about people's actions, this new field of research suggested, was that their behavior was not consistently rational. Behavioral economists assume that the reason for this must be that people were influenced by different kinds of cognitive bias (Haselton, Nettle, and Andrews 2005). For many scholars associated with behavioral economics, self-interest thus continues to play an important role: Although they do not believe that people's actions are predominantly rational, they believe in the distinction between rational and irrational behavior, and many of them seek to increase the rational components in people's actions by reducing cognitive bias (Kahneman 2011; note that Kahneman, although associated with behavioral economics, is a psychologist).

In summary, while criticism of rational choice coming from behavioral economics and other fields has challenged the assumption that people are typically rational actors, the idea that individual action is the core unit that structures social and political space, and that this action is or should normally be rational (self-interested), is still dominant. This view is so deeply engrained in our social and political institutions, our legal frameworks, and our personal ways of thinking that it is difficult to conceive of an alternative. And the question of how to account for the important role that people around us—and our considerations for them—play in shaping our emotions, habits, and ultimately, our personhood, is a notoriously difficult problem to address. The works of social anthropologists such as Marcel Mauss (1966 [1925]) or social policy scholars like Richard Titmuss (1970), both strongly influenced by Durkheim, are important illustrations of what we can gain, both analytically and politically, by acknowledging the importance of concern for others in the practices of people and in the emergence and practice of social institutions. The work of these two scholars is very different in that Mauss wrote about "archaic societies," while Titmuss focused on the Western world in the twentieth century. The work of both, however, illustrated how self-interest and concern for others overlap. In the words of Marilyn Strathern, people are not individuals first who then form relations to others. Instead, connections to and with others are always already part of who we are (Strathern 1988).

Given the long history of relational understandings of personhood, and the apparent interconnectedness of concern for ourselves and concern for others (see also Christakis and Fowler 2009), why is the assumption that we can separate between the two still so deeply engrained in norms and values governing the practice and research of medicine?[2] Exemplified by three cases—end of life decision making, organ donation, and health data governance—the next section of this chapter will illustrate some of the problems that this assumption has created in the domain of medicine. Despite their differences, all three cases show how impactful different understandings of personhood can be for medical practice and research. They also illustrate the importance of clarifying what notion of personhood we employ when we speak of personalization. In the final section of this chapter I will argue that solidarity—a concept that overcomes the distinction between self-interest and concern for others—can help address some of the problems that a focus on self-interested independent individuals has brought to the field of medicine.[3]

## The Comfort of Kin? Decision Making at the End of Life

The principle of informed consent stems from a rights-logic that treats individuals as the primary unit of agency. It has been the ethical gold standard within Western medical practice since the second half of the twentieth century, despite the fact that it has also attracted a lot of criticism. This criticism has ranged from the technical—namely that it is impossible for consent to be fully informed and specific—to the conceptual, arguing that informed consent does not automatically enhance autonomy in a meaningful way (see, for example, Koenig 2014; Manson and O'Neill 2007; O'Neill 2003). Over the decades, this critique has fuelled improvements and new practical solutions around consent procedures (Dove et al. 2011; Kaye et al. 2011; Prainsack and Buyx 2013).

The point I wish to make here, however, relates to a different aspect of informed consent, namely the assumption that it expresses a decision that will normally have been made by *one* person. Conjoined with this assumption—this is the baggage that the dominant conception of persons as rational actors tacitly brings along—is that this person will regularly make decisions on the basis of what is best for her. There are, of course, mechanisms and protocols in place for persons incapable of giving consent, because they are unconscious, too young, mentally too frail, or in another situation that compromises or abolishes their capacity to make or express an autonomous decision. But even here, the default rule is that only one person needs to consent to treatment that is done on her body.

One of the areas where the limits of this approach have become apparent in a particularly painful manner is health care at the end of life. It is probably not a coincidence that these issues were first addressed in the United States, the heartland of individual autonomy (R. Fox and Swazey 2008), yet in a region that is culturally very diverse, the San Francisco Bay area. In an impactful article published in 1995, medical anthropologists Barbara Koenig and Jan Gates-Williams, drawing upon ethnographic fieldwork with patients at the end of their lives, described several situations where dying patients, their families, or the medical professionals treating and caring for them suffered because existing guidelines and protocols clashed with the beliefs and wishes of patients. As the authors argued, "[I]t is useful to bear in mind that in many Asian societies, ideas about 'selfhood' vary from the western ideal of an autonomous individual" (Koenig and Gates-Williams 1995: 247; see also Searight and Gafford 2005; Strathern 1988; C. Taylor 1985b; for a similar discussion on the situation in the United Kingdom, see, for example, Gunaratnam 2014; Kai, Beavan, and Faull 2011).

Koenig and Gates-Williams recognize, of course, that cultural and social norms are never entirely fixed, and that we cannot assume that somebody's ethnic background or religion determines how she will feel or decide in a given situation. Nor do these authors suggest that there is a dichotomy between community-based understandings of selfhood in the East and individualistic understandings in the West, which would be far too simplistic. Instead they show that an understanding of personhood that also sees people as shaped by their relations with others is in tension with most of the ethical and legal instruments that govern medicine in the West (see also Dodds 2000).

Also on the other side of the Atlantic, Swiss bioethicist Kathrin Ohnsorge and a European team of colleagues (2012), on the basis of 116 interviews with dying patients, their caregivers, friends, families, and physicians, demonstrated that dying patients' thoughts and wishes regarding their own death were inseparably linked to their relationships with others. What patients considered important to them included "what their surroundings or the persons they talk to [ . . . ] suggest, the ideas they pursue (or are believed to pursue), how they react to them or what they assume to be morally or rationally permissible" (Ohnsorge et al. 2012: 632). What some see as "ambivalence" in dying patients' wishes—namely that they express a wish to die but ask for life-prolonging interventions at the same time—could also be a reflection of the simultaneous consideration of their own and other people's needs. For example, while a person in great pain may want to die, she may, equally, want to hold on to life a little bit longer to make it easier for her loved ones to say goodbye. Both goals could be equally important to her. The idea that people's actions and desires are underpinned either by self-interest or concern for others, rather than these two dimensions being intertwined, contributes to these patients being seen as confused or ambivalent (Ohnsorge et al. 2012; see also Valentine 2008).

The notion of relational autonomy can be helpful here. Catriona Mackenzie and Natalie Stoljar (2000) introduced this notion drawing upon feminist critique of the dominant liberal, "atomistic" understanding of autonomy (see also Downie and Llewellyn 2011; Nedelsky 1990, 2011). Not only do our human, natural and artefactual environments (Vickers 1983; Cook 2005) influence how we express our autonomy, but they make up who we are as people. By doing so they also shape our identities and interests. In the words of public health ethicists Françoise Baylis and colleagues, we "develop within historical, social, and political contexts and only become persons through engagement and interaction with other persons" (Baylis, Kenny, and Sherwin 2008: 201).

In health care at the end of life, the employment of the notion of relational autonomy, instead of liberal autonomy, has already led to policies and protocols that acknowledge the social nature of decision-making processes (see also Priaulx and Wrigley 2013). Shared decision making, for example, is now seen as best practice in end of life situations in many parts of the world. It acknowledges that decision-making processes are social in at least two respects: First, in the sense that many patients' wishes of where and how they want to die are shaped by conversations, values, and practices shared with, family, friends, or even clinicians. Second, decision making is social also in the sense that considerations for other people shape an important part of our own identity and our interests (Strathern 1988).

For legal and practical reasons, informed consent for competent adults needs to be recorded as if it were based on the decision of only one individual, even if it is preceded by shared decision making. There is currently no way of avoiding this; especially in medicine, where people's bodies are so immediately and visibly at stake, requiring the consent of the person who has and is in that body is not something that could or should be overcome. What institutions *can* do, however, is to acknowledge explicitly that the process leading up to the recording of informed consent is a social process rather than a situation of isolated decision making based on rational reasoning of individuals. They could treat collective decision making as a normal and valuable human practice, and not as something that reflects a deviation from standard protocols. The adoption of shared decision making makes big strides toward this goal; it provides room for dialogue in the process leading up to the expression of the decision, the outcome of which is then recorded in the form of consent. Further solutions can entail that a patient can ask for another person close to her to be adopted as a full member of the clinical care team, as increasingly practiced in institutions with focus on patient-centered care. Finally, protocols for decision making at the end of life, and in health care more generally, should include the consideration of aspects that are meaningful to those involved, rather than corresponding to a narrowly defined notion of rationality, safety, or clinical utility (I have referred to these as "social biomarkers," Prainsack 2014c; see also Gawande 2014; NHS Scotland 2016). This would make medicine more personal in the deep sense of the word.

## Altruism versus Self-Interest: A Troubling Distinction in Live Organ Donation

Practices and regulations in the field of live organ donation are also underpinned by the assumption that it is possible to distinguish clearly between self-interest and care for others. That the feelings, motivations, and practices of many people do not map neatly onto the categories that rules and protocols operate with is not specific to organ donation: Written rules are always "amended" by the practical judgments of the people enacting them (Wagenaar 2004; see also Woolgar and Neyland 2013). What makes the misfit between the legal and institutional categories and the reality on the ground so troubling in transplantation medicine is that decisions over life and death are left to informal ways of bridging such misalignments.

While such informal ways of bridging exist in many countries, Marie-Andrée Jacob's (2012) ethnographic study on live organ donation in Israel provides a rare insight into the practice of such bridging work. Jacob carried out interviews and observed the work of patients, health care providers, administrators, and informal-sector workers including transplant "brokers." Because Orthodox Judaism defines death as the cessation of aerobic activity (breathing), many members of strictly Orthodox communities have not accepted brain death as a valid criterion of death, which in turn has rendered cadaveric organ transplantations impossible in these cases. As a result, the rate of organ donations in Israel is very low compared to Western countries: While in the United States, for example, almost half of all adults have agreed to become organ donors,[4] in Israel, only 16 percent of adult Israelis have signed donor cards. In the mid 2010s fewer than half of all requests for post mortem organ donations were approved by the family of the deceased (Siegal 2014: 2). In 2015, Israel's cadaveric organ donation rate was at 9 per million people, compared to 40 per million in Spain, 29 per million in the United States, and 26 per million in France.[5] The shortage of available cadaveric organs for donation has had two main consequences: First, it led to the flourishing of alternative supply channels, which used to attract considerable negative attention from international media (see, for example, Brimelow 2009) and also led to the issuing of the Transplantation Act by the Israeli Parliament in 2008. This law, which went into effect in 2010, outlawed organ trafficking, organ brokerage, and the giving and receiving of financial "rewards" for organs given to first-degree relatives.[6]

The second consequence of the shortage of cadaveric organs in Israel is that live donations now compose the bulk of organ donations in Israel. The only organs suitable for live donation are kidneys and parts of a liver, which means that many transplantation needs cannot be met in this manner (Boas 2009; 2011; Transplant Procurement Management 2010). For live donations, Israeli regulations differentiate between donations within close family, within remote family, friends, and "unrelated donations" (Jacob 2012: 35). There are different bureaucratic procedures for each of these groups. This sets Israel apart from countries such as the United States, where regulations do not rely on such classifications. Israeli hospitals run "family committees" tasked with separating donations within families into two groups. One is "first-degree relative donations" from siblings, parents, children, spouses, grandparents, uncles and aunts, or cousins, where donations are assumed to be motivated by love. Live donations to "second-degree relatives" and people with whom potential donors have no family relations form the second group. For this latter group, a special committee is set up to ensure that the motivations of donors in this group are "truly altruistic" (Jacob 2012: 37). Donors and applicants are interviewed separately by the committee to weed out those arrangements that people enter due to social coercion or the expectation of payment. In fact, one of the committee's explicit tasks is to filter out donors who secretly receive financial compensation from the prospective recipient.

Even at the outset of Jacob's study it becomes apparent that the reality of "matching organs with patients," as she calls it, does not fit into the categories that the system operates with. Perhaps the most pronounced example of how even the most "altruistic" motivations also have a self-affirming component is the story of Sandra, a Christian American woman who decided to donate a kidney to an Israeli Jewish recipient, Yitzhak. Sandra did not know Yitzhak when she decided to donate a kidney to him. In Sandra's words,

> It all began three years ago [ . . . ] my husband is a pastor in a church, we're from Michigan [ . . . ] we've always been attached to the God of the Jewish people. I didn't understand the Jewish people, though, I mean, I knew of their persecution. I met a Russian man, when I told him I didn't understand, he gave me this book, look I have it here [ . . . ] Then I understood and the scriptures came to life. Then I began my journey, I started to love the Jewish people; my husband and I, we got to know this organization "Chosen People." (quoted in Jacob 2012: 38)

In a newsletter from this organization Sandra learned about an Israeli man with a kidney disease who was in urgent need of a donor. For Sandra, the moment of deciding to donate her kidney to this man was one of divine inspiration: "I was at home alone; I was praying, and as I was, God interrupted me, and said: 'I want you to give your kidney'" (quoted in Jacob 2012: 39).

Sandra's decision, which was approved by the committee of the Israeli hospital as genuinely "altruistic," not only saved Yitzhak's life but also was a source of profound happiness for Sandra, a way of enacting her faith. Thus, although what Sandra did was not purely altruistic, it would be ironic to argue that this latter situation detracted from the value of her gift. Sandra's donation to Yitzhak helped them both. Moreover, through the donation, a part of Sandra literally became part of Yitzhak's body, and Yitzhak became part of Sandra, if only for what he symbolized for her. A similar argument could be made in response to the frequently heard claim that the supposed "sacrifices" that people make for others mostly serve their own needs. Irrespective of whether this argument has any merit, if we assumed it were true, this would not detract from the other-regarding value of the practice or action. Being part of others, typically in less physical, but sometimes also in very physical ways, is the default state for human beings.

From this perspective, it is puzzling that in many contexts, health law and regulation operates *as if* humans were deciding in isolation from others. The dominant understanding of individual consent as a decision made by one person independent of others thus requires a person to step out of the social fabric that she is part of and assume responsibility for her decision by herself. As Jacob (2012: 160) put it, "the person [ . . . ] has to be individuated by the consent form."

Jacob's fieldwork also included observations and interviews with organ brokers, whose role it is to put people in need of organs in contact with potential donors. An important, yet informal and illegal role of some brokers is to help prospective paid donors and organ recipients build stories that will pass as proof that the donation is altruistic. Brokers do this, among other things, by helping donors and recipients develop a so-called "shared history" (*historia meshutefet*). This shared history typically starts with actual connections such as siblings who may have gone to the same high school, or spouses who may know each other through work contexts. The potential donor and recipient then add fictitious details to strengthen the appearance of a bond. Jacob's work shows that these shared histories, rather than being entirely made up, emerge in parallel to prospective donors and recipients becoming more familiar and sometimes very close to each other. In this sense, they become real. By the time the story is told to the committee, both parties tell their shared history as they experienced it during the time of preparing for the committee hearing. They do not do this in the same manner as one would recall a history that actually happened. But it seems that in many cases, these imagined shared histories and commonalities have become a part of the people telling them. It is one of the fascinating insights of Jacob's study that some kind of personal bond between organ donors and recipients can be an outcome of the process that was intended to pretend its existence in the first place.

Jacob's work shows that while regulatory and bureaucratic categories assume that unrelated people donate organs *either* because they care for others *or* they are driven by selfish motivations, most people's practices include elements of both. It illustrates in fascinating detail how this misconceived dichotomy is overcome by informal practices. Paid donors, whom the system goes to so much trouble to set apart from altruistic donors, often care about the people who will receive their organs, especially as their relationship deepens in the process of making up a "shared history." It is ironic that emotional bonds emerge as a result of a joint effort to bend the very rules that prescribe that only those who act out of "pure" altruism may donate, while everybody else needs to be protected from donating.

## What Does "Personal" Mean in the Context of Health Information?

The two previous case studies have discussed problems with ethical and legal instruments that assume people to be self-interested and autonomous individuals. The first case, decision making in health care at end of life, highlighted the problems created by the tacit assumption that decisions are made by one person (see also Widdows 2013). In the second case, live organ donation, the idea that people act either out of self-interest or out of "altruism" has led to the emergence of an entire apparatus to help people bypass legal provisions.

In connection with the use of personal health data, the predominant Western understanding of personhood poses a number of problems. The most obvious one is the assumption that such data are personal for only one individual. This, as scholars have pointed out, has led to gaps in data sharing and data-protection provisions. People who could have legitimate interests in health information stemming from other people—for example, biological relatives—do not normally have a say in how these data will be used, and often there are no legal remedies available to them if something goes wrong. Legal scholar Mark Taylor, in his book *Genetic Data and the Law* (2013), criticizes that "secondary" data subjects—that is, people who are not the originators of the physical source of genetic data but with whom the information can be associated (such as family members or individuals associating themselves with a group identified in published work)—are treated as less worthy of privacy protection:

> Even if you define the phrase "relate to" to mean "is capable of impacting upon an individual's privacy," then the range of potentially relevant transactions has still been limited by the fact that the data must bear this relation to a particular identifiable person. Data that relates to a group of persons, even if it has an impact upon multiple identifiable individuals, would thus appear to fall outside of the scope of "personal data" and legal protection (M. Taylor 2013: 98).

More equality between primary and secondary data subjects, for Taylor, would represent an important step toward better data-protection frameworks in the context of genetic research. Such an approach would also capture the stakes of genetic discrimination more adequately. Because most biological data pertain to characteristics that are shared between biological relatives, the same set of genetic data can contribute to the identification of more than one individual and can lead to the discrimination of more than one individual.

Although Taylor himself focuses on genetic data, his argument can be applied to other types of data as well. My mother's hypertension, my neighbor's mental health problems, and my friend's breast cancer all disclose information that can be used to make probabilistic inferences about their families and relatives. Regarding genetic relatives, such as parents, siblings, or children, this is possible because genetic dispositions to diseases often "run in families." In some cases probabilistic inferences can also be made about nonbiologically related people, because health problems are known to correlate with socioeconomic status, racial or ethnic groups, or sexual orientation (see, for example, Institute of Medicine 2014). The broader and wider the types of data that we use for analyses in all walks of life, the more urgent is Mark Taylor's call for regulatory frameworks that accommodate the social nature of data (M. Taylor 2013; see also Widdows 2013). Such frameworks would support uses of individual-level data for common benefits and recognize the stakes and interests of multiple data subjects. Taylor is conscious, of course, that such frameworks would also need to provide rules about how to decide whose preferences are to prevail in case of conflicting interests (M. Taylor 2013).

That personal data are personal only to the individual they came from is a direct outcome of the problematic yet predominant understanding of persons as bounded individuals. And there is another problem that the understanding of people as *self-interested* individuals brings to the field of medicine. It tacitly implies that people participate in research because they hope to benefit personally, even if the benefit is not immediate or direct. This not only contradicts evidence from many empirical studies (for example, Facio et al. 2011; Marcantonio et al. 2008; Williams et al. 2008), but it has led to the mushrooming of measures to minimize risks to participants even in contexts where the risks are already very low. If participants cannot benefit personally, they at least should not need to worry about any risks. While the minimization of risks—wherever this is meaningfully and reasonably possible—is a worthy goal and clearly an ethical and moral obligation for researchers, it has, at times, taken on a life of its own. It has turned into a goal in its own right, suggesting that the task of research ethics is to abolish risks to participants altogether. But this goes against the very idea of research participation. Participants agree to give something of themselves—time, effort, pain, tissue, and sometimes dangers to their health and lives—to support a goal they consider worthy.

For people who contribute "only" data to biomedical research, the most substantive risks are the risk of discrimination in the case of re-identification of their data and the risk that their data will be used to pursue goals they do not approve of. Although stricter data-protection standards seem necessary to prevent data misuse, critics have argued that this should be done without unduly hindering research that is likely to have public benefit (see, for example, Science Europe 2013). Leading scholars have also argued that benefiting from medical research is a human right (Chapman 2009; Donders 2011; Knoppers et al. 2014). If we accept this argument, then the point where we draw the line between data protection on the one hand and making data more easily and more widely accessible for research purposes on the other would need to shift in favor of the latter. But perhaps privacy and data use for research aiming to create public benefits need not be pulling in different directions. In fact, several projects are currently under way that seek to develop tools and instruments to enable individual-level data to be used while keeping the risk to data donors to a minimum. Solutions include systems enabling researchers to use data without allowing them to export them: An example is the "lending library" model of Genomics England, where those wanting to use data need to go to a specific building and can only use data there. Another solution is to allow researchers to search data sets for relevant characteristics without granting access to the full data set itself (for example, matchmakerexchange.org; Philippakis 2015).

Besides the reduction of risks where it is meaningfully and reasonably possible, however, we also need to acknowledge much more openly that research participants can experience harm and to strengthen instruments for harm mitigation. We should also broaden our understanding of harm: It does not include only physical or financial aspects but also the increase of power gaps between citizens and corporations. Regardless of the safeguards in place, it is obvious that the collection and use of personal data is embedded in profound power asymmetries between citizens as data donors on the one hand, and corporations using personal data on the other. One implication of an approach to data governance that does not treat people as atomistic self-interested individuals is that we should strengthen collective control and oversight of data use in our societies. For example, we need to ensure that people who are harmed by data use—irrespective of whether they were harmed by the use of their own or other people's data—receive adequate support. We have proposed the establishment of harm-mitigation funds as a way to provide such support (Prainsack and Buyx 2013; 2017). This is based on the observation that legal remedies often are not available or do not provide adequate support, in such cases: When people are harmed by data use, they often do not have access to legal remedies because they cannot prove that the entity that has used their data has done something wrong, or because they have no legal standing as they are not the originators of the data that were used to harm them. An example is the practice of predictive analytics, where large data sets are mined for patterns. If it turned out people who watch daytime television and buy children's clothes online—to use two random, seemingly innocuous examples— have a higher risk of defaulting on their mortgage, this information could be used to discriminate against anybody who watches daytime television and buys their kid's clothes online. In many cases people will not be aware of the reasons for being treated differently, so they would not even know who caused the harm that occurred. Moreover, relatives and others who experience harm by association with this person would not have access to legal remedies. These people could appeal to harm-mitigation funds.

Harm-mitigation funds could be established at institutional levels— for example, by individual biobanks or organizations who process data—or at regional or national levels. A certain proportion of the over-all budget—the funding received by a research project, a company's net income, or a particular proportion of tax revenue—would equip harm-mitigation funds to make payments to people who can make a plausible case for having experienced harm as a result of data use. But financial payouts would not be the only way in which harm-mitigation funds can respond to appeals by people: In some cases, the most adequate response could be to acknowledge that harm has occurred and to issue an apol-ogy, even if the organization using the data is not culpable in the legal sense. And they could feed back information on what has gone wrong to the organization processing the data.

Such solutions treat data protection and the right to benefit from sci-entific research as personal and collective rights at the same time (see also Wilson 2016). An understanding of people not as bounded inde-pendent individuals but as relational beings with porous boundaries helps us to see that there is no inevitable tension between the collective and the personal levels in this regard. If we stop focusing on the sup-posed antagonism between individual rights and collective benefits, we will, in turn, be able to turn our attention to a much more worrisome and damaging tension, namely the one between societal welfare and the interests of giant transnational corporations.

## Solidarity and Personalized Medicine

The idea of harm-mitigation funds is rooted in what bioethicist Alena Buyx and I called solidarity-based governance. We have used the notion of solidarity to address governance challenges in a way that takes *interactions* between people as its unit of analysis, instead of treating social reality as reducible to the actions of single individuals (Prainsack and Buyx 2017). We also proposed a definition that sees solidarity first and foremost as a practice, and not merely as a sentiment or an abstract principle. In their most bare-bones form, solidaristic practices are those by which people or groups express their willingness to accept "costs" to assist others with whom they recognize similarity in a relevant respect. By costs we do not only mean financial contributions, but any kind of support that people provide for somebody else. Solidarity practiced between individuals (tier 1 solidarity) can become so common that it develops into a social norm within a group or community (tier 2 solidarity). If group-based solidarity solidifies further into contractual or legal norms, we speak of tier 3 solidarity (Prainsack and Buyx 2012; 2017). This latter, most formal level of solidarity is characteristic of European welfare states.

Besides improving the governance of personal health information in medical practice, a solidarity-based perspective would also have implications on ethical and regulatory instruments used in many other contexts of health care. For health care at the end of life, shared decision making has already started to address some important issues (see also NHS Scotland 2016; Mulley et al. 2017). And *institutionalized* acknowledgment that decision making is a collaborative process could also entail that people designated by a patient for such a role become full members of her care team. More broadly, decision making at the end of life should provide adequate time and spaces for conversations between the patient and others she wants to include in the decision making process.

While this suggestion for decision making at the end of life results from the relational understanding of personhood and autonomy underpinning the solidarity-based approach, and not from the concept of solidarity itself, the concept of solidarity has very direct implications in the field of live organ donations: It requires that we cease operating with the distinction between altruistic and nonaltruistic donations. Self-interest cannot be separated strictly from care for other people; this is not only true among family members and very close friends. Giving up the distinction between altruistic and "selfish" motivations for organ donation, in turn, has consequences for how we think about donations involving financial exchanges. Marie-Andrée Jacob (2012: 109) reported cases of family members who volunteered to donate a kidney because they felt they had to.[7] But is this latter scenario categorically different from one in which somebody is willing to sell a kidney for money? Both cases involve acts emerging from contexts of hardship; is the fact that one scenario involves a financial transaction and the other does not sufficient justification for why the former scenario is often tolerated and the latter one is illegal? It is clear that people who are ready to give away a part of their body for money can be assumed to do so out of a situation of desperate need, and they thus need to be protected by law. But this begs the question of what exactly they need to be protected from. If we feel that by outlawing paid live donations we protect people from their own judgment, which is compromised by hardship, we need to ask whether there are other contexts where people's decisions based on hardship can have serious effects on their health, and thus mandate being overturned. Is somebody who decides to forego treatment for her cancer, for example, because she lacks adequate health insurance and the funds to pay out of pocket, *less* in need of society's protection from acting upon her own judgement than a person ready to sell her kidney?

I am not making a case for the legalization of the sale of organs here; my point is that the same reasons that make us outlaw paid live organ donation should make us "outlaw" situations where people do not have access to health care. This is the most important objective that a solidarity-based framework brings to the table. A solidarity-based perspective cannot provide easy solutions for all complex problems. What it can do, however, is to shift the central questions being asked in the process from formulaic assessments of voluntariness, or from trying to find out whether a particular decision was motivated by "true" altruism, toward considerations of a person's personal, economic, and social situation. Moreover, a solidarity-based perspective can help foreground what people have in common, and not what sets them apart. It can increase the space for personal meaning. And the shift in the kinds of questions that we ask by viewing problems through the lens of solidarity can facilitate new ways of thinking. Why do some of us who can afford to pay for expensive treatments not recognize sufficient similarity with less-privileged people to support publicly funded universal health care? If we accept that humans do not exist in an isolated space, and thus that others are part of how we form, understand, and articulate ourselves and our interests, questions such as this one need to be asked in the process of personalizing medicine.

## Conclusion

At the crossroads of personalized and participatory medicine, it is particularly important to overcome the binary opposition between self-interest and care for others. Relinquishing this dichotomy has several benefits. One of them is that it helps to avoid a common fallacy in discussions about personalization, namely that personalization is synonymous with a kind of individualization that destroys social bonds and solidarity. Although the latter *can* be the outcome if public actors take personalization as an excuse to devolve onerous responsibilities from the collective level to individuals, this is not inevitable.

An understanding of the term "personal" in medicine that acknowledges that people are inseparably linked to others, that they rarely ever act purely out of self-interest, could lead to a more humane, more socially just, and perhaps even more cost-effective medicine. It would be one that focuses both on subjective needs of people and on systemic measures to ensure that systems are fair and affordable. In the next chapter, I will discuss several ways that could bring us closer to achieving a personalized medicine committed to these goals. Perhaps counterintuitively, personalization can help this process, if we broaden our understanding of what counts as "evidence." By focusing not only on the somatic characteristics but also on the subjective needs and values of individual patients, it could help people bring their own terms, notions, and values to the table, and could contribute to agenda setting. This would require that we take patients seriously as contributors of information and knowledge for personalization, and that we find ways to systematically include their knowledge, values and preferences into our "tapestries of health data" (Weber, Mandl, and Kohane 2014).[8] I will argue that the inclusion of what I call social biomarkers would provide a useful step in this direction.

7

# The Social Life of Evidence in Personalized Medicine

## High Tech or High Touch—or Both?

Frequent comparisons of big data to natural resources or natural forces suggest that big data are just "out there" waiting to be used; and that they are too powerful to be controlled by humans. This has led to the concern that big data analytics could become the new truth machine (I borrow the term from Lynch et al. 2008) in personalized medicine, pushing out human experience and dialogue.

This need not necessarily be so. In this chapter, I will discuss initiatives and ideas that can help us to work toward a kind of personalized medicine that foregrounds what matters to patients and that treats people as more than mere doppelgangers of their data. If we uncritically pursue the ideal of ubiquitous data capture and predictive analytics, we lose something in the thicket of observation that we should win back for the sake of patients and the good of our society. I will thus argue for a new understanding of personalization that is less focused on high tech than are dominant images of personalized medicine (for example, National Research Council 2011; Topol 2015). Such a new understanding of personalized medicine utilizes some of the potentials of digital technologies, but it also broadens the remit of what we understand as health information, bringing in more "subjective" factors that matter to patients. Most importantly, such a new understanding does not assume that the most pressing problems in health care can be solved by digital or even technological means. This applies also to reducing cost: In the words of a London-based clinician, "you have no idea how far an encounter with another human being goes in making people feel better. It's a fallacy to believe that costs will go down if people diagnose themselves with their smartphones" (personal communication to author, London, May 2016).

I will start this chapter by discussing ways in which we can broaden our understanding of evidence in medicine. It hinges on greater attention being given to *meaning*, namely to what makes life valuable for people and within the societies we live in. Meaning is, for example, what Atul Gawande (2014) refers to when he asks patients what matters to them at the end of their lives (see also Cribb, in press). What makes life meaningful clearly has a physical dimension for all patients, but it goes beyond that, and it does so in different ways for each one. Health, illness, and decisions about diagnosis, treatment, and the arrangements regarding care and dying, all carry meanings that are deeply personal to each individual. At the same time, these meanings are part of the social fabric of our societies. I will introduce the notion of "social biomarkers," that is, information reflecting nonsomatic characteristics of patients that matter to them in connection with their health care, to bring personal meaning into the realm of evidence used for decision making in personalized medicine. Bringing social biomarkers to the forefront of medicine requires changing many of our practices and ideas, including who should be the gate keeper of personal health data, who should have access to our information, or who should be allowed to benefit from it. Giving a greater role to social biomarkers also foregrounds the importance of human relationships and meaning-making practices: Meaning cannot be ascertained by handing out questionnaires to patients about what matters to them and what they believe in. Knowing what is important to patients, and supporting them in making decisions that are meaningful to them and their significant others, requires that patients are treated by people and in institutions that know them, see them, and listen to them.

At the same time, it must be recognized that discussions about how to improve health care also need to consider cost. Cost can be contained by imposing external restrictions, typically by limiting what services are reimbursed for patients (insurer- or government-led rationing), or by making it de facto dependent on what patients can afford (socioeconomic rationing). Recently, more attention has been paid to a third way of rationing, namely self-rationing by people who decide that although they would be eligible to receive a service, they decide not to. To be clear, I am not referring here to instances where people forego health care out of personal financial considerations; I mean situations where people decide against an intervention or a treatment that is accessible and affordable to them on the basis that this intervention or treatment would have little value for them, or because it would go against their most important goals. An example would be a painful intervention that requires hospitalization for a patient at the end of her life who would like to stay at home with her family. Empirical evidence suggests that many people go for interventions not because they really want them, but because they were never asked (Kaufman 2015; see also Kaufman 2005). Exploring what meaning and value certain interventions have for individual patients serves two goals at once: Reducing suffering and harm, and cutting cost.

In this chapter I will discuss these and other ideas designed to reduce waste and cut cost and at the same contribute to the aim of providing good health care. Reducing waste is not only a way to bring down the cost of medicine and health care, but it also helps us in pursuing exactly the goal that I described above, namely to give meaning and relationality in health care a more prominent role. I will conclude this chapter by challenging the promise that big-data analytics will solve the most pressing issues in medicine and contribute to making medicine more personal at the same time. For health care systems to become sustainable, and for personalized medicine to help patients and health care practitioners make meaningful decisions, we need more human touch and more emphasis on personal and collective meaning, not just better algorithms.

## Personalization in Deep Water

Somewhat ironically, the idea that data-rich medicine will contribute to better health outcomes is accompanied by the fear that we will not be able to manage all the data that we have generated and collected. Metaphors such as "lake," "ocean," "tsunami," or "drowning" make frequent appearances in discussions on data-driven medicine, and big data more broadly (Lareau 2012; Khoury et al. 2013; Roski, Bo-Linn, and Andrews 2014). Such watery metaphors, as Deborah Lupton argues, refer to "uncontrollable entit[ies] possessing great physical power [ . . . ] as well as their unpredictability and the difficulty of control and containment" (Lupton 2013). Oceanic metaphors in particular also convey the smallness of humans in the face of a supposedly awesome force.

Such metaphors suggest that no matter how hard we try, we will never be able to control the flow of data completely. Comparisons of big data to water and other natural resources thus convey to us that data have a life of their own, and that their power is bigger than ours. Humans can alleviate the dangers and mitigate the harms of oceans and tsunamis, but we can never fully master them (see also Dean 2014; Neff 2014). And the metaphors we use are not merely a matter of semantics. As George Lakoff and Mark Johnson (1980) famously argued, the metaphors we use structure our experience of the world. For the field of medicine, such portrayals of the intrinsic and natural "force" of data have several implications. First, because the very function of medicine is to alleviate or even cure people's suffering, metaphors that highlight the inexorable intrinsic power of data can, in turn, articulate a moral obligation for individuals to harness this power in order to reap clinical benefits.

For data to be useful in the health domain, they first need to be discoverable and usable. Recently, an increasing number of scholars and activists refer to Article 15 of the *International Covenant on Economic, Social and Cultural Rights* (United Nations 1966), which defines a human right to "enjoy the benefits of scientific progress and its applications" (Knoppers et al. 2014). If people have a right to enjoy the benefits of scientific research, does this mean that there is an obligation for research to "open up" and use all available data sets in medical research institutions? Do we also need to "open" clinical data? Do people have a moral, if not a legal, obligation to allow others to use their personal health information if used for research with likely public benefit? And what does opening data sets mean in this context: Does it mean that we need to make these data available to bona fide researchers, or to everybody? While we are deliberating these questions, we may be unlikely, at this point, to wonder about what meaning these data sets have in a wider context of a person's well-being and whether we should have created them in the first place.

## Making Medical Evidence More Social: The Clinic

Physician and health care policy scholar Trisha Greenhalgh and colleagues (2014) voiced an important call for a more holistic understanding of evidence in the context of evidence-based medicine. The current focus on "hard" evidence in clinical decision making, so Greenhalgh and colleagues (2014) argue, has created a tacit hierarchy between different practices and kinds of knowledge. Digital and computable data in centralized systems and repositories have been the focus of our attention, at the cost of the practical experience of patients, nurses and doctors. In the words of the authors,

Well-intentioned efforts to automate use of evidence through computerised decision support systems, structured templates, and point of care
prompts can crowd out the local, individualised, and patient initiated elements of the clinical consultation. [ . . . ] Inexperienced clinicians may
(partly through fear of litigation) engage mechanically and defensively
with decision support technologies, stifling the development of a more
nuanced clinical expertise that embraces accumulated practical experience, tolerance of uncertainty, and the ability to apply practical and ethical judgment in a unique case. (Greenhalgh et al. 2014)

According to these authors, one challenge that is addressed particularly
poorly by evidence-based medicine in its current form is multimorbidity. Multimorbidity refers to patients suffering from several health
problems at the same time. Their symptoms, as well as the remedies used
to treat them, often compound each other and lead to further problems.
Because every patient experiences a different combination of diseases
and symptoms and has different somatic and psychological characteristics, multimorbidity expresses itself uniquely in everybody. This defies
efforts "to apply [supposedly] objective scores, metrics, interventions, or
guidelines" in the context of evidence-based medicine (Greenhalgh et al.
2014). The solution to this problem, according to Greenhalgh and colleagues, is to change the way we understand evidence. We need to find
better ways to systematically consider patients' experiences with their
illness and "the real life clinical encounter for different conditions in
different circumstances" (Greenhalgh et al. 2014; see also Glasziou et al.
2013; Timmermans and Mauck 2005; E. Nelson et al. 2015; NHS Scotland
2016; Mulley et al. 2017).

Such a more inclusive understanding of evidence also requires and
produces new knowledge paradigms. For a long time, randomized controlled trials have been considered the "gold standard against which
all other sources of clinical evidence are measured" (Longhurst, Harrington, and Shah 2014: 1229; see also Kaufman 2015; Timmermans and
Berg 2003b). In the past, they have been criticized for oversampling particular groups of the population, mainly white men; its findings are thus
not applicable to women, children, and minorities. But in the context
of personalized medicine, this is not the only problem that they pose:
The more we know about differences between people, the less accept-

able it becomes to lump people together into large groups. The computational (*in silico*) modeling of physiological and pathological processes has been suggested as a possible alternative to randomized controlled trials; another one is to equip clinical decision makers with data from electronic health records, observational data, and "deep phenotyping" data. These data give answers to questions such as: How are proteins expressed in the diseased cells of this particular patient? What gut bacteria does the patient have? Does she have problems that seem unrelated but might share a common pathway (Delude 2015; see also Jensen, Jensen, and Brunak 2012; P. Robinson 2012)? In addition, greater use of patient-generated information, including diaries, or information that they collect via sensors or digital tools, has been proposed in order to obtain insights into the expression and effects of diseases and treatments in individual patients (Wehrlen et al. 2016).

It could be argued that moving away from the randomized controlled trial as the gold standard of evidence-based medicine is long overdue: To date, it is estimated that less than one fifth of published clinical guidelines are based on randomized controlled trials (Longhurst, Harrington, and Shah 2014). This is the case partly because evidence from randomized controlled trials does not generalize well to real-life clinical situations, a challenge that is known as the "external validity" problem (see also chapter 2 in Kaufman 2015). Experts suggest that much stronger use should be made of observational data, which has become better in quality. As Christopher Longhurst and colleagues argue,

> for most clinical questions the only relevant data available to aid decision making are observational. Historically, this type of data has been administrative in nature, creating the potential for misleading interpretations of findings. However, the rapid adoption of information technology is creating large new clinical data sets and argues for a reconsideration of the role that observational studies can play in evidence-based medicine, particularly in comparative effectiveness research. (Longhurst, Harrington, and Shah 2014: 1231)

The so-called Green Button initiative was established to foster this goal: It aims at helping clinicians to access aggregate clinical data from other patients similar to those they are treating. This could be particularly useful in situations where few or no published studies are pertinent (Longhurst, Harrington, and Shah 2014: 1231).

But even if such Green Buttons were widely available in hospitals, there would still be a number of challenges to address. These challenges range from the technical to the practical to the ethical. Imagine a surgeon who is about to operate on a patient. This surgeon wants to know what patients have in common who are similar to one she will operate on next week and who have undergone the same type of surgery and recovered particularly well. Did they all rest for a specific period of time after surgery? Did they take a particular drug? Are they in a specific age range? Even if this surgeon has access to relevant data sets—for example, if she can search the data of all patients treated by the same hospital group—she first needs to know what patients are "similar" to hers. Should she look at all patients who underwent the same surgery? Or only those who are in the same age range? Or those within the same age range who also have a similar combination of symptoms? In addition, will the system even allow her to search for these aspects? Patient similarity criteria are one aspect that needs to be defined and measured in a standardized and consistent manner, and results need to be made available in ways that they are useful to clinicians (Longhurst, Harrington, and Shah 2014: 1232).

Another major challenge for the use of aggregate clinical data to aid decision making is that electronic health records were designed for clinical management, not research. This means that the classifications and formats used in these records may not "speak to each other"; they represent different aspects of a phenomenon, do not adhere to the same standards, or are stored in incompatible formats (see also Doods et al. 2012). Moreover, as Isaac Kohane puts it, electronic health records "provide only the exposures that clinicians have been routinely trained to gather." Other factors that could have bearing on the situation, such as toxin exposure, workplace milieu, or exercise history, are not normally included in electronic health records (Kohane 2011: 425).

And there are, of course, privacy challenges. When data cannot be fully anonymized, existing privacy regulations, such as HIPAA in the United States, may need to be amended to allow frontline clinicians to access aggregate patient data (Longhurst, Harrington, and Shah 2014: 1233; see also El Emam, Rodgers, and Malin 2015). Similarly, the current drive to include social and behavioral data, such as information about lifestyle and living conditions, in a person's medical records is laudable in the sense that these factors are known to affect health outcomes. But because these data include highly sensitive information such as sexual orientation or exposure to partner violence (Institute of Medicine 2014), if such information were included in electronic health records this would require us to think very carefully about ways to mitigate harm following unauthorized reidentification. It will be impossible to ensure that nobody will be harmed as a result of the use of these data.

Another important concern pertains to how the increasing use of observational and other patient-generated data to inform individual health care decisions will affect underserved populations. Because certain groups—older people, children, women, members of minorities— are underrepresented in, or even excluded from, clinical trials, some people hope that greater use of observational instead of experimental study designs could help gather evidence on people in those groups. While this may hold true for elderly people or children who, despite being excluded from clinical trials, are regular recipients of health care, observational studies cannot solve the problem of missing data on under- or nonserved populations. A health insurance company or a group of hospitals that uses aggregate patient data to inform the treatment of individual patients is inevitably restricted to using data from people who are on their patient register. Thus, there is a risk that the greater use of observational and patient-generated data will make underserved populations even less visible than they are now.

Countries with easily accessible universal health care are in the unique position to have access to data from almost the entire population.[1] Countries with publicly funded health care systems where patient information has been stored centrally for decades are particularly well placed in this respect. Besides being broadly representative of the population, they provide longitudinal, "real life" data, as well as opportunities for follow-up. Epidemiologist Arlene Gallagher at al. (2011), for example, analyzed data from the UK General Practice Research Database to evaluate the association between the time when patients received warfarin—a blood thinner—and the risk of stroke and mortality. They found that coagulation control was indeed associated with a reduced risk of stroke. Another example are researchers working with the Danish Multiple Sclerosis (MS) Registry to estimate incidence rates of bone fractures in MS patients, finding that specifically fractures of the tibia, hip, and femur occurred more often in those patients than in other groups (Bazelier et al. 2012).

Moving from clinical to other health care data, in the United States, the Center for Medicare and Medicaid Services makes aggregated privacy-protected data available on its websites in machine-readable form. These data include previously unpublished statistics on Medicare spending or quality performance in hospitals (Brennan et al. 2014: 1199). Such initiatives for the opening and repurposing of health care data have already had impacts on policy debates as well: Following the release of data on average hospital charges for the one hundred most common Medicare inpatient admissions in the United States, a national debate on variation in hospital charges ensued.[2]

## Making Medicine More Social: Patients' Experience and Knowledge

Personalized medicine has great potential to help broaden the notions of evidence further. The idea that symptom-based disease taxonomies will be replaced by data-rich characterizations of individuals at various stages of health and disease can help create room for the consideration of dynamic, collaborative, and "subjective" patient-centered information. Some commentators consider patient-centered medicine as a countermovement to personalized medicine because of personalized medicine's specific focus on technological solutions (Busse 2015: vi; see also Dickenson 2013). Indeed, medicine can only be patient-centered in a deep sense if patients are not treated as mere data sources but we also consider what these data actually mean to people, and how they can improve health care—and more broadly their lives—from their perspective (see also Bardes 2012). A great example for this approach is the "Realistic Medicine" approach pioneered by the Scottish doctor—and now Scotland's chief medical officer—Catherine Calderwood. Realistic Medicine encourages health professionals to convey to patients and their families a realistic understanding of what is possible, and it poses a lot of emphasis on listening to patients to understand what is important to them. It also promotes the development of new metrics that capture value in health care better and in a truly patient-centered manner.[3] In a short time the approach has become a movement far beyond the borders of Scotland (NHS Scotland 2016). And initiatives with similar goals—to acknowledge that more medicine does not always lead to better health and to place much more emphasis on listening to what patients really want and value—are emerging in other regions (see, for example, Mulley et al. 2017).

While approaches like Realistic Medicine advocate a notion of patient-centeredness that is indeed sensitive to the subjective, personal needs and values of patients, it is important to keep in mind that not everything that carries the label "patient-centered" actually is patient-focused in a deep sense. Terminology can be misleading, because some types of information that have "patient" in the title are not controlled by patients: often patients have not been involved in deciding how information about them would be collected and used, other than giving "consent" by signing a paper or ticking a box. Also, some so-called patient-reported outcome measures (PROM), which were initially introduced by the U.S. Food and Drug Administration (FDA) to collect data on side effects (and other outcome measures) directly from patients, can be patient-centric only in a superficial sense. Historically, PROM have "focused on tightly controlled, structured data elements intended to meet the expectations of a specific audience (such as the FDA)" (Howie et al. 2014: 1222–1223). In other words, patients have had little if any say in what information is collected and what measures and criteria are used.[4]

To illustrate this, Lynn Howie and colleagues at Duke University give the example of a patient named Joe, who suffers from lung cancer and emphysema. PROM require Joe to quantify his symptoms. Rather than recording what is meaningful to Joe, his narrative is translated into a preexisting matrix of questions and gradients. "A qualitative story is transformed into discrete data that can be efficiently managed using the principles of informatics and information science" (Howie et al. 2014: 1223). Other aspects of Joe's life and health are not considered under the PROM remit on this occasion, because they do not lie within the area of interest demarcated by regulatory authorities. What remains left out here are questions that could make an important difference to Joe's quality of life, such as: Would he prefer a potentially more effective, but also more invasive, disease management plan? What activities or aspects give meaning to Joe's life and should thus be taken into consideration when making treatment decisions? Personalized medicine, if put to use in a deep patient-centered manner, could provide an opportunity to help support patients in maintaining the parts of their lives that are most meaningful to them. Patients would need to have a say in what type of information about them will be included in their records, who gatekeeps this information, and how it will be used. Experts can make suggestions, but patients need to have a say in what will be collected about them specifically, and they need to be able to suggest additional data that matters to them. Fortunately, recent advances in PROM methodologies and use have broadened out to wider ranges of patient experiences, including how patients perceive shared decision making (see, for example, Elwyn et al. 2013)

## Bringing in the Person and Her World: The Value of Social Biomarkers

One way to give patients more say in how information about them is used to personalize their health care would be to complement the range of somatic biomarkers—that is, different kinds of data characterizing a person's physiology and pathologies, such as cancer markers, cholesterol values—by "social biomarkers." Such social biomarkers would indicate a person's most important social bonds, her preferences, and, if the person wants to include these, also her spiritual or religious commitments, as well as other types of information that the patient considers relevant. Social biomarkers would thus include information not only about what a person wants to be done in situations where she would be unable to give consent (for example, emergency treatments), but also regarding who the people closest to her are and what religious representatives, if any, should be consulted. Information on what the person wants to be done in situations where she cannot speak for herself are not limited to medical treatments, but to wider aspects of care. These data would not need to be set in stone; like other health-related data that change over time, such as gene expression, blood pressure, or weight, they could be modified over time to adjust to changes in the patient's circumstances or preferences.

The types of personal information that visionaries of personalized and precision medicine envisage including in medical decision making are mostly data that are already digitally available (Weber, Mandl, and Kohane 2014). The inclusion of social biomarkers, in contrast, requires information that is not available in digital format, or that has not been recorded at all. Here again, a deep patient-centered approach would entail that people have a say in what kinds of information are included about them, and that they can make decisions together with people and within institutions they know and trust (and vice versa). If a patient can, and wants to, do this herself, she can become the gatekeeper for her own health information; otherwise she can name a designated person to do this on her behalf. The designated person could be a family member, a treating physician, or an organization (see also Hafen, Kossmann, and Brand 2014).

## People as Gatekeepers to Their Own Health Data?

Although many visions of personalized medicine emphasize the importance of patient-centered research and practice, they typically leave out the question of how patients can decide what information about them is used in medical decision making. The question of what data and information to include is still seen as an issue best decided by experts. At the same time, the increasing push toward open data and transparency has prompted clinics and hospitals in many countries to provide patients with access and control over their health data. Several hospitals in the United States, for example, offer "MyChart" (see, for example, Cleveland Clinic 2016), a free and ad-free online system to view test results after they were released by the treating physician. The system also includes information about medication, past and upcoming appointments, health reminders and suggestions for preventive care, as well as prescription renewals. MyChart also has a dedicated portal for caregivers. It does not, however, allow patients to upload any information that they would like to see included, and it is far from the idea of embracing social biomarkers. At present it includes only data and information that were generated and collected in the context of care received by the medical institution using the MyChart service. This is yet another instance of the notorious problem of health information fragmentation: many electronic health record systems emerged within single institutions or organizations and do not "speak" to other systems. Moreover, some institutions do not have electronic health record systems at all, because they have insufficient resources, inadequate IT infrastructures, personnel shortages, workflow issues, or security concerns (Horning 2011; Hufstader et al. 2014; Maust 2012; T. Mills et al. 2010). This problem has been found to be particularly acute in rural areas (more in the United States than in Europe; for a discussion of the latter, see Jensen, Jensen, and Brunak 2012). Moreover, in some places, clinicians resist the adoption of electronic health records because they fear that their contact with patients will become less personal, or that health records could be used to monitor or control them (Lluch 2011).

To make electronic health records easier to use in the clinic, software developers look to create tools that can process natural language and use machine learning to "detect" relevant information from widely dispersed sources and integrate them at the point of care. IBM's Watson or Apixio's Hierarchical Condition Category (HCC) Profiler are examples of such software: While IBM's Watson focuses on mining the medical literature, the HCC Profiler brings clinical information locked away in institutional files together with billing data to calculate risk scores for patients, allegedly to support health care providers to decide where and what care is needed (Apixio 2015). This, however, would move decisions over what data are used for their care even farther away from patients.

In Europe, similar initiatives to MyChart exist. In England, for example, all patients need to be given the opportunity to access their doctor's records electronically in the very near future (NHS England 2012; 2014; 2015), and several software systems have been developed for this purpose.[5] The Dutch platform Mijnzorgnet.nl (lit. "My care network") also offers access to health data to patients and clinicians. Initially launched by a university hospital in Nijmegen in the eastern Netherlands, Mijnzorgnet.nl differs from MyChart in several respects. In contrast to MyChart, Mijnzorgnet.nl encourages the use of the platform not only as an access point for medical records, but also as a discussion forum. Moreover, Mijnzorgnet.nl allows patients to upload medical and other health-relevant information. In fact, at Mijnzorgnet.nl, patients, not clinicians, are gatekeepers: Patients decide what information to upload—ranging from diary entries to blood test results—and who to share them with. In short, although both MyChart and Mijnzorgnet.nl are set up as secure personal medical information databases, the former is exclusively linked to a specific institutional setting, and the latter is intended to be managed by patients.

These differences between the two platforms, MyChart and Mijnzorgnet.nl, illustrate a seemingly inevitable trade-off between patient-centeredness and ease of access and use. With Mijnzorgnet.nl, patients can decide what types of data and information to include. MyChart, in contrast, is relatively restrictive regarding what it allows to be imported into the system, and the process is largely driven by medical professionals. By putting clinicians, rather than patients, in charge of data curation, and by allowing carers to access records on behalf of patients, MyChart is attractive to a wider range of people, including very elderly or severely disabled patients. Mijnzorgnet.nl allows patients to do much more; the way that the platform is set up in terms of design and visualization facilitates encounters between patients and medical professionals at eye level. However, for patients who cannot or do not want to be the kind of active and communicative patient that the platform envisages, Mijnzorgnet.nl is not of much use.

I already mentioned the Green Button initiative that aims at giving clinicians access to aggregate patient data. Another, complementary initiative, "Blue Button," is geared toward patients: The U.S.-government initiative seeks to give people better access to their own health data. Having emerged out of the Veterans Administration, it cashes in on the legal right of all U.S. citizens to access their health records in whatever form they are stored, in paper form or electronically. While the initiative considers access to health records as particularly important for people whose care is complex to manage, or who want or need to change doctors, its wider goal is to give everyone "more [ . . . ] control of your health and your personal health information" (Department of Health and Human Services 2014). Because some hospitals or doctors are still not aware that access to health information is a legal right of patients, the Blue Button initiative provides patients with a letter to print out and show to their doctors or hospital staff. The organization also provides guidance for institutions wanting to join the movement. New members must commit to making up-to-date personal health information (either the complete record, or a subset) available to patients or to designated caregivers in a secure and user-friendly manner.

## Making Medicine More Social: Research

MyChart, Mijnzorgnet.nl, and the Blue Button initiative all aim to give patients better control over the data and information stored and processed about them in the clinic. Some of them move patients a step closer to being gatekeepers for the data and records used for their health care. Other initiatives try to make it easier for people to make their health data available for research. Portable Legal Consent is an example. It is an initiative conceived by Sage Bionetworks, a nonprofit research organization based in Seattle. It was set up in 2009 with funds from disease-specific research foundations, anonymous donors, and the commercial health care company Quintiles (quintiles.com). An important substantial contribution to the launch of the organization came from the pharmaceutical company Merck (Sage Bionetworks 2014a). The key problem that the initiative sought to address are so-called health data silos, that is, the reality that a lot of data are held at institutions that do not want to, or that do not know how to, make them accessible to external researchers. As Stephen Friend, a director of Sage Bionetworks who now works at Apple, put it, their mission was to help such organizations and institutions get their data out of silos without needing to worry about IT (Davies 2009).

The basic idea of Portable Legal Consent is that patients sign up to a central registry once, deposit their (broad) consent to how their data can be used, and then decide what data they upload. Once they have uploaded their data, the data are available to a wide range of researchers worldwide. Researchers using data must also accept the terms and conditions of Portable Legal Consent and confirm that they will not attempt to reidentify individuals, even if they have the mathematical capacity to do so. They also need to commit to avoiding other types of harms (see also Wilbanks 2013).

Potential participants of the first phase of Portable Legal Consent were directed to an online tutorial that included information about the project's mission, an overview of how data that volunteers uploaded would be used, and a discussion of potential harms that could result from the participation. The tutorial also included a warning that it was impossible to foresee exactly what the consequences of participating would be. People who had doubts about whether their participation could have unintended consequences for them were discouraged from participating.[6] Participants were also informed that the possibility of re-identification could not be excluded entirely. They were told that their data would be treated as a "gift" and therefore they would not receive compensation or any direct benefits.[7] Since the conclusion of the first phase of its activities, Sage Bionetworks has launched new projects and partnerships (Doerr, Suver and Wilbanks 2016; Dolgin 2014a; 2014b).

In recent years, a range of other initiatives and infrastructures have been created for people who are seeking to make their personal data available to biomedical research. Spurred by the increasing availability of genome-testing services directly to consumers, a number of not-for-profit services have emerged that support people in interpreting their DNA information and making these data available for researchers at the same time. On sites such as OpenSNP (openSNP.org), Open Humans (openhumans.org), and DNAland (dna.land), for example, volunteers can upload their DNA information and other data, such as from microbiome analyses, or data from activity trackers, to see how their data compare to others', and to create a publicly available database to facilitate discovery.

Such initiatives not only collapse the distinction between medical research and practice, but also tie data and information about people's bodies and lives more closely to both. This process has two effects: It "datafies" people's bodies and lives and makes information about them usable in the medical domain. At the same time, it gives people a better understanding of data and information used for these purposes. Often it also gives people more control over their data. At the same time, even some initiatives that explicitly serve the aim of giving patients more control over their health data do not give them a lot of say over what data and information are collected in the first place. In other words, people participate mostly by uploading data, and not by governing the project. Some initiatives are also relatively restrictive in terms of the data and information that can be uploaded onto their platforms; unstructured, nondigitized, narrative information in particular does not have a place in most data repositories. How can we change this situation?

## Facilitating Meaningful Personal Decisions on Therapies and Treatments

Currently only the most informed and assertive of patients routinely bring their own preferences and values to the table. Many do not dare to complement or reject the choices presented to them by their physicians. Although the number of physicians who support shared decision making is growing, it can be risky for them to suggest unorthodox options to their patients. It is often safest to stick to established protocols and customs. This situation needs to change if we want to tailor health care more closely to the values and needs of patients—and to reduce waste as well.

In this section I will give a brief overview of initiatives that have a few things in common: They all put people with relevant experience in the center of decision making—patients as experts on their needs and values, and doctors as experts on where "ordinary medicine" (Kaufman 2015) wastes resources and causes harm. Moreover, all these initiatives share the conviction that health care decisions should not be driven purely by supposedly "rational" reasoning. Instead, they assume that decision making should include people's experiences, feelings, and needs. Rather than challenging the idea that medical practice should be evidence-based, they employ a broader understanding of evidence. They work with traditional statistical and quantitative evidence, for example, in the form of cost-effectiveness measures, or epidemiological data, while equally encouraging people to make their own, deeply personal assessments of risk, harm, and benefit. Finally, they seek to tie these "subjective," personal assessments into medical decision making in a way that is systematic, transparent and accountable.

Choosing Wisely is one such initiative dedicated to this goal. It was launched by the American Board of Internal Medicine Foundation (ABIMF) in collaboration with Consumer Reports, an independent nonprofit organization in the United States, in 2011. It is committed to the primary goals of patient welfare, patient autonomy, and social justice (Wolfson et al. 2014). To reach these goals, the people behind Choosing Wisely believe that it is necessary to tackle the problem of wasteful oversupply in health care head-on. As a first step, Choosing Wisely invited societies of medical specialists to each submit the five diagnostic and therapeutic measures with the lowest value—meaning interventions with a significant cost but low or no benefit to patients (Good Steward-ship Working Group 2011; Morden et al. 2014;).[8] It was very important that doctors, not payers, should decide which interventions to drop, and that they should provide scientific evidence to back up their recommendations (see also Berenson and Docteur 2013).

It turned out that doctors in each discipline named services provided by medical specialties other than their own as low value (Morden et al 2014: 590). But despite this, the exercise has been a success. Physicians were "willing to make recommendations to improve health care value even against their own financial interests" (Morden et al. 2014: 589). Choosing Wisely now discourages the use of imaging in certain contexts, as well as the performance of routine general health checks for healthy adults, or feeding tubes in patients with advanced dementia (Wolfson et al. 2014). In addition, Choosing Wisely emphasizes the importance of good communication between physicians and patients, which it considers serving both the goal of patient welfare and cost savings.

Choosing Wisely is continuously expanding its remit; it offers a range of resources for patients and doctors, including videos to teach doctors how to convey to patients that in some cases, "doing more" can be harmful instead of helpful. It is also expanding its activities to other parts of the world (see, for example, Frühwald 2013; Levinson et al. 2015).

Another initiative that tries to bring personal meaning to decisions regarding health care is Death over Dinner (deathoverdinner.org). It aims to do so by encouraging people to make meaningful decisions about what they want, and what they do not want, at the end of their life. When its founder, Michael Hebb, learned that three quarters of Americans would like to die at home, but that only about a quarter do, he decided that something needed to be done to change this. Hebb, a self-professed "food provocateur" from Oregon (Hochman 2007), believed that the dinner table is the best place to start removing the taboo of talking about death. He believed that it would be good for patients, their families, and society as a whole if people thought about what they would want at the very end of their lives, and also told others. It would result in less pain inflicted on people, and in saving costs by foregoing expensive and invasive interventions that people did not want.

Discussions about how we would like to die, Hebb believes, should not be seen as something morbid. On the contrary, such conversations can be life-affirming by bringing people closer together. And they can help us to avoid harm and useless interventions for people who do not really want them. The initiative provides online materials for people willing to host Death over Dinner meals for friends, family, coworkers and even for strangers to discuss the end of their lives, hoping that people will understand better their own and others' feelings and preferences related to their death—and deepen their social relationships at the same time. The materials provided include conversation prompts and suggestions for addressing particularly sensitive and difficult aspects, as well as "homework" for dinner participants to complete before they attend. The movement just opened a chapter in Australia and is expanding to other countries of the world.

Bringing subjective meaning to health care decision making is hoped to have the positive side effect of reducing costs. Another movement worth noting in this context is Preventing Overdiagnosis (preventingoverdiagnosis.net; see also Moynihan, Doust, and Henry 2012; Welch, Schwartz, and Woloshin 2011). It comprises people from various disciplines and fields of expertise who are united by the belief that "too much medicine" causes harm and wastes resources. Researchers estimate that in the United States, between 158 and 226 billion dollars were wasted on unnecessary treatments in 2011 alone (Berwick and Hackbarth 2012); a 2017 report by the Organisation for Economic Co-Operation and Development (OECD) concluded that a staggering 20 percent of the money spent on health care in OECD countries is currently being wasted (OECD 2017). While unnecessary treatments do not account for all of the 20 percent, of course—some goes to correcting medical mistakes, excessive costs for drugs and administration, and fraud committed by medical providers, for example—unnecessary treatments play a big role in increasing the cost burden. Unnecessary treatments are those that do not benefit patients, and where it is possible to foresee that they will not. A surgery with good chances of success that goes wrong is not an unnecessary treatment according to this definition; but many of the low value interventions singled out by Choosing Wisely fall into this category. An important cause for unnecessary treatments is overdiagnosis, meaning that a problem is diagnosed that will never trouble the person during her lifetime. This could be a tumor that disappears by itself, or a malignancy in a very elderly person where it can be foreseen that the person will not experience symptoms during her lifetime. Some experts also speak of overdiagnosis when people are diagnosed with a problem that is unlikely to have an effect on mortality because there are no effective treatments available (see, for example, Carpenter, Raja, and Brown, 2015; see also Carter et al. 2015).

Preventing Overdiagnosis organizes annual conferences for health practitioners and patients. These conferences are becoming increasingly popular as awareness of the emotional, societal, and economic costs of overdiagnosis are growing. The influential *British Medical Journal* launched a series discussing the effects of "Too Much Medicine" in 2013, and similar initiatives are emerging in other parts of the world.

All three initiatives, Choosing Wisely, Death over Dinner, and Preventing Overdiagnosis have in common that they broaden the range of factors to be considered when health care decisions are made. Anthropologist Sharon Kaufman argued that in the United States, the question of whether there is a medical indication for a treatment that renders a patient eligible for cost reimbursement is central in today's health care decisions. As a result, many invasive, expensive, and onerous interventions have become "ordinary" in the sense that patients are expected to ask for them, and get them, if they are eligible (Kaufman 2015). The initiatives discussed in this section add an important set of questions to be asked when making treatment decisions: As a patient, even if I am eligible, do I want this treatment? Does it have value for me? What am I gaining by it? What am I giving up? As a doctor or health professional, how can I help my patient make a decision that is in line with her values, needs and desires? These initiatives increase space for patients and health care practitioners to consider goals that go beyond clinical parameters and include what is meaningful to individual patients, even if, in some cases, this could shorten their lives (see also Gawande 2014; NHS Scotland 2016). They promote personalization on the basis of a wider notion of evidence than mainstream visions of personalized medicine envisage. Last but not least, they seek to enhance the "high touch" content of medicine, meaning that health care professionals and patients interact with each other as people with bodies, souls, and minds that are more than their medical records and digital data doubles.

Having said this, high-touch medicine need not be seen in competition with high-tech solutions: They can both serve the same goal of increasing human contact and creating more room for personal meaning. Technologies have always occupied an ambiguous space between facilitating social detachment and attachment. The telephone is a good example: Telephones can bring people closer together by enabling communication in cases where no communication would take place otherwise, but they can also lead to detachment if people use them as a replacement for face-to-face interaction. In the context of personalized medicine, we need to enlist technology more strongly into the service of high-touch medicine, and not see it as a silver bullet to cut costs, or as an end in itself (see also Lock 2013).

## How Technology Can Help Support High-Touch Medicine

How can technologies be used to support high-touch medicine? Think of Google Glass, the smart glasses prototype that the company rolled out in 2014 and discontinued a year later to improve the model. Smart glasses, which are transparent computers with displays that are worn on one's head like glasses, can enable doctors to maintain eye contact with their patients while reading and dictating information, instead of needing to spend long periods of time looking at their computers (see Meskó 2014: 29). And they can enable clinicians to "touch" patients who are not in the same room (Chu 2014). Health entrepreneur Zen Chu calls this "scalable medicine": Technology can help expand interactions between health care professionals and patients into wider contexts and new media. New forms of interaction range from the stereotypical "the doctor will Skype you now" consultation via video-link (Eisenberg 2015) to remote robotic surgeries for patients in areas that would not normally have access to specialists.

With some technological devices getting cheaper, their use is no longer restricted to wealthy people or world regions. In this sense, digital health technologies follow the trajectory of many other information and communication technologies. Let us return to the telephone for another moment: When telephone communication was first introduced, it was not accessible to the masses. And this was intended. Elites argued that making telephone communication available to "ordinary" people could lead to trouble. The masses could organize themselves to riot or engage in otherwise undesirable behavior. Enabling only elites to communicate over long distances faster and more easily was considered one of the very functions of telephones: "[T]he utility of the telephone could not be preserved without restricting its availability," as it was argued in the British Parliament in 1895 (Marvin 1988: 101). Line rentals remained unaffordable for many people until deep into the twentieth century. Nowadays, access to telephone communication is no longer a means of class distinction. On the contrary: Being glued to one's phone and being available around the clock is increasingly seen as a sign of not being very high up in the social pecking order.

Many digital health technologies will follow a similar trajectory; they turn from an expensive good that only the richest can afford into something available to anybody. But this does not mean that everybody will be able to use them in the same manner. In rich areas, smart glasses may be used to enable doctors to maintain better eye contact with their patients while entering information or checking files. People in low-income countries, in contrast, may be used as data sources, such as for the exploration of "natural" disease trajectories. In rich countries, we no longer know how diseases evolve if left untreated, because they always get treated. Smart glasses could be handed out to poor people for "free" in return for their consent that their data can be used to improve treatments and technologies for the rich.

It should also be noted that in the era of data-driven medicine, it is often not technology, but interpretation, that is the luxury item. In many instances, such as genetic analysis, or imaging, technology use has already ceased to be the cost bottleneck—interpretation is. Although much wider strata of people will be able to afford a genome sequence or a proteome profile in the near future, very few people would be able to afford the interpretation of this information. And the cost for interpretation is not going to drop in the same manner as the cost for technology has. There are several reasons for this: Interpretation of data in medicine always requires the knowledge of organisms in vivo (Leonelli 2014); it cannot be modeled in its entirety. Moreover, as long as computers cannot separate between meaningful information and "noise," the interpretation of data cannot be fully automated. The time and effort of human experts is required to make data meaningful, and differences in access to this resource will be an important manifestation of inequity in the era of personalized medicine—unless we manage to avoid that such inequities emerge, which is what I will turn to next.

## Personalized Medicine Requires More Solidarity, Not Less: Why Personalized Medicine Requires Universal and Affordable Health Care

Rising expenses are a notorious problem in health care systems. Reasons for this include the development and proliferation of new and expensive technologies, increasing longevity, and—partly related to the latter— the growing prevalence of chronic diseases. Rising administrative costs, which are partly a result of managed care, are also to blame. Last but not least, in some parts of the world, including the United States, the highly fragmented nature of the demand side of health care also contributes to rising costs: A fragmented demand side means that suppliers can more or less dictate prices (see, for example, Angell 2015).

Rising costs mean that we either need to spend more money on health care or we ration health care more strongly than we do it at present. Rationing as such is not controversial; every health care system in the world does it. What differs are the types of criteria that are used for this purpose. Most of us are so used to clinical indications being used to determine access to services that we do not even consider them rationing criteria. But they are: Without clear indications that a lung X-ray may provide clarification as to the cause of a person's persistent cough, for example, a person may not have access to a lung X-ray other than as part of preventive checkups or boutique medicine services paid out of pocket. Few would disagree that clinical indications are a useful and meaningful rationing criterion. Without it, anybody could merely demand whatever they think may benefit them, irrespective of experience, expertise, and evidence.

A second type of rationing uses economic criteria: People get what they can afford. Systems where people "choose" what services to spend money on, or what type of health insurance to buy, are examples. What somebody's insurance does not cover, she cannot get unless she pays out of pocket. Economic criteria are controversial, and most countries mitigate or even eliminate the effects of economic rationing. The United

Kingdom, with its tax-funded system of universal health care that is free at the point of use, is the most "extreme" example, but even countries without publicly funded health care, such as Switzerland and the United States, have programs in place to help people who cannot afford to pay their insurance premiums.

A third type of rationing looks at person-centric criteria. Person-centric criteria can be objective, such as chronological age; some countries restrict the publicly funded services available to people above a certain age limit, for example in the domain of assisted reproduction. Others relate to people's behavior. For example, people who "choose" unhealthy lifestyles by eating too much or by smoking are excluded from certain services, or they have to pay higher premiums. In the private insurance sector, such decisions are made on the basis of actuarial reasoning: If smokers or obese people are likely to suffer from more, and more expensive, health problems, they need to pay more into the system. In the publicly funded health care sector, the suggestion to penalize people with unhealthy lifestyles has been supported mostly on the grounds of the alleged moral responsibility of people for their lifestyle "choices": Those who impose the likelihood of higher costs on society by not looking after themselves well enough, so the argument goes, are not deserving of societal support to the same extent as those who lead healthy lives (for a summary see Buyx and Prainsack 2012). In the context of personalized medicine, there is the risk that differences in behavior obtain yet another role in health care rationing: Differences in people's lifestyles could be used as a justification for the exclusion of certain groups from interventions they would be likely to benefit from. This would be the case not because they are seen as less deserving, but because certain lifestyle characteristics are found to be "objectively" associated with worse prognoses. People who smoke, drink too much, or are overweight—all of which are characteristics that are linked with distress and poverty, of course—could be excluded from access to certain interventions due to their seemingly objective likelihood to respond less well to them than other people. Or people who suffer from "accelerated aging" due to their genetic heritage, or due to stressful life events leaving their epigenetic marks, could be denied a hip replacement, a kidney transplant, or another expensive intervention once their biomarkers indicate that their biological age is above a certain limit.

Again, it is not that exclusion per se is a problem. Excluding patients on the basis of a high likelihood that they will not benefit from treatment—or may even be harmed by it—is in the interest of the patient. Such knowledge or likelihood can come from "objective" indicators such as a genetic predisposition (somatic biomarkers), or from a person stating her preferences (social biomarkers). For example, if a patient whose genetic makeup shows that she would not benefit from a particular drug is not given said drug, this does not seem to be an issue. Or if a person in the final stages of cancer were excluded from life-prolonging treatment because she did not want such treatment, then this exclusion would correspond with her explicit wishes.

But excluding patients from interventions is problematic when individual characteristics such as somatic biomarkers, personal or demographic characteristics, or lifestyle "choices" are used to justify exclusion *against* the interests and needs of patients. Health is a basic need of every person. Whatever key function we see political communities as fulfilling, providing accessible and affordable health care must be one of them. To justify this, it is not necessary to go as far as to refute arguments about the danger of an alleged "nanny state" making decisions on behalf of its citizens. A national system for the financing and provision of health care has clear economic advantages as well: A nationally organized system of health care for all ("universal health care") puts payers in a much stronger position in the negotiation of prices than in situations in which payers are small and fragmented and where the suppliers call the shots and set prices (Angell 2015; Relman 2014). Moreover, countries with universal health care have been found to provide the most cost-effective health care (Karen Davis et al. 2014; Britnell 2015). State-run universal health care also makes health care provision easier to regulate, and it is thus harder for big corporate actors to abuse the system for the sake of profit maximization. For these reasons, it seems economically, politically, and ethically preferable to provide universal health care that is affordable for and accessible to all people living in a given country.

Within a system of universal health care, a good basket of services needs to be affordable to all, and no further stratification according to risk should be carried out that limits access to services, other than risks that have a direct connection to prognosis (such as cardiovascular health as a consideration in decisions on the use of surgery requiring general anesthesia). Instead of resorting to antisolidaristic measures, efforts to save costs should focus on voluntary self-rationing, on the elimination of waste, and on the reduction of administrative, non-frontline costs, examples of which have been discussed in this chapter. Only against such a background could personalized medicine be realized without increasing inequalities.

## Personalized Medicine Needs to Be Based on More than Predictive Analytics

In the previous section I mentioned the possibility that lifestyle characteristics can be used to identify patients who are less likely to benefit from an intervention. Such measures would be based on predictive analytics, that is, on analyses of large data sets aiming to discern patterns in these data—such as what characteristics people have in common who live the longest after a particular kind of heart surgery. These characteristics do not need to be limited to lifestyle characteristics; in principle, any type of data can be used for this purpose. The use of algorithm-based predictive modeling using information from patients' electronic health records is currently promoted as a silver bullet for cost containment. In the words of Boston-based patient safety scholar David Bates and colleagues, "[E]ven in the short term, it will be possible for health care organizations to realize substantial benefits from deploying predictive systems. [ . . . ] Such tools are important because many potential outcomes are associated with harm to patients, are expensive, or both" (Bates et al. 2014: 1124).

The development of predictive models typically takes place in the following manner: first, patient data are obtained from electronic health records, or from patients directly—for example, via "observations of daily living" (ODL) metrics (Robert Wood Johnson Foundation n.d.). Sometimes data from electronic health records are also linked with data in large biomedical databases, public health databases, or databases used for insurance or reimbursement (Jensen, Jensen, and Brunak 2012: 397; Kohane 2011: 420). Genotyping data, imaging data, or data on prescription drugs can also be used. These data are then "cleaned," which means that incorrect, incomplete, or corrupt files are removed. This can be a very long, onerous, and resource-intensive process. As a next step, a predictive algorithm is developed and then validated using different data sets than the one on the basis of which it was developed. The resulting model is then tested and monitored so that it can be modified and adjusted if necessary (G. Cohen et al. 2014: 1140).

The algorithm's success will depend on whether the data used for the development and testing of the algorithm are the right kind, and sufficient amounts of, data (Amarasingham et al. 2014; Kohane 2011). This, in turn, often depends on whether a big enough number of health care providers are willing to contribute data to a shared platform, or make their devices interoperable. Currently there are strong disincentives for health care organizations to allow their data or devices to be accessed or used by others. These disincentives include legal and ethical restrictions that would need to be changed or bypassed, as well as a lack of resources. In the case of organizations that are accountable to shareholders, there may also be concerns about competition. A consequence of this situation is that clinical data sets in particular remain fragmented and of relatively low value to support clinical decision making; patterns that are found in these data sets are likely to suffer from biases. Any conclusions drawn from the analysis of these data would need to be validated in larger data sets (see also Jensen, Jensen, and Brunak 2012).

A social and ethical rather than technical challenge relates to the fact that decision making according to algorithm-based predictive modeling would rely on criteria that were not set by, and may not even be transparent to, the people affected by it. This entails the risk that aspects that are meaningful to patients could be blackboxed to an even greater extent than is the case today (see also Tutt 2016). Moreover, the adoption of algorithm-based predictive modeling into routine health care introduces a new decision maker into the system that is not accountable to anyone. The increasing power differential between those who are using personal data and the people from whom these data come is an important political problem (see also Stalder 2009). Besides this, there are a number of regulatory and ethical questions to be answered. For example, if people are excluded from a particular health care intervention on the basis of an algorithmic decision that the treating clinicians do not understand, do they need to be informed of this (Amarasingham et al. 2014)? And should complex algorithmic recommendations that cannot be understood by the people involved in health care decision making ever justify somebody's exclusion from an intervention? I suggest that we answer this latter question negatively. Predictive analytics drawing upon a broad set of data and information in such a way that the individual steps of decision making are not open to scrutiny should only be used to stratify patients into groups to optimize their treatment. They should not be used to exclude patients from services.

And if modes of predictive analytics are intransparent, even their use to stratify patents for different treatment paths is not without problems. Consider, for example, a hospital that has offered fourteen-day follow-up appointments to every patient discharged. Imagine that this hospital plans to use predictive analytics to identify high-risk patients to be seen much earlier than the two-week mark, while low-risk patients need not be seen at all (Bates et al. 2014: 1125). How can we be sure that these high-risk patients are not treated differently in other respects too? High-risk patients are often high-cost patients as well. Can such risk-related classifications be kept confidential so such patients avoid facing discrimination in other respects? And should there be an obligation on the side of institutions to inform patients of their risk score, so that they can take precautions or take steps to correct false information? The U.S. Centers for Medicare and Medicaid Services (CMS), for example, already use a probabilistic risk-scoring system that, although it is not used to make treatment decisions, could have negative consequences for people even if they are innocent: The CMS Fraud Prevention System monitors 4.5 million Medicare claims every day. If a fraud is suspected, providers are supplied with a "risk score" for the patient suspected of fraud so that they can monitor her claims more closely (Brennan et al. 2014). The "suspect" is typically not aware of it.

While predictive analytics in the health care domain have so far focused on electronic health records or payment data kept within the health care domain, some authors suggest that other types of information such as online shopping, Internet use, and other personal information should be analyzed to inform health care as well (Weber, Mandl, and Kohane 2014; see also Massachusetts General Hospital 2016). This means that asymmetries in information and accountability will increase further. Citizens are increasingly held accountable for things they have done, or that they have not done but should have, to prepare for the future. Predictive analytics pose additional challenges for our daily conduct: For example, a study found that there is a correlation between buying sports goods online and the "overuse" of emergency rooms (Dixon and Gellman 2014). If you are a person who buys sports goods online and you know that this puts you at a higher risk to be profiled as a costly patient, should you, as a responsible partner or parent, stop doing this in order to improve your and your family's health credit score? Although you may be accountable for whatever decision you make, privately owned companies in particular are not accountable for the types of information they use to make probabilistic assessments of your future that could have tangible effects on you.

## The Accountability Vacuum

We do not have good solutions to date to counterbalance this accountability vacuum. Frank Pasquale makes an important start by suggesting stricter regulation of scoring systems used by digital companies and those that rate or score citizens. He also argues that stronger measures to prevent the monopolization of online services should be undertaken, and that the fines for companies who lie to their customers, or who process or disclose false information about individuals, should be much harsher than they currently are (Pasquale 2015).

The requirement that every data processing entity should sign up to a harm-mitigation fund would be another important measure to help limit or remediate the negative effects of power asymmetries (see chapter 6). Funders or database owners would pay into such a fund that would be governed by an independent body. People who were harmed by data use within the remit of a database could turn to the harm-mitigation fund, even if they had no legal case because they cannot prove any wrongdoing (Prainsack and Buyx 2017).

The accountability vacuum of predictive analytics exists not only in the relationship between citizens and corporations but also at the level of decision making in health care. As noted, if decision aids for patients or clinicians are underpinned by predictive analytics, these tools become de facto decision makers without being accountable to anybody. This can be the case because device manufacturers refuse to share the algorithms used, or because the assumptions and algorithms that are designed into a clinical tool are not understood by anybody and thus not open to scrutiny (similar to the trading software that contributed to the economic crisis in 2008; see also Tutt 2016). Predictive models built into decision-support systems thus give greater power to commercial providers who make it practically impossible for users to "open up" and tinker with their model. To mitigate this problem, Glenn Cohen and colleagues (2014: 1139) recommend the inclusion of patients and other stakeholders from the earliest phases of development of predictive analytics methods. In the words of the authors: "Physicians and other clinical decision makers cannot evaluate a 'black-box model' that simply provides instructions for its implementation and use. Instead, they need to know how a model is making its decisions" (G. Cohen et al. 2014: 1142). They argue that the development of predictive analytics models should always be transparent, and no exemptions from this should be made on grounds of business interests to keep algorithms proprietary (G. Cohen et al. 2014: 1140).

While the inclusion of patients and other stakeholders in the development of predictive analytics methods and protocols would be a welcome step, it is not a satisfactory solution for the problem that these methods pose, especially not where machine-learning methods are used. When the software learns how to make decisions on the basis of previous patterns or evaluations, the lack of transparency and accountability can be particularly pronounced if the method by which the machine learns is black-boxed.[9] This is a pressing issue not only because of the dangers that this poses to patients, but also because it could become a problem for health care professionals: if doctors, for example, deviate from the suggestions made by the predictive analytics, they may be personally liable.[10] They would also be putting themselves at risk by tinkering with predictive analytics models underpinning software or other tools by commercial providers; in the past, U.S. case law has used such interferences with computer decision software "as a reason to shield the software vendor from liability" (G. Cohen et al. 2014: 1144).

## Conclusion

The vision of personalized medicine understood as data-rich, high-tech medicine in which algorithms increasingly replace human experience, intuition, and human contact (see also Greenhalgh et al. 2014), is concerning. An example is the promotion of technology-mediated personalization as the main way to reduce costs and make medicine more effective (e.g. Meskó 2014; Topol 2012). Such visions are, however, not the only way to understand and enact personalization. Working toward a personalized medicine that makes medicine more meaningful and useful to patients requires us to do two things. First, we need to think about ways to use technologies and data-rich approaches to foreground "subjective" needs and values of patients, as well as collective responsibility. Second, we need to find ways to give information that is meaningful to patients a more important role in medical decision making, even if the value of this information is not commensurable with the metrics of clinical utility and clinical outcomes. Including social biomarkers in the body of evidence that we use for medical decision making would be a step in the right direction. This would require institutions and processes that acknowledge and accommodate the importance of human relations within and outside of medical institutions. The potential societal and economic benefits of a vision of personalized medicine that foregrounds human contact and durable social relations, instead of merely outsourcing medical consultations to smartphones, have not yet been explored sufficiently. "Patient work" in such a system would be embedded in strong relationships with people and institutions who know and see patients with their needs and preferences, rather than reducing them to digital doppelgangers.

In addition to the foregrounding of social relations, we should also ensure that the realization of personalized medicine is embedded in a system of universal and affordable health care that excludes as few people as possible (see also Prainsack and Buyx 2017). Giving solidaristic practices and arrangements a more important role would also help ensure that participatory medicine does not become a synonym for a type of medicine that devolves all decision making—and thus responsibility—to individual patients (Prainsack 2014b). For Don Berwick, a famous physician and proponent of patient-centered medicine, giving the personal meaning that interventions and situations have for individual patients a more prominent place in health care is one of the key missions of "truly" patient-centered medicine. At the same time, Berwick warns of a situation where decision-making responsibilities are devolved to patients in such a way that medical professionals merely implement what patients have decided. Berwick suggests that we need to create "flexible systems that can adapt, on the spot, to the needs and circumstances of individual patients" (Berwick 2009: 563). This clearly precludes any tools and instruments that would divert the attention of medical professionals or patients away from meaningful human interaction. And it rules out any decision aids that cannot be overruled by humans. Patient-centered and family-centered care, Berwick argues, should count "as a dimension of quality in its own right, and not just through its effect on health status and outcomes, technically defined" (Berwick 2009: 563; see also Elwyn et al. 2013). The best way of giving personal meaning a more prominent place in medicine is to support shared decision making where data and algorithms are seen to support, rather than dominate, decision making. Patients and those who patients would like to include in this process should have the opportunity to bring in aspects and information that are meaningful to them. To reach this goal, we need to appropriate the concept of personalized medicine for the interests and needs of patients, regardless of their class, gender, or ethnicity. In the next and final chapter of this book I will discuss what understandings of participation and empowerment will help us in this quest.

# 8

## Conclusion

*Patient Work in the Context of Personalization*

Medicine was personal long before personalized medicine became popular as a concept. Health professionals have long taken into consideration individual characteristics of their patients when diagnosing, treating, and caring for them. The work done by patients who cared for themselves and for each other also made health care "personal." Given this long history of medicine being personalized, it is surprising that this notion has gained so much traction at the beginning of the new millennium.

I have argued in this book that one of the developments that brought about the renewed interest in personalization has been a shift in our understanding of what counts as evidence in the context of medicine. Medical practice informed by digital, quantified, and computable information about individual patients is now seen as more precise and effective than previous practice based on unstructured data, narratives, and embodied experience. Now that we have a much better understanding of individual differences and can measure these differences in objective ways, proponents of contemporary personalized medicine argue, it is time to say farewell to the "hit and miss" medicine of the past. Some also advocate a shift from reactive and symptomatic medicine toward continuous and presymptomatic medicine underpinned by monitoring patients as comprehensively and continuously as possible (Agus 2016; Ausiello 2013; Topol 2015). Just like the physical spaces that we navigate with the help of Google Maps and other geolocation apps, personal health is to be rendered suitable for navigation; based on what has happened in a person's past, personal health maps are predicted to offer interpretations ("diagnoses") of the present and make probabilistic predictions about the future. Personal health maps are designed to "know" things before we do: Avoid this route as there will be a traffic jam. See your doctor as a heart attack is on its way (see, for example, Hein 2015).

What is implicit in such visions is that some data are seen as more useful than others, and some are not seen as relevant evidence at all. Visions of personalized and precision medicine are based upon a tacit hierarchy of utility, with digital and computable data on top, and unstructured, narrative, and qualitative evidence at the bottom. This hierarchy was not created by public deliberation, and not even by discussions among professional experts; instead it is a hierarchy that was brought about with the technological tools and practices that we, as a society, have decided to invest and trust in, and that corporations see as profitable. This strategy is not committed to finding out what exactly a patient wants and needs, and what is meaningful to her. Instead, it seeks to collect and utilize large amounts of data that are necessary to create and test workable algorithms for medical decision making in the first place. These algorithms are then used to "personalize" the health care of individual patients.

This notion of personalization stands in clear tension with an approach that focuses on the lived experiences and the personal needs and preferences of patients. As I have argued throughout this book, letting this former understanding of personalization dominate our policies and practices would have tangible effects and costs for patients. Such a personalization of medicine and health care requires more and wider types of contributions from patients while their influence in what information about them is used and to whose benefit is decreasing. Whereas scholarship in the social studies of medicine has helped make "patient work" more visible (Strauss et al. 1982; 1997; Kickbusch 1989), the types of work that contemporary articulations of personalized medicine expect from people have remained largely unquestioned. Such "patient work 2.0" often takes place in people's homes and in other places outside the clinic. It requires that people interact with organizations and institutions whose commercial and political stakes and interests are often difficult to fathom. It also creates new patterns of exclusion. People who cannot, or will not, make use of digital tools to collect, view, and share data and information about themselves literally become "missing bodies" (Casper and Moore 2009). For one, they are structurally disadvantaged within health care systems that are increasingly set up for online-people—for example, by requiring that people check symptoms or arrange appointments or consultations online.

Offline-people are also missing from the data we use to make decisions about population and individual health. The private personal genome testing company 23andMe, for example, which I discussed in several contexts throughout this book, now holds one of the largest DNA databases in the world. It attracts public funding and partnerships. But it represents a very specific sub-set of the world's population: The majority among the company's user base are wealthy and educated Caucasians (Aicardi et al. 2016). Similar biases exist in other resources for disease genomics research (Popejoy and Fullerton 2016).

I have also argued that patient and public participation in medicine today take place in a situation of profound power asymmetries between corporate actors who "see" and know a lot about citizens who in turn see and know relatively little about the former (see also Stalder 2009). As a result, the traditional goalposts of participation in clinical medicine, as they are found in methodologies for public and patient involvement (PPI), for example,[1] are of only limited use for a critical assessment of participatory practices in medicine.

## A Fresh Look at Empowerment

How, then, are we to make sense of participatory medicine in the era of personalization? Let us return to the notion of empowerment. In chapter 4 I discussed different dimensions of power and the distinction between "hard" and "soft" power. Hard power refers to situations of conflict with power being exercised openly and visibly, whereas soft power refers to the less visible and more subtle forms of influencing people and agendas. I argued that technological practices at the heart of personalized medicine shift power between different actors and bring new ones to the scene. Being cognizant of the different forms of power helps us to avoid an unduly simplistic analysis of personalized medicine as either empowering patients or not. And it sensitizes us to the cultural and other structural characteristics that influence the meaning and effects of participation and empowerment. In North America and increasingly in other parts of the world too, empowerment is closely associated with the notion of individual autonomy and choice. Individual autonomy is seen as strongest where people are able to choose freely among a wide variety of options. This close discursive link between empowerment and individual autonomy and choice is also the reason that those who refuse to see patients first and foremost as autonomous consumers are considered empowerment "skeptics" (see, for example, Berwick 2009). But what these critics are skeptical of is not empowerment as such. Instead they challenge an idea of empowerment that treats patients as independent decision makers who will choose what serves them best if supported by accurate and comprehensive information. Many so-called empowerment skeptics are, in substance, critical of treating people as bounded, atomistic, and self-interested entities. Often they are also skeptical of the idea that health care should be commodified and commercialized.

Given the wide use of empowerment-rhetoric in current health care policy and practice, it is particularly important to take a closer look at what values and goals underlie specific calls or instances of empowerment. The Italian philosopher Luca Chiapperino takes an important step in this direction by distinguishing claims to patient empowerment according to the different intentions and values underpinning them:

> What needs to be clarified is whether [a concrete instance or ideal of] empowering citizens has an *intrinsic value* (e.g. it is the right thing to do for reasons of democracy, freedom and justice), an *instrumental value* (e.g. allows policy choices to be coproduced with publics in ways that authentically embody diverse health outcomes, values and meanings), or is animated just by *economic motivations* (e.g. it fosters social responsibilities for the management and improvement of health with consequent reduction of national health costs). (Chiapperino 2014: 12, emphasis added; see also Chiapperino and Tengland 2016)

Looking at the social and political assumptions and goals of those who call for empowerment directs our gaze toward the social, political, and economic stakes in concrete calls for, and instances of, empowerment. Moreover, by distinguishing between the political and social goals and assumptions of a speaker or discourse we also make visible the different roots of the current empowerment rhetoric in the health domain (see also Del Savio, Buyx, and Prainsack 2017).

As noted, one important root of empowerment lies in the value of individual autonomy and choice (see also Latimer 2007). Empowerment that serves the goal of increasing individual autonomy and choice follows what I call the *individualistic* model. A second tradition of understanding empowerment judges empowerment projects in terms of their expected *instrumental,* often economic value. Empowerment has instrumental value when it is thought to generate better outcomes and solutions, or when it legitimizes specific processes, decisions, or institutions. And it can have economic value when it moves expensive or otherwise onerous tasks from the collective level to individuals (see also Thorpe 2010). This is the case when onerous or expensive tasks that were typically carried out in the clinic are shifted to the homes and within the personal responsibility of patients, or when volunteers are being enrolled in data collection projects in the name of advancing science.

A third root of empowerment lies in ideals of democratization, often understood as "injecting politics" into processes and organizations. We inject politics when we widen the space for deliberation and increase the range of possibilities for formulating, framing, and solving a problem. In the medical domain, an example of empowerment with such deliberative value would be to increase the space within which patients can make decisions that are meaningful to them, irrespective of whether or not they correspond with clinical or economic rationalities. Another example would be patient advocacy for funds being shifted to areas of research that are different from what other professional experts had envisaged. Here, the value of empowerment lies primarily in the process of deliberation and inclusiveness, not in a particular outcome. For this reason, I call it the *democratic* model of empowerment. Here, enhancing the agency of patients does have intrinsic value.

A fourth and final understanding of empowerment is the *emancipatory* model of empowerment. In this understanding, empowerment is seen as pushing back or resisting the power that others have over a person or group of people. This notion of empowerment, which is strongly anchored in feminist, civil rights, and LGBTQ movements, fosters the goals of emancipation and liberation from political, economic and cultural hegemonies (see, for example, Bell 2009; Klawiter 2008; see also Chiapperino 2014: 73). The emancipatory model of empowerment is politically the most "radical" notion of empowerment. It has the biggest potential to bring about innovation that improves the lives of people who are excluded or marginalized. It is also most likely to restore health care as an institution and a practice that primarily serves the well-being of patients and not corporations. In sum, in order to assess claims of empowerment in the context of personalized medicine, we need to look at the values that a specific practice or ideal of empowerment embodies. In the context of personalized medicine it is important that we promote an understanding of empowerment that goes beyond individualistic or individual-centered practice. If we accept that human beings are relational, then empowerment is regularly a collective endeavor and always relevant to more than one person. This does not mean that empowerment is a zero sum game where doctors lose power to the same extent that their patients gain it, or where the disempowerment of clinical research institutions is proportional to the empowerment of patients who organize their own medical studies (see also Laverack 2009). Instead, empowerment is a collective, cooperative practice. Patient empowerment that is in line with genuinely emancipatory participation will increase the range of meaningful practices that patients can engage in. Such genuinely emancipatory empowerment can challenge the rationales embedded in our political and health systems. It can change the focus of ethical and regulatory debates, such as by broadening discussions about data protection from individual privacy to collective stakes in the good use and protection of patient data. And it could lead to integrating social biomarkers into processes of medical decision making for individual patients.

| TABLE 8.1. Four models of empowerment | |
|---|---|
| Model | Example |
| Individualistic empowerment | Calls for greater patient choice |
| Instrumental empowerment | Suggestions that health care systems need to listen to patients to increase the (cost-) effectiveness of service provision |
| Democratic empowerment | Patient and consumer rights movements in the 1960s and 1970s, when discourse focused on collective action and not individual choice |
| Emancipatory empowerment | Women's health movements |

## Participation

In contrast to the notion of empowerment, which is strongly anchored in a discourse of individual choice, the concept of participation has a different and more explicitly political history. Sherry Arnstein, in a much-cited article published in 1969, argued "that participation without redistribution of power is an empty and frustrating process for the powerless" (Arnstein 1969: 2016). The lowest rung of Arnstein's "ladder of participation" refers to instances where people are acted upon while the highest rung has citizens in control of processes and agendas. Arnstein's work has been highly influential in diverse fields such as planning, technology development, and medicine.

Within the current discourse on participatory practices in science and medicine, including the enthusiasm around "citizen science," the political connotations of the concept of participation seem to have largely disappeared. Instead, participation is seen as a tool to make medicine and science faster, cheaper, or otherwise more effective (Prainsack and Riesch 2016). A notable exception is the work of Chris Kelty and colleagues, who proposed seven criteria according to which participatory projects can be assessed (Kelty et al. 2015). These seven dimensions, developed by analyzing more than one hundred case studies and a wide range of literature on participatory projects, include characteristics such as the educational benefit for participants or how easy it is to opt out (see box 8.1; see also box 2.1 in chapter 2). Kelty and colleagues' approach includes criteria that go beyond the merely instrumental. But their approach does not go quite far enough. Because these authors refrain from engaging with the explicitly political arguments in the literature on democratic participation, their criteria do not allow us to distinguish between participatory projects that primarily aim at commercial gains and those whose main goal is to create wider social and societal benefits.

---

**BOX 8.1. "Seven dimensions of contemporary participation" by Kelty et al. (2015: 475)**

1. The educative dividend of participation
2. Access to decision-making and goal setting in addition to task-completion
3. The control of ownership of resources produced by participation
4. Its voluntary character and the capacity for exit
5. The effectiveness of voice
6. The use of metrics for understanding or evaluating participation
7. The collective, affective experience of participation

## Is There a Participation Paradox?

How can we obtain a richer, more political understanding of participation in medicine, one that will help us to redefine personalization? Similar to what I argued in connection with the notion of empowerment, one strategy is to look at the goals that specific calls for and practices of participation serve, and what political, social, and economic circumstances they are embedded in. Participation is not always synonymous with increasing deliberation, diversity, and democracy. Most participatory practices have both disruptive and conservative effects. They challenge some established narratives, practices, and institutions and reinforce others. They empower and disempower different groups of people in specific situations or contexts. The field of biohacking is a good illustration of this: Many biohackers see themselves as striving for an alternative to institutionalized science, which they see as compromised by commercial and corporate interests (see also Tocchetti 2014; 2015). Many biohackers employ their knowledge, their tools, and their experience outside the confines of established[2] research institutions and thus "disrupt" the quasi-monopoly of institutionalized science. They also unsettle established modes of academic credit and quality control. At the same time, the biohacking movement has been criticized as being pro-market and conserving existing hegemonies and hierarchies. For the American historian of economics Philip Mirowski, the open source movement symbolizes the kind of false consciousness that is typical for the neoliberal era:

> One of the most fascinating technologies of faux rebellion [ . . . ] is the construction of situations in which [a person] is led to believe she has opted out of the market system altogether. There is no better simulation of contumacy [*refusal to obey authority*] than the belief that you have removed yourself from the sphere of the market, itself then subordinated to the process of market engagement. (Mirowski 2014: 141)

For Mirowski, the way that open-source movements, for example, engage people bears striking similarity to neoliberal marketing technologies. In open-source initiatives, he argues, people are lured into providing free labor "in the guise of a rebellion against the market system" when what they do is in fact contribute to an exploitive system. Instead of liberating themselves and others from oppressive power structures, participants thus help to create new ones, with the only difference being that different corporations profit from their labor. Mirowski considers such a "hybrid of voluntary unpaid labor and hierarchical control and capitalist appropriation" so commonplace that it amounts to a new form of economic organization (Mirowski 2014: 142–143). Following this rationale, the open-source and biohacking movements could be seen to illustrate the paradoxical situation of our contemporary political economy: We are without a feasible alternative. Even those of us who try to create a way out find ourselves in the same trap that we sought to escape from. A solution outside the current market hegemony is not conceivable.

Even if we do not, as Mirowski does, ascribe some kind of false consciousness to those engaging with participatory practices in science and medicine, we would still have to ask the question: Are patient empowerment and participation in medicine trapped in this very dilemma? Can we avoid that participation always also means reinforcing the values and structures of the institutional setting within which participation takes place?

"Emancipatory" empowerment—the last of the four kinds of empowerment discussed earlier—aspires to avoid that situation by freeing people from oppressive structures. When biohackers, for example, move labs out of established institutions that they see as dominated by corporate interests, or when women's health activists push back against the medicalization of their bodies and lives, these seem clear instances of emancipatory empowerment. But can "participation" do the same? Can greater patient participation in medical decision making, or in deciding what data and information will be held about them in their electronic health records, liberate patients from oppressive structures?

## The Political and Economic Context of Participation

In order to answer this question, let us take a look at the importance of the social, economic, and political context that concrete instances of participation are embedded in. This helps us to understand how nationally or regionally dominant beliefs about how collective decisions should be made, or what tasks individuals or families should be responsible for, influence formats of participation. Late in the first decade of the 2000s, political theorists John Dryzek and Aviezer Tucker compared consensus conferences on genetically modified food in Denmark, France, and the United States (Dryzek and Tucker 2008). They found that the ways in which public participation was organized in these three countries corresponded with dominant governance models in each country. Following earlier work by Dryzek (1996; Dryzek et al. 2003), the authors distinguished between three main types of deliberative systems. The first are *passively inclusive* nations, such as the United States, that allow a wide range of interests to enter into policy-making processes if they are strong enough to make themselves heard. Within this model, participation often takes the form of advocacy and lobbying (Dryzek and Tucker 2008). The second type comprises *actively inclusive* states—such as Denmark—that *proactively* identify and invite social movements and interests into policy-making processes. Here, the idea is often that widening the range of people who participate in decision making is valuable as such. The third type, exemplified by France, are *exclusive states* that "offer few points of access to interests and movements beyond a privileged few" (Dryzek and Tucker 2008: 866). Societies of the third type are often ruled by elites who try to nip any articulation of disruptive interests, such as those of labor unions, in the bud. Public participation in such "exclusive" states, according to Dryzek and Tucker, is typically organized in a managerial fashion, where the limits of the influence of the participating stakeholders are carefully drawn before participation starts. Strongly resonating with the model of "instrumental empowerment" discussed earlier, in exclusive states participation is often seen as a necessary evil in order to know what "the public" wants (Dryzek and Tucker 2008: 869; see also Laurent 2000: 132–133). In sum, societal and political values shape where the participation of new actors is seen as fruitful, and for what purposes.

This example only covers participation that was invited by public bodies. What about uninvited participation? What about people joining forces to tackle a problem without having been "invited" to do so by corporate actors? Also here, the macro-level of societal institutions, values, and traditions is an important aspect to consider. It helps us to understand why such uninvited, "emancipatory" participation faces a lot of resistance in some places and less in others. Jay Katz, in his classic book on the doctor-patient relationship, showed that the idea of patient participation in medical decision making has long been considered alien to the ethos of physicians. Patient participation has encountered a lot of resistance throughout the history of professional and institutionalized medicine everywhere in the world (Katz 2002). It is not a coincidence that the main impetus for change eventually came from the United States, where the historically strong emphasis on individual autonomy provided a strong counternarrative to the benign paternalism that had dominated the professional ethos of doctors until then. Today, the idea that patients should be given an important role in decision making about their own health care is almost universally accepted.

Does this mean that participation, both invited by established institutions and emerging spontaneously and "bottom-up," can avoid the trap of reinforcing the values of the institutions that it is embedded in? Can participation be "emancipatory" for patients and their families? Can it enhance their agency to change the goalposts and terms of an interaction?

I argue that it can, but not every instance of participation that takes us closer to a desirable goal is emancipatory. What do I mean by this? Let me give an example. In the United States, about 80 percent of long-term care is provided by family members. This places great burdens on carers, many of whom are women (see also Blum 2015; Hill 2003; J. Wolf 2010; see also C. Stacey 2011 for a discussion of the burdens on paid caregivers). And although these strains are becoming more severe and affect ever wider ranges of people due to the aging of our societies, public responsibility for the provision of long-term care in particular is not on the political agenda. Sociologist Sandra Levitsky sees one of the causes for this in the societal belief that caregiving is a family responsibility. This, in turn, means that it typically rests upon the shoulders of women. This conviction is so strong that even many carers do not consider themselves as fulfilling an important societal role; they see themselves as doing merely what they ought to do as spouses, daughters, or parents (Levitsky 2014). Calling the unpaid work of these women and men "participation" in health and social care would be ironic. It is labor that remains unpaid because society does not assume collective responsibility for it. This is what I mean when I say that not each instance of participation that brings us closer to a desirable goal is emancipatory. The "participation" of women and men in providing care for their family members ensures that such care is provided—which is a desirable goal.

But such "participation" is not emancipatory, because it reduces pressure to find alternative solutions that may be even more desirable.

In short, a step on the path to repoliticize the notion of participation is to stop using this term for instances where people do what public or other collective actors should be doing. This also helps avoid the possibility that politically conservative rhetoric can present the unwillingness or inability of public actors to provide education, health care, or social services as an opportunity for citizen or patient "empowerment." In the era of digital health, the dumping of expensive and onerous tasks on the shoulders of patients and their families under the guise of participation and empowerment is a common cost-saving strategy: We are told that by wearing monitoring devices—which we have to, because our doctor has no time to call to see how we are doing—we are empowered to be more proactive and informed patients. Moreover, if more patients are engaging in self-monitoring, doctors will be asked to do many more other things to fill the time that was supposedly "freed up" by not having to talk to their patients. Here, resisting not only the empowerment rhetoric but also the temptation to refer to such instances of patient work as "participation" can help to expose, and in turn address, systemic issues and challenges. Instead, the words that we use to describe such practices should be sensitive to the power structures that they are embedded in. We should speak of responsibilities devolved to patients, invited participation, and, again, of "patient work."

*Ways to More Meaningful Participation: What Do "Good" Participatory Initiatives Have in Common?*

The quest to redefine personalization requires a repoliticized understanding of patient participation. What do such "politicized" participatory initiatives have in common? What do participatory practices look like that enhance the agency of patients and other people in meaningful ways, without losing sight of the needs of all people in our societies?

I argue that there are three things that unite practices and initiatives (see box 8.2): First, even if they focus on addressing a specific practical issue, they invite reflection on the political and cultural meaning of the participatory practices that they include or promote. They are conscious of the larger societal consequences these practices are likely to have. Such initiatives do not end, for example, with getting more people to sign advance directives, or using crowd-sourcing to solve a scientific question; they also consider the systemic effects of the practice, and the values that underpin it. Do we want people to sign advance directives only to save the cost of unwanted treatments, or also to prevent suffering? How can we support people in making these decisions, and ensuring that they get all the care they need? Similarly, if we use the unpaid labor of volunteers to collect data for medical research, does this push out other forms of (paid or unpaid) expertise? Questions like these are important concerns.

Second, participatory practices and initiatives that are capable of re-defining personalization emphasize meaning and interaction, not individual choice. If, as I argued in chapter 6, we understand humans to be first and foremost relational beings, we need to conceive people's agency as shaped by social relations too. In this spirit, a person's accessing her electronic health records is not a choice made by an atomistic individual but an act also shaped by the person's family ties and social relations, and her connection to others. For example, the person may want to share and discuss this health information with her spouse, friend, or children. The same applies to participation in medical decision making. As Jay Katz famously argued, we need to focus more on what goes on between doctors and patients, and not assume that they are each independent decision makers:

> Greater patient participation in the disclosure and consent process requires an exploration of the complex caretaking and being-taken-care-of interactions that develop between physicians and their patients. Appeals to "patient self-determination" and "physician discretion" [ . . . ] focus too much on what goes on inside the actors' separate minds and not on what should go on between them. (Katz 2002: 84)

If we treat patients as independent decision makers, medical professionals become mere executors of supposedly autonomous decisions of patients (Berwick 2009). This, in turn, would reduce the notion of patient participation to a cover for the lobbying of individual interests.

The third feature that participatory initiatives and practices capable of redefining personalization have in common is that they carefully consider what groups are excluded from participating, and what effects this will have on them. Exclusion could be voluntary: Despite having the possibility to do so, a patient may not want to look at her own health records, choose between different types of surgery, or videoconference with her doctor. Or it could be involuntary, for example, because some people lack the skills or tools necessary for participation. Initiatives, people, and organizations who understand participation as a way for people to make decisions that are meaningful to them will try to reduce instances of involuntary exclusion and ensure that people who are excluded voluntarily do not suffer undue negative consequences. In practice, it will be difficult to distinguish participatory initiatives that consider the larger societal and political consequences of the practices that they promote from those that do not. There are at least two reasons for this. The first reason is that the goals people pursue when engaging in a particular participatory practice are not homogenous. In addition, their understandings of what they are doing by engaging in a particular participatory practice may differ from the understandings of people who invited their participation, and from those of other participants. For example, a person downloading her electronic health records could be doing this for merely instrumental reasons, without any kind of political agenda. She may, for example, want to change her doctor, and not care at all about whether it is important for patients or their caregivers to hold a copy of their health records. Not every instance of participation is aimed at political or emancipatory change, or seeks to make a political point—and it would be patronizing to assume that it has to. But even in cases where it is difficult to assess how reflexive an organization or initiative is about the types of participation that it invites or promotes, such participatory practices could still contribute to a larger change in culture.[3] In other words, even if individual initiatives are not "deeply" participatory in an openly political or emancipatory sense, they can still amount to something that is bigger than the sum of their parts. They can change the dominant discourse. And they can show that there is a way out of the "empowerment trap" that provides us with the choice of either being content with the status quo or contributing to yet another exploitative system.

> **BOX 8.2. Characteristics of participatory practices and initiatives that are capable of redefining personalization**
>
> Participatory practices capable of redefining personalization
>
> — are reflexive of the political and cultural meaning of the practices they promote or facilitate;
> — focus on (personal and collective) meaning, and interaction, not individual choice
> — ensure that people who cannot or will not participate will not suffer serious disadvantages

## Patient Work 2.0 in a Changing Landscape of Data Use

Why does the emancipatory and "democratic" quality of participatory practices matter so much in the context of personalized and precision medicine? I have argued in this book that the notion of difference underpinning more recent understandings of personalized medicine assumes that every person is unique in health and disease. In such visions, attention to differences between people is seen not as a political choice but as a scientific and ethical requirement. Because of how much we know about individual differences, so the argument goes, it would be irresponsible to ignore these. From there it is only a small step to conclude that we have an obligation to actively obtain as much information about individual difference as we can. It has thus become a moral duty—of medical professionals, of patients, and of healthy "patients-in-waiting" (Timmermans and Buchbinder 2010)—to know what is knowable about our own unique admixture.

Such a view has profound implications not only for the realization of personalized medicine but also for how we organize medicine and health care. Attempts are already being made to replace traditional symptom-based disease taxonomies with data-rich characterizations of individuals at various stages of health and disease (National Research Council of the Academies 2011). Experts call for new ways to complement and in some contexts, replace traditional group-based clinical studies. What they demand is not that different groups of people should be represented more accurately in clinical trials but that the idea of putting people together in groups be given up altogether. Instead it is suggested that we improve and expand our methods to study small populations of people who are similar in whatever respect is relevant to a specific question. This includes computer (*in silico*) modeling, or in-depth N=1 studies (Schork 2015). Such in-depth studies of individual patients often combine longitudinal clinical data with lifestyle data and data from genomic analysis; sometimes data from handheld or wearable sensors are included as well. In the words of researchers at the Scripps Research Institute in California, N=1 studies explore patient variability "in an objective way while simultaneously leading to an informed decision about the best way to treat an individual patient using his or her own data" (Lillie et al. 2011: 163–164). The hope is that N=1 studies will help identify interventions that are of low value, or even harmful, at the level of individual patients. And the more N=1 studies have been carried out, the better underlying dynamics will be understood that can also be extrapolated to wider groups.

Patient work will be needed here as well. The need for data and information to personalize health care cannot be satisfied with what is available in the clinical and research domains alone. It will also have to come from people, from their homes, lives, and workplaces. And it will not come only from people who are already patients, but from everybody. Only a few years ago, science writer Carina Dennis called the idea that people make themselves available for detailed in-depth study "the rise of the narciss-ome" (Dennis 2012). Today, such people are no longer seen as self-obsessed nerds. They are considered the spearhead of a paradigm shift from symptomatic, reactive medicine toward continuous and presymptomatic medicine (see, for example, Ausiello 2013; Topol 2015). In the era of patient work 2.0, the governance of data use has become a collective concern.

## Rethinking Data Use

The abolition of the dividing line between medical research and health care is no longer the stuff of a handful of visionary activists, but it is part of the mission of personalized medicine (National Research Council of the Academies 2011; see also Moloney, Tambor, and Tunis 2016; Weber, Mandl, and Kohane 2014). And there is another dividing line that is dwindling: the one between medical research and other types of research. Data produced and collected for the diagnosis and treatment of individual patients is not used only for medical research but also for research outside of the medical domain. As I argued in the course of this book, patients are becoming digital data sources and research contributors by default.

Against this backdrop it is a fallacy to believe that we can assess risks for patients by separating different types of data and information, as we have done for decades: We have separated medical data from non-medical data, personal from nonpersonal information, identified from nonidentified information, and so on. Today it is not data types, but types of data *use*, that are problematic. For this reason, I propose that we should decrease the risk for unauthorized reidentification for all sets of data, and then distinguish between two main types of data use: data use in the public interest and data use that is not in the public interest.[4] Data use is in the public interest when it can be plausibly assumed that it will have clear benefits either for many patients, for society as a whole, or for future generations, and no person or group will experience significant harm. Public interest is particularly pronounced if the benefits are likely to materialize for underprivileged groups.[5] An example for data use in the public interest is the analysis of clinical data sets to see what the patients who recover particularly fast after a specific surgery have in common. An example for data use not in the public interest is the use of medical insurance data for targeted marketing.

Here I should emphasize again that I am talking about data *use* here, not different kinds of data; the question of public interest is not a property of the data themselves, but of the practical use of them. In chapter 3 I made the case that certain types of data collection (namely those where people are not actively involved in the collection) and data handling (namely instances where data can be used for individual-level health-related purposes) are more problematic than others and thus require closer public scrutiny. Here I complement this analysis by arguing that different types of data use should be treated differently. Where data use is in the public interest, we should make it easier to collect, share, and use data. This means that in cases where regulatory frameworks require the consent of the originators of the data, preference should be given to "light touch" consent frameworks such as broad consent, or the consent to be governed (Koenig 2014) combined with trustworthy and independent governance mechanisms. Where data use is not in the public interest, a tax or levy could be introduced to ensure that some of the profits made on the basis of citizens' personal data flow back into the public domain. If we are serious about personal data being the new currency in our societies, we need to start treating them as assets in every respect.

I have suggested two more measures to improve data use in the course of this book; these are applicable independent of whether data is used for public benefit. The first is the introduction of harm-mitigation funds (Prainsack and Buyx 2013; 2017). As outlined in chapter 6, harm-mitigation funds can be established at the level of individual institutions—for example, a biomedical database or a university—or regionally or nationally. They would be supplied by a certain proportion of the institution's funding, or by tax contributions. Harm-mitigation funds would be governed by people who are independent of the institution or corporation using the data, and anybody who considers herself to have been harmed by data use could appeal to the fund. Such funds should exist in parallel to, and not as a replacement for, legal systems of compensation and redress. Their role is not only to mitigate harm with financial means but also to provide feedback on what could be improved in how data are used in the first place.

Second, scholars such as Graeme Laurie, Mark Taylor, and Heather Widdows have argued that personal data are not personal only to one individual (Laurie 2002; M. Taylor 2013; Widdows 2013). Drawing upon their work I have argued in this book that the realization of personalized medicine needs to be accompanied by new regulatory approaches that acknowledge the rights and interests of secondary data subjects. It is very clear that people can be harmed by data use not only if the data come from themselves but also if they come from other people. For example, it could be established on the basis of data set A that people who watch daytime television are statistically more likely to suffer from a chronic disease than people who do not. This probabilistic assumption could then be used to identify my partner, who loves to watch cookery shows when he is off work, as a likely sufferer of chronic diseases, even though thankfully he does not suffer from one at present. Being considered an expensive patient, he could be refused insurance or other purchases. I, as his spouse, could suffer harm on the basis of such practices that clearly do not derive from the use of my own data. Profiling in this manner is not radically new; what is new, however, is the volume and breath of data sets available for such purposes, and the relative ease with which they can be used. Harm-mitigation funds would give me an opportunity to seek redress in such a situation.

Table 8.2 provides a summary of measures that should be undertaken to improve data governance when data use is in the public interest, and when it is not in the public interest, respectively.

| TABLE 8.2. Replacing risk-based data governance with new principles for the governance of data use | | | | |
|---|---|---|---|---|
| | Make it easier to collect, share, repurpose data | Establish harm-mitigation funds | Acknowledge rights and interests of secondary data subjects | Tax corporate data use |
| *Data use in the public interest* | Yes | Yes | Yes | No |
| *Data use not in the public interest* | No | Yes | Yes | Yes |

## Conclusion: Patient Work at the Time of "Radical Difference"

The narrative of personalization—namely that people make, or are expected to make, contributions in terms of data, information, effort, and time for the purpose of personalizing their health care—aligns patient work even more closely with the subject position of a neoliberal entrepreneurial self. Personalized medicine does not only imply the ideal of "radical" individual difference (Prainsack 2015a); it also shifts the focus from presumably stable genetic and genomic information to the inclusion of wider ranges of often malleable data such as information about lifestyle, or on epigenetic markers seen to correspond with behaviors such as smoking or exercise. This widens the space for individual self-optimization (see also Elliott 2004).

Here, the notion of individual risk that personalized medicine relies on so prominently is the fuel that biomedical entrepreneurial selves run on (Mirowski 2014: 92; Petersen and Lupton 1996). Individual risk is the seemingly value-neutral, objective, scientific evidence that tells people where they should focus their self-improvement (read: health promotion and disease prevention) efforts. And the toolbox of personalization makes self-optimization efforts more easily measurable: By changing our diet or exercise levels, for example, our proteome profile may improve or deteriorate—and data visualization technologies can make these changes traceable. By focusing not only on genomic data, which are stable and thus beyond our control, but by including characteristics that vary with behavior, personalized medicine produces visible evidence of successful or failed self-optimization. As I have argued in this book, no aspect of our lives is exempt from being health relevant, at least potentially. The increasing datafication of our lives and bodies means that anything can become health data, and any data can be used for or against us. When experts suggest that hospitals and doctors should use predictive analytics to identify patients who, after a surgical intervention, have a particularly high risk of experiencing complications and offer them extra care, the profiling of this group as high risk will not necessarily remain contained within the clinical sphere. These scores are recorded and thus become readable and usable by other actors, outside the health care field. People with undesirable scores may not be offered certain services, or may be denied certain types of insurance, without even knowing why, and without having any redress (Prainsack 2015b).

There are at least two lessons to draw from this. First, privacy and data protection should no longer be treated merely as rights or needs of individuals. They need to be seen as collective (Casilli 2014) and social concerns as well. They have become collective concerns because health data are personal to a wider range of people than the person they come from, and because they are produced and used in social settings and for collective purposes. And they have become social concerns because they represent a fundamental interest of people in light of the strong power asymmetries that we live in. In societies where more and more public institutions are in the service of business interests, data use is no longer a technology of *govern*mentality but one of *econo*mentality. Because states are too invested in economic interests to curtail the power of large multinational corporations, the solution to the problem of surveillance cannot come from states alone: They will continue to enact data protection legislation, but they are often not willing or able to hit large transnational corporations where it hurts. In chapter 2 I argued that solutions must thus also come from patients and other citizens: from people who demand to know what kind of information is held about them in public and private repositories, from people who refuse to "share" data with corporations that are secretive or deceptive about how they use them, and from people who instead donate their data to "information commons" that use data for public benefit (Evans 2016). Last but not least, we, as citizens, need to resist systems that increase ethnic, racial, and gender discrimination and make the most vulnerable of us even harder to see.

A solidarity-based perspective can help us to reach these goals. An important implication of a solidarity-based perspective is that it tells us to use characteristics that people have in common as a guide for practice and policy wherever meaningfully possible. This means that we should refrain from using individual difference as a justification for exclusion in cases where it unduly harms those who are excluded. This has direct implications for the organization of health care provision. One of the key lessons to draw from the cases and arguments discussed in this book is that publicly funded universal health care, based on various layers of solidaristic insurance and exchange, is the best precondition for personalized medicine to be realized in a socially just and sustainable manner. Such a system will be faced with financial challenges. It will be impossible to pay for everything that would benefit patients, but these questions would at least not be decided by how much individuals can afford. I have discussed a number of initiatives that address the problem of health care overuse and cost constraints by other means. Many of them do so by supporting patients in making decisions about what interventions are useful to them and which ones are not, thus encouraging self-rationing on the basis of personal and social meaning. Some initiatives also enlist health care professionals in this quest—for example, by asking medical specialists what interventions and treatments are of low value, and then trying to stop offering them. What all these initiatives have in common is that they consider the value of an intervention according to a wide range of factors, including personal and "subjective" ones (see also NHS Scotland 2016, Mulley et al. 2017). Evidence shows that asking people what interventions they actually want can be very effective in bringing down health care costs (Hatkoff, Kula, and Levine 2014; Institute of Medicine 2015).

The current mantra is that personalized medicine will be data-driven. But what we need is a personalized medicine that is driven not only by data about people's bodies and behavior but also by information that is subjectively meaningful to patients. This book has discussed a number of ways in which meaning at the personal level can be worked into the types of evidence that we use when making decisions about the treatment of individuals and about the organization of health care. Such a personalized medicine requires a commitment to a different political economy than is dominant today. It departs from a commitment to cost-effectiveness defined according to purely clinical and managerial paradigms. It is committed to technological practice in the service of medicine that sees people as relational beings, and not self-interested decision makers. And it is a collective endeavor in the interest of those who cannot, or will not, participate in the personalization of their health care.

# NOTES

## CHAPTER 1. SETTING THE STAGE FOR PERSONALIZED MEDICINE

1 The term "stratified medicine" is also often used to refer to existing practices of assigning patients to different diagnostic or treatment groups (on the basis of their gender, age, the particularity of their symptoms within a disease group, or on the basis of their genetic or other molecular characteristics). The term "stratified biomedicalization," introduced by Adele Clarke and colleagues, refers to something more specific: Rather than signifying the idea of personalizing medicine in general, it foregrounds the "cooptative and exclusionary tendencies" of medicalization, and the fact that these mechanisms of coopting and excluding are becoming more complex (see Clarke et al. 2003: 170–171; Clarke et al. 2010c).

2 By "the Internet" I mean the assemblage of materials, technologies, and practices that create and enact electronic networks of communication. I do not mean to imply that "the Internet" is a homogenous entity that has intrinsic agency.

3 To use the appearance of the term in journal articles as an (of course imperfect) indicator, the term "participatory medicine" appeared only once in the title, abstract, or key words of published papers in all disciplines between 2000 and 2005, but it appeared fifteen times between 2006 and 2010, and sixty-four times between 2011 and 2016 (source: scopus.com; analysis by the author). Moreover, since 2010, a number of organizations such as the U.S.-based Society for Participatory Medicine (participatorymedicine.org) were set up, and journals have started series on participatory medicine (such as *Genome Medicine:* https://www.biomedcentral.com/collections/participatory).

## CHAPTER 2. THE PATIENT RESEARCHER

1 Some authors attribute the distinction between "lean back" and "lean forward" technologies to Jakob Nielsen, the Danish-born founder of a movement advocating inexpensive ways to improve user interfaces for web-based tools. Note that the "lean forward" argument disregards the early days of the Internet when users and producers of content and infrastructure overlapped greatly, due to the limited and esoteric nature of the net (Thomas and Wyatt 2000). As the early days of the Internet did not include health-related applications in a prominent manner, however, in the specific context of health-related use of the Internet an overall trend from lean back to lean forward forms of online engagement seems accurate. Lean-forward technologies are closely associated with the social media revolution

of the late 2000s and early 2010s. The focus of most recent technological development, such as remote sensing and monitoring, caters to passive use again.

2 For a discussion of the difficulty of defining "content" see Brake (2014).

3 Self-tracking refers to various practices of recording, and sometimes also analyzing, data that people collect about themselves. Data can be recorded manually (by measuring blood pressure and entering it in an Excel file), or automatically with the help of smartphones, pedometers, or other devices.

4 Parts of this subsection draw upon Prainsack (2014a), where I first developed the classification of different types of participation. In fact, the static way in which participatory projects are treated in the literature on citizen science represents a shortcoming of otherwise very useful typologies of citizen science projects according to the degree of participation. Shirk and colleagues (2012), for example, distinguish between contractual, contributory, collaborative, cocreated, and collegial projects (see also Ely 2008).

5 Research studies indicate a negative correlation between financial incentives and drop-out rates in web-based studies. Other factors that were found to correlate with lower attrition rates are user-friendly web-page design, faster loading time, high reputation of the institution or organization carrying out the study, the perception of "true" voluntariness, high medical or social utility of participation, shorter questionnaire length, and higher levels of education and socioeconomic status on the side of the participants (Christensen, Griffiths, and Jorm 2004; Eysenbach 2005; Frick, Bächtiger, and Reips 2001; Reips 2002; Wu et al. 2005). Eysenbach (2005) also found that early adopters were less likely to drop out than later adopters. See also Christensen and Mackinnon (2006).

6 The inclusion and exclusion criteria for this study are listed here: www.nature.com/nbt/journal/v29/n5/full/nbt.1837.html#methods (accessed November 7, 2016).

7 It should be kept in mind, however, that data collection and data analysis also varies significantly between different "participatory" initiatives. In the case of PatientsLikeMe, for example, both the collection and analysis of data are very complex and require considerable amounts of time and effort from the side of the platform (Kallinikos and Tempini 2014; Tempini 2015).

8 For Europe, see, for example, the French carenity.com, or the Spanish saluspot.com, medtep.com—which operates in English, Spanish, and German. Diagnosia.com operates in fourteen languages but does not include discussion forums.

## CHAPTER 3. ALWAYS ON

1 *Gattaca* is the title of a 1997 movie by Andrew Niccol that portrays a dystopic future of genetic determinism. It has since become shorthand for societal visions of genetic essentialism and genetic determinism.

2 The hybridity between human and nonhuman materials is reminiscent of Donna Haraway's *Cyborg Manifesto* (1991), in which she famously challenged the distinction between natural and artificial life (and much more) with the notion of the

"cyborg." Haraway's cyborg is "a hybrid of machine and organism, a creature of social reality as well as a creature of fiction" (2013 [1991]: 274). In addition, the fluid boundaries of humanness have become particularly topical again in recent years due to the surge of attention to the role of microorganisms for our health, which has heightened the sense of hybridity of human bodies and lives. Not only have "artificial" organs and parts, such as prostheses, tooth fillings, and implanted defibrillators, become parts of our bodies, but other nonhuman entities, such as microbes, that are necessary for our survival, have also received increasing attention. The question of what it means to be human remains high on the agenda in scholarship in the humanities and social sciences in particular. Haraway did this in a quest to move feminist debate beyond traditional categories such as gender, nature, and identity, and beyond traditional boundaries such as natural and artificial, human and animal, physical and nonphysical. Drawing attention to the material hybridity of humans, however, is not the point I wish to make here; instead, I want to highlight the extent to which artifacts and machines have become a template for human practices.

3 Vitores (2002: 4) refers to the process of shifting more tasks from the clinic into people's homes as the "extitutionalization" of medicine. It is " a kind of virtualization [ . . . ] used to account for the resultant of reversing the centripetal strengths that characterize institutions, that is, to describe the way this strengths become centrifuge: from in to ex." Vitores attributes the notion of extitutionalization to Michel Serres (1994).

4 Data from other countries are scarce. For England, Clark and Goodwin (2010: 4) state that "it is estimated that between 1.6 million and 1.7 million people [. . . of a population of 53 million, BP] have some form of remote monitoring support, primarily in the form of telecare," and "more than 5,000 people in England are benefiting from home-based vital signs monitoring." No current data from the United States are available (but see Kinsella 1998; Whitten and Buis 2007).

5 I did not conduct interviews as part of a systematic study on this topic; instead, I talked to the first people I encountered who I saw using FuelBand and who were willing to talk to me about it. Thus, the group of people I talked to cannot be taken as representing the users of FuelBand in any particular area or age group. Jesper (not his real name) has given his explicit consent for these quotes to be used in this chapter, and he has read and commented on drafts. I changed certain details (such as dates or places) to reduce the risk of reidentification.

6 That we do not understand exactly how they work is not unique to activity trackers, of course. It also applies to other tools, electronic or not. The difference is that with my car or my television, I could find out how exactly it worked if I put my mind to it. But I cannot find out how FuelBand works because Nike treats the algorithms as proprietary information.

7 I am grateful to Hendrik Wagenaar for very helpful discussions on this point.

8 For more information see www.semanticweb.org/wiki/Main_Page (accessed November 8, 2016).

9  See also Evgeny Morozov's (2013) discussion of the "ryanairation of privacy"—a notion that he borrows from Glen Newey to refer to the breaking down of cash-free practices into "severally billable units of account." Ryanair is an Irish airline (in)famous for offering "cheap" airfares and then adding a wide range of additional charges. See also Sandel (2012).

10  The e-mail sent to the company via its customer services' website read as follows: "I am thinking of buying a FuelBand but can't find information on who owns my data once it's synced/analyzed with the software. Could you let me know what the policies are?" (sent on November 25, 2013).

11  This was the response (received on November 27, 2013):

Hi Barbara, It's great to see that you are interested in purchasing a Nike+ FuelBand. This is a great device for tracking daily activity. I understand that you want to know what happens to personal data captured by Nike, please be assured that I can help you with this. Barbara, I have included a link to our Privacy Policy in this e-mail. Its [sic] quiet [sic] long but it covers everything that you would need to know. www.nike.com. I trust that this information is useful to you. If you have any other questions please let me know. "Make it Count." Jared, Nike+ Support

12  I am grateful to Sabina Leonelli for helpful conversations on this point.

13  Some types of data use—such as data use for scientific research—are exempt from some of the Regulation's requirements, given that the use of personal data for scientific research is covered by more specific rules.

14  See also Peppet 2012: 85, arguing that these privacy vaults should operate as trusts, and not be accountable to citizens directly. See also Prainsack and Buyx 2013.

## CHAPTER 4. BEYOND EMPOWERMENT

1  The vignette is a composite of real stories that I encountered during my research on direct-to-consumer (DTC) genetic testing between 2007 and 2015. All details that could identify individual test takers were left out or altered. In spring 2016 the DTC company 23andMe stopped offering health-related information to customers in certain countries, including Austria; thus if Milena had decided to take a test after that date she would only have had access to information about her genetic ancestry.

2  Saying that human life is never devoid of power does not imply that it is everywhere; that power can be exercised requires, for example, the presence of an interaction (see Heiskala 2001: 248; Kusch 1991). It should be noted also that because of the understanding that power is virtually everywhere, the Foucauldian notion of power is sometimes referred to as a notion of "distributed power." This is not to be confused with Max Weber's "distributive" concept of power. Weber envisages power as a kind of zero sum game where an increase in power for one person means a decrease in power for another.

3  By "technologies" Foucault did not refer to material devices as we commonly understand the term today, but to practices and strategies that people use to form themselves into the kind of people they want to be.

4 See, for example, Anis et al. 2010; Birmingham et al. 1999; Cawley and Meyerhoefer 2012; Colagiuri et al. 2010; Levy et al. 1995; Lobstein 2015; Schmier, Jones, and Halpern 2006; Suhrcke et al. 2006; Tsai, Williamson, and Glick 2011; Wolf and Colditz 1998.

5 Thaler and Sunstein define nudges as "any aspect of the choice architecture that alters people's behavior in a predictable way without forbidding any options or significantly changing their economic incentives" (Thaler and Sunstein 2008: 6). See also Prainsack and Buyx 2017.

6 These variations at the level of single nucleotides are called SNP (single nucleotide polymorphism). SNP-based tests do not sequence an entire gene or genome; rather, they look at certain nucleotide combinations that indicate particular genetic variants. In other words, SNP-based tests are a more "superficial" yet much cheaper and faster way of carrying out genome analysis. With the cost of DNA sequencing decreasing, SNP-based tests are being replaced by more comprehensive sequencing methods in many contexts.

7 "Clinical validity" is commonly seen as a test's ability to consistently and correctly identify a clinical status. Clinical utility refers to the use that a test has for clinical decision making (for example, diagnosis, treatment, and monitoring).

8 This and the next two paragraphs draw upon an unpublished work written jointly with Lea Lahnstein, whose contribution is gratefully acknowledged. I am also grateful to Ingrid Metzler for helpful conversations on this topic.

9 The conflation of access and ownership in this quote is noteworthy, but not exceptional; see also the discussion on the Nike fitness tracker FuelBand in chapter 3.

10 This is not to say that the "manual" assessment of radiologists is consistent either; in the absence of reliable results from imaging devices, however, many radiologists need to keep quantifying "manually."

CHAPTER 5. JUST PROFIT?

1 The Open FDA initiative in the United States (open.fda.gov), for example, also grants commercial actors access to data on adverse drug reactions and other data. The Explore Data initiative (catalog.data.gov/dataset) is another example of data flowing from the public to the private domain.

2 "Impact investing" is another instantiation of the idea that profit making and the creation of social value mutually reinforce each other. Impact investors put their money in organizations or companies that promise measurable positive social change on top of financial returns. See Bugg-Levine and Emerson 2011.

3 Other nonprofit initiatives dedicated to "using Internet technology and data for humanitarian ends" (Lohr 2013) include DataKind (datakind.org), Ushahidi (ushahidi.com), Crisis Mappers (crisismappers.net), and InSTEDD (instedd.org), as well as Crowdrise (crowdrise.com), GDACS (portal.gdacs.org), and Humanitarian Kiosk (humanitarianresponse.info/applications/kiosk).

4 A note on the relationship between the concepts of philanthropy and CSR may be helpful here. Although some authors use the two terms interchangeably, others treat CSR as a necessary part of running a business while philanthropy is merely

an additional extra for those who can afford it. Leisinger, for example, speaks of a "hierarchy of corporate responsibilities" consisting of three tiers. The basic tier is what a company "must" do, such as obey laws, minimize emissions, and improve health and safety in the work place. The second tier—what a company "ought to" do—includes corporate social responsibility and other "citizenship beyond legal duties." The third and highest tier—what Leisinger calls the "nice to have" tier—is corporate philanthropy (Leisinger 2005: 584).

5 The related term "philanthrocapitalism" (Bishop and Green 2008) explicitly denotes the situation that "altruism is a useful business strategy" (McGoey 2012: 187).

6 New companies offering personalized analysis and advice on the basis of microbiomes include the American Gut Project (microbio.me/americangut/), the British Gut Project (britishgut.org), UBiome (ubiome.com), and SweetPeach (sweetpeachprobiotics.com); a company offering personalized nutrition advice on the basis of photos of meals and activity tracking data is Rise (rise.us). Interestingly, by looking at the websites alone it is often impossible to discern between for-profit and nonprofit projects.

7 In the survey, these data ranged from exercise and fitness data to blood sugar to data on sleep, weight, and menstrual cycles.

8 For a discussion of how biohacking and DIY-biology communities fund their activities, see Gewin 2013.

## CHAPTER 6. BEYOND INDIVIDUALISM

1 The understanding of rationality described here—strategic rationality aimed at the fulfillment of individual interests—is not the only understanding of rationality. For example, rationality can refer to *logos* in the philosophical sense; this meaning is not in the center of my argument. Instead I mean a type of rationality as it is understood and employed in many Western societies. In Charles Taylor's words, "we have a rational grasp of something when we can *articulate* it, that means, distinguish and lay out the different features of the matter in perspicuous order" (C. Taylor 1985b: 137, emphasis in original). In such an understanding, rationality is inseparably linked to normative values, e.g. regarding a presumed meaningful order of society or societal teleology. Thus, rationality is more than a prescription to be logically consistent. At the same time, many authors, especially those who understand human beings as relational rather than bounded and self-interested ones, have proposed alternative understandings of rationality than the one that is discussed here as dominant in Western societies. I am grateful to Christoph Rehmann-Sutter for very helpful discussions on this aspect.

2 An exception to this is public health ethics. Due to the prominent role that binding and coercive measures play in this field, which routinely have the capacity to infringe on individual autonomy for the sake of collective benefit, the tension between these two goods has received explicit attention. Perhaps because of the latter, conceptualizations of personhood that accommodate noninstrumental, nondeliberate, and sometimes also the unconscious nature of social relations and

attachments have been more pronounced in public health than in other areas of medicine (see also Baylis, Kenny, and Sherwin 2008; Prainsack and Buyx 2011).

3 I borrow the title of the following section from Monika Schreiber's (2014) book *The Comfort of Kin: Samaritan Community, Kinship, and Marriage.*

4 This includes people who agreed to donate on their driver's licenses and those who signed donor cards or signed up to organ donor registries; Department of Health and Human Services 2016.

5 Data were taken from the irodat.com database, which offers continuously updated information on organ donation from many countries around the world.

6 The major change introduced by the Transplantation Act (2008) was that it imposed penalties on organ brokers and Israeli medical professionals who are involved in organ trading within and beyond Israel's borders. The Transplantation Act made only minor changes to already existing regulations for living and cadaveric donations, for example, by suggesting a steering committee to determine criteria for adequately compensating living organ donors. Expanding the pool of organ donors was the target of yet another law: In the same year (2008) in which the Transplantation Act was published, the Knesset issued the Brain Respiratory Death Act, which specified protocols to determine neurological death. This law was aimed at mitigating the opposition of many religious Jews to the standard definition of brain death, indicating the loss of the stem-brain, responsible for respiratory functions, as the moment of death. Furthermore, the law surrenders the final rule in determining death to the patient's relatives, thus allowing greater leverage for those who oppose brain death definitions (Jotkowitz and Glick 2009). Although it is difficult to attribute this increase to any specific factor, the number of deceased organ donors have increased in Israel after these two laws have come into effect (from 8 to 11 donors per million population; Lavee et al. 2013: 780).

7 Jacob (2012) reports that in cases where it was apparent that a donor had volunteered due to pressure from her family, the hospital committee tasked with approving donors then found a "medical excuse" for them not to do it, away from the scrutiny of the family (thus the committee did fulfil its mission to protect donors, albeit in perhaps unintended ways).

8 The next chapter's title is inspired by Corinna Kruse's book *The Social Life of Forensic Evidence* (Kruse 2016; which she in turn borrows from Appadurai 1986).

## CHAPTER 7. THE SOCIAL LIFE OF EVIDENCE IN PERSONALIZED MEDICINE

1 This is, in fact, an argument in favor of opt-out solutions for the use of clinical databases for research (such as proposed in the care.data context in the UK): If people had to opt in to their clinical data being used for research, this would skew the data set. Possibly a good solution here would be to implement opt out for data that can be used for very narrowly defined health research with very plausible public benefit. Wider data use would need to be opted in.

2 Releasing such data as such is not new; the National Center of Health Statistics in the United States has released aggregate date from a range of areas for a long time, ranging from mortality data to data on reproductive health (see Centers for Disease Control and Prevention 2016). What is new is the scale of the data sets available, and the ability to establish links between data sets much more easily.

3 Proponents of Realistic Medicine differentiate between three types of value: First, allocative value, which is determined by how resources are distributed within the population; second, technical value, which relates to how well resources are used to improve outcomes with particular attention to over- and underuse; and third, personal value, which is "determined by how well the outcome relates to the value of each individual" (NHS Scotland 2016: 12)

4 Patient-reported outcomes can range from very specific questions asking patients to quantify their responses (for example, pain "scores") to answers to open questions. Not all patient-generated data can be considered PROMs.

5 Amir Hannan, a general practitioner in Haughton Vale near Manchester, England, is a pioneer in this regard. Updates on his activities, including his blog, are available here: http://www.htmc.co.uk, last accessed November 26, 2016.

6 The video can still be accessed at www.vimeo.com/38239245, last accessed July 1, 2015.

7 The Portable Legal Consent framework is thus oriented toward the "open consent" framework developed by Lunshof et al. (2008); see also Sage Bionetworks 2014b.

8 This suggestion had already been made earlier by physician and ethicist Howard Brody (Brody 2010; see also Berwick and Hackbarth 2012; Frühwald 2013; Morden et al. 2014).

9 Jensen, Jensen, and Brunak (2012: 401) discuss several scenarios of machine-learning on electronic health records data.

10 U.S. case law on electronic health records has established that "physicians can be held liable for harm that could have been averted had they more carefully studied their patients' medical records" (G. Cohen et al. 2014: 1144; see also Hoffman and Podgurski 2009).

## CHAPTER 8. CONCLUSION

1 "Patient and public involvement" (PPI) has been firmly established within the British National Health Service (NHS) since the early 2000s. Any research in the NHS context needs to consider PPI and involve patients and publics wherever meaningfully possible. See, for example, Mockford et al. 2012.

2 By "established" I mean science that is carried out by professionally trained people and published in peer-reviewed journals.

3 I am grateful to Thomas Palfinger for helpful discussions on this point.

4 A survey by the British Wellcome Trust in 2016 showed that the purpose for which their data are used matters a great deal to people (Wellcome Trust 2016; see also Prainsack 2016).

5 I will discuss the specifics of how public interest in the context of data use can be ascertained in another place: McMahon, Prainsack, and Buyx, work in progress.

# REFERENCES

23andMe. 2017. "23andMe." Accessed April 5, 2017. https://www.23andme.com/research/.

Access to Medicine Index. 2014. Bi-Annual Report 2014. Accessed May 10, 2016. www.accesstomedicineindex.org.

Agus, David B. 2016. *The Lucky Years: How to Thrive in the Brave New World of Health.* New York: Simon and Schuster.

Ahmed, Sara, Richard A. Berzon, Dennis A. Revicki, William R. Lenderking, Carol M. Moinpour, Ethan Basch, Bryce B. Reeve, and Albert Wu, on behalf of the International Society for Quality of Life Research. 2012. "The Use of Patient-Reported Outcomes (PRO) Within Comparative Effectiveness Research: Implications for Clinical Practice and Health Care Policy." *Medical Care* 50 (12): 1060–1070.

Aicardi, Christine, Maria Damjanovicova, Lorenzo Del Savio, Federica Lucivero, Maru Mormina, Maartje Niezen, and Barbara Prainsack. 2016. "Could DTC Genome Testing Exacerbate Research Inequities?" *Bioethics Forum*—The Blog of the Hastings Center Report, January 20. Accessed May 10, 2016. www.thehastingscenter.org.

Albrechtslund, Anders, and Peter Lauritsen. 2013. "Spaces of Everyday Surveillance: Unfolding an Analytical Concept of Participation." *Geoforum* 49: 310–316.

Amarasingham, Ruben, Rachel E. Patzer, Marco Huesch, Nam Q. Nguyen, and Bin Xie. 2014. "Implementing Electronic Health Care Predictive Analytics: Considerations and Challenges." *Health Affairs* 33 (7): 1148–1154.

Andersson, Gerhard. 2009. "Using the Internet to Provide Cognitive Behaviour Therapy." *Behaviour Research and Therapy* 47 (3): 175–180.

Angell, Marcia. 2005. *The Truth About the Drug Companies: How They Deceive Us and What to Do About It.* New York: Random House.

Angell, Marcia. 2015. "Health: The Right Diagnosis and the Wrong Treatment." *New York Review of Books*, April 23. Accessed November 26, 2016. www.nybooks.com.

Anis, Aslam, W. Zhang, N. Bansback, P. D. Guh, Z. Amarsi, and L. C. Birmingham. 2010. "Obesity and Overweight in Canada: An Updated Cost-of-Illness Study." *Obesity Reviews* 11 (1): 31–40.

Apixio. 2015. "Apixio Iris Platform Powers Accurate Patient Risk Adjustment for Improved Healthcare." Press Release, November 19. www.apixio.com.

Appadurai, Arjun. 1986. *The Social Life of Things: Commodities in Cultural Perspective.* Cambridge, UK: Cambridge University Press.

Arendt, Hannah. 1978 [1973]. *The Life of the Mind.* San Diego: Harcourt.

Armfield, Greg G., and Lance R. Holbert. 2003. "The Relationship Between Religiosity and Internet Use." *Journal of Media and Religion* 2 (3): 129–144.

Arnstein, Sherry R. 1969. "A Ladder of Citizen Participation." *Journal of the American Institute of Planners* 35 (4): 216–224.

Auletta, Ken. 2009. *Googled: The End of the World as We Know It.* London: Virgin Books.

Ausiello, Dennis. 2013. "From Symptomatic to Pre-Symptomatic, Continuous Care." *YouTube,* March 26. Accessed May 10, 2016. www.youtube.com/watch?v=X9wZKCLtujE.

Ausiello, Dennis, and Stanley Shaw. 2014. "Quantitative Human Phenotyping: The Next Frontier in Medicine." *Transactions of the American Clinical and Climatological Association* 125:219–228.

Bachrach, Peter, and Morton S. Baratz. 1962. "Two Faces of Power." *American Political Science Review* 56 (4): 947–952.

Bachrach, Peter, and Morton S. Baratz. 1963. "Decisions and Nondecisions: An Analytical Framework." *American Political Science Review* 57 (3): 632–642.

Bainbridge, Lisanne. 1983. "Ironies of Automation." *Automatica* 19 (6): 775–779.

Bannan, Christine. 2016. "The IoT threat to privacy." *TechChrunch,* August 14. Accessed August 17, 2016. www.techcrunch.com.

Bardes, Charles L. 2012. "Defining 'Patient-Centered Medicine.'" *New England Journal of Medicine* 366 (9): 782–783.

Basch, Ethan. 2009. "Patient-Reported Outcomes in Drug Safety Evaluation." *Annals of Oncology* 20 (12): 1905–1906.

Basch, Ethan. 2013. "Toward Patient-Centred Drug Development in Oncology." *New England Journal of Medicine* 369 (5): 297–400.

Basch, Ethan, Xiaoyu Jia, Glenn Heller, Allison Barz, Laura Sit, Michael Fruscione, Mark Appawu, Alexia Iasonos, Thomas Atkinson, Shari Goldfarb, Ann Culkin, Mark G. Kris, and Deborah Schrag. 2009. "Adverse Symtpom Event Reporting by Patients vs. Clinicians: Relationships With Clinical Outcomes." *JNCI Journal of the National Cancer Institute* 101 (23): 1624–1632.

Bates, David W., Suchi Saria, Lucila Ohno-Machado, Anand Shah, and Gabriel Escobar. 2014. "Big Data in Health Care: Using Analytics to Identify and Manage High-Risk and High-Cost Patients." *Health Affairs* 33 (7): 1123–1131.

Battersby, Christine. 2007. *The Sublime, Terror and Human Difference.* London: Routledge.

Baylis, Françoise, Nuala P. Kenny, and Susan Sherwin. 2008. "A Relational Account of Public Health Care Ethics." *Public Health Ethics* 1 (3): 196–209.

Bazelier, Marloes T., Frank de Vries, Joan Bentzen, Peter Vestergaard, Hubert G. M. Leufkens, Tieerd-Pieter van Staa, and Nils Koch-Henriksen. 2012. "Incidence of Fractures in Patients with Multiple Sclerosis: The Danish National Health Registers." *Multiple Sclerosis Journal* 18 (5): 622–627.

Beato, Greg. 2014. "Growth Force." *Stanford Social Innovation Review,* Spring. Accessed May 10, 2016. www.ssireview.org.

Beaulieu, Anne. 2002. "Images Are Not the (Only) Truth: Brain Mapping, Visual Knowledge, and Iconoclasm." *Science, Technology & Human Values* 27 (1): 53–86.

Beck, Ulrich. 1992. *Risk Society: Towards a New Modernity.* London: Sage.

Bell, Susan. 2009. *DES Daughters. Embodied Knowledge and the Transformation of Women's Health Politics in the Late Twentieth Century.* Philadelphia: Temple University Press.

Bengtsson, Linus, Xin Lu, Anna Thorson, Richard Garfield, and Johan Von Schreeb. (2011). "Improved Response to Risasters and Outbreaks by Tracking Population Movements with Mobile Phone Network Data: A Post-Earthquake Geospatial Study in Haiti." *PLoS Medicine* 8 (8): e1001083.

Benkler, Yochai. 2006. *The Wealth of Networks: How Social Production Transforms Markets and Freedom.* New Haven, CT: Yale University Press.

Berenson, Robert A., and Elizabeth Docteur. 2013. *Doing Better by Doing Less: Approaches to Tackle Overuse of Services. Timely Analysis of Immediate Policy Issues.* Princeton, NJ: Robert Wood Johnson Foundation/Urban Institute.

Berger, John, and Jean Mohr. 1967. *A Fortunate Man. The Story of a Country Doctor.* Edinburgh: Canongate.

Berwick, Donald M. 2009. "What 'Patient-Centered' Should Mean: Confessions of an Extremist." *Health Affairs* 28 (4): 555–565.

Berwick, Donald M., and Andrew A. Hackbarth. 2012. "Eliminating Waste in US Healthcare." *Journal of the American Medical Association* 307 (14): 1513–1516.

Beurden, Pieter van, and Tobias Gössling. 2008. "The Worth of Values—A Literature Review on the Relation Between Social and Financial Performance." *Journal of Business Ethics* 82 (2): 407–424.

Bilgin, Pinar, and Berivan Elis. 2008. "Hard Power, Soft Power: Toward a More Realistic Power Analysis." *Insight Turkey* 10 (2): 5–20.

Biomarker Definitions Working Group. 2001. "Biomarkers and Surrogate Endpoints: Preferred Definitions and Conceptual Framework." *Clinical Pharmacology and Therapeutics* 69:89–95.

Birch, Kean, Edward S. Dove, Margaret Chiapetta, and Ulyi K. Gürsoy. 2016. "Biobanks in Oral Health: Promises and Implications of Post-Neoliberal Science and Innovation." *OMICS: A Journal of Integrative Biology* 20 (1): 36–41.

Bird-David, Nurit. 2004. "Illness-Images and Joined Beings: A Critical/Nayaka Perspective on Intercorporeality." *Social Anthropology* 12 (3): 325–339.

Birmingham, C. L., J. L. Muller, A. Palepu, J. J. Spinelli, and A. H. Anis. 1999. "The Cost of Obesity in Canada." *Canadian Medical Association Journal* 160 (4): 483–488.

Bishop, Matthew, and Michael Green. 2008. *Philanthrocapitalism: How the Rich Can Save the World.* London: Bloomsbury Press.

Blum, Linda M. 2015. *Raising Generation Rx: Mothering Kids with Invisible Disabilities.* New York: New York University Press.

Boas, Hagai. 2009. "The Value of Altruism: The Political Economy of Organ Supply." PhD thesis, Tel Aviv University.

Boas, Hagai. 2011. "Where Do Human Organs Come From? Trends of Generalized and Restricted Altruism in Organ Donations." *Social Science and Medicine* 73 (9): 1378–1385.

Boero, Natalie. 2012. *Killer Fat: Media, Medicine and Morals in the American "Obesity Epidemic."* New Brunswick, NJ: Rutgers University Press.

Boggan, Steve. 2001. "'We Blew It.' Nike Admits to Mistakes Over Child Labor." *Independent UK,* October 20.

Bouchelouche, Kirstin, and Jacek Capala. 2010. "'Image and Treat': An Individualized Approach to Urological Tumors." *Current Opinion in Oncology* 22 (3): 274–280.

Boyle, Elizabeth A., Thomas M. Connolly, Thomas Hainey, and James M. Boyle. 2012. "Engagement in Digital Entertainment Games: A Systematic Review." *Computers in Human Behavior* 28 (3): 771–780.

Brake, David R. 2014. "Are We All Online Content Creators Now? Web 2.0 and Digital Divides." *Journal of Computer-Mediated Communication* 19 (3): 591–609.

Bratteteig, Tone, and Ina Wagner. 2013. "Moving Healthcare to the Home: The Work to Make Homecare Work." In *ECSDW 2013: Proceedings of the 13th European Conference on Computer Supported Cooperative Work,* edited by Olav W. Bertelsen, Luigina Ciolfi, Maria Antonietta Grasso, and George A. Papadopoulos, 143–162. 13th European Conference on Computer Supported Cooperative Work, Paphos, Cyprus, September September 21–25.

Brawley, Otis W., and Paul Goldberg. 2012. *How We Do Harm: A Doctor Breaks Ranks About Being Sick in America.* Basingstoke, UK: Macmillan.

Brennan, Niall, Allison Oelschlaeger, Christine Cox, and Marilyn Tavenner. 2014. "Leveraging The Big-Data Revolution: CMS is Expanding Its Capabilities to Spur Health Systems Transformation." *Health Affairs* 33 (7): 1195–1202.

Brimelow, Adam. 2009. "Israel Organ Donors to Get Transplant Priority." BBC News, December 17. Accessed May 10, 2016. news.bbc.co.uk.

Britnell, Mark. 2015. *In Search of the Perfect Health System.* London: Palgrave.

Brody, Howard. 2010. "Medicine's Ethical Responsibility for Health Care Reform—The Top Five List." *New England Journal of Medicine* 362 (4): 283–285.

Brown, Nik, and Andrew Webster. 2004. *New Medical Technologies and Society: Reordering Life.* Cambridge, UK: Polity Press.

Brown, Phil. 2013. *Toxic Exposures: Contested Illnesses and the Environmental Health Movement.* New York: Columbia University Press.

Brunton, Finn, and Helen Nissenbaum. 2011. "Vernacular Resistance to Data Collection and Analysis: A Political Theory of Obfuscation." *First Monday* 16 (5). Accessed April 12, 2017. doi: dx.doi.org/10.5210/fm.v16i5.3493.

Buck, David, and David Maguire. 2015. *Inequalities in Life Expectancy: Changes Over Time and Implications for Policy.* King's Fund. www.kingsfund.org.uk.

Bugg-Levine, Antony, and Jed Emerson. 2011. "Impact Investing: Transforming How We Make Money While Making a Difference." *Innovations* 6 (3): 9–18.

Busse, Reinhard. 2015. "Geleitwort (Preface)." In *Dienstleistungspotenziale und Geschäftsmodelle in der Personalisierten Medizin* [Business and service opportunities in personalised medicine], edited by Elisabeth Eppinger, Bastian Halecker, Katharina Hölzle, and Martin Kamprath, v–vi. Wiesbaden, Germany: Springer.

Butler, Judith. 1990. "Gender Trouble, Feminist Theory, and Psychological Discourse." In *Feminism/Postmodernism,* edited by Linda Nicholson, 323–347. New York: Routledge.

Buyx, Alena, and Barbara Prainsack. 2012. "Lifestyle-Related Diseases and Individual Responsibility through the Prism of Solidarity." *Clinical Ethics* 7 (2): 79–85.

Byrne, Katherine. 2014. "Adapting Heritage: Class Conservatism in Downton Abbey." *Rethinking History* 18 (3): 311–327.

Caball, Marc, Soulla Louca, Roland Pochet, Daniel Spichtinger, and Barbara Prainsack. 2013. "The Best Open Access Policies Put Researchers in Charge." *Impact of Social Science Blog,* December 18. Accessed May 10, 2016. blogs.lse.ac.uk/impactofsocialsciences.

Canguilhem, Georges. 1989. *The Normal and the Pathological.* New York: Zone Books.

Carpenter, Christopher R., Ali S. Raja, and Michael D. Brown. 2015. "Overtesting and the Downstream Consequences of Overtreatment: Implications of 'Preventing Overdiagnosis' for Emergency Medicine." *Academic Emergency Medicine* 22 (12): 1484–1492.

Carter, S., W. Rogers, I. Heath, C. Degeling, Jenny Doust, and Alexandra Barratt. 2015. "The Challenge of Overdiagnosis Begins With Its Definition." *British Medical Journal* 350:h869.

Casilli, Antonio A. 2014. "Four Theses on Mass Surveillance and Privacy Negotiation." *Medium,* October 26. Accessed May 10, 2016. medium.com/@AntonioCasilli/four-theses-on-digital-mass-surveillance-and-the-negotiation-of-privacy-7254cd3cdee6.

Casper, Monica J., and Lisa J. Moore. 2009. *Missing Bodies: The Politics of Visibility.* New York: New York University Press.

Caulfield, Timothy, M. N. Ries, N. P. Ray, C. Shuman, and B. Wilson. 2010. "Direct-to-Consumer Genetic Testing: Good, Bad or Benign?" *Clinical Genetics* 77 (2): 101–105.

Cawley, John, and Chad Meyerhoefer. 2012. "The Medical Care Costs of Obesity: An Instrumental Variables Approach." *Journal of Health Economics* 31 (1): 219–230.

Centers for Disease Control and Prevention. 2016. "National Center for Health Statistics." www.cdc.gov/nchs.

Centre for Effective Altruism. N.A. "Doing Good Better." www.effectivealtruism.org.

Cetina, Knorr K. 2005. "The Rise of a Culture of Life." *EMBO Reports* 6 (S1): 76–80.

Chadwick, Ruth, Mairi Levitt, and Darren Shickle. 1997. *The Right to Know and the Right Not to Know.* Aldershot, UK: Avebury.

Chadwick, Ruth, Mairi Levitt, and Darren Shickle. 2014. *The Right to Know and the Right Not to Know: Genetic Privacy and Responsibility.* 2nd edition. Cambridge, UK: Cambridge University Press.

Chadwick, Ruth, and Udo Schüklenk. 2004. "Bioethical Colonialism?" *Bioethics* 18 (5): iii-iv.

Chapman, Audrey R. 2009. "Towards an Understanding of the Right to Enjoy the Benefits of Scientific Progress and its Applications." *Journal of Human Rights* 8 (1): 1–36.

Charisius, Hanno, Richard Friebe, and Sasha Karberg. 2014. "Becoming Biohackers: The Long Arm of the Law." BBC Online, January 24. Accessed May 10, 2016. www.bbc.com.

Cherkas, Lynn F., Abraham Aviv, Ana M. Valdes, Janice L. Hunkin, Jeffery P. Gardner, Gabriela L. Surdulescu, Masayuki Kimura, and Tim D. Spector. 2006. "The Effects of Social Status on Biological Aging as Measured by White-Blood-Cell Telomere Length." *Aging Cell* 5 (5): 361–365.

Cherkas, Lynn F., Juliette M. Harris, Elana Levinson, Tim D. Spector, and Barbara Prainsack. 2010. "A Survey of UK Public Interest in Internet-based Personal Genome Testing." *PLoS ONE* 5 (10): e13473.

Chetty, Raj, Michael Stepner, Sarah Abraham, Shelby Lin, Benjamin Scuderi, Nicholas Turner, Augstin Bergeron, and David Cutler. 2016. "The Association Between Income and Life Expectancy in the United States, 2001–2014." *Journal of the American Medical Association* 315 (16): 1750–1766.

Chiapperino, Luca. 2014. "From Consent to Choice: The Ethics of Empowerment-Based Reforms." PhD thesis, European School of Molecular Medicine, Milan, Italy.

Chiapperino, Luca, and Per-Anders Tengland. 2016. "Empowerment in Healthcare Policy Making: Three Domains of Substantive Controversy." *Health Promotion Journal of Australia* 26 (3): 210–215.

Chiu, Cindy, Chris Ip, and Ari Silverman. 2013. "The 'Social' Side of Chinese Health Care." *McKinsey Quarterly*, June. Accessed May 10, 2016. www.mckinsey.com.

Chodorow, Nancy. 1980. "'Gender, Relation, and Differnce in Pyschoanalytical Perspective.'" In *The Future of Difference,* edited by Hester Eisenstein and Alice Jardine, 3–19. Boston: G. K. Hall.

Choudhry, Nauman S., Ashish H. Shah, Nicholas Ferraro, Brian M. Snelling, Amade Bregy, Karthik Madhavan, and Ricardo J. Komotar. 2013. "Predictors of Long-Term Survival in Patients with Glioblastoma Multiforme: Advancements From the Last Quarter Century." *Cancer Investigation* 31 (5): 287–308.

Christakis, Nicholas A., and James H. Fowler. 2009. *Connected: The Surprising Power of Our Social Networks And How They Shape Our Lives.* New York: Little, Brown and Company.

Christensen, Helen, Kathleen M. Griffiths, and Anthony F. Jorm. 2004. "Delivering Interventions for Depression by Using the Internet: Randomised Controlled Trial." *British Medical Journal* 328 (7434): 265.

Christensen, Helen, and Andrew Mackinnon. 2006. "The Law of Attrition Revisited." *Journal of Medical Internet Research* 8 (3): e20.

Christman, John. 2015. "Autonomy in Moral and Political Philosophy." In *The Stanford Encyclopedia of Philosophy,* edited by Edward N. Zalta (Spring 2015 edition). Accessed April 18, 2017. https://plato.stanford.edu/archives/spr2015/entries/autonomy-moral/.

Chu, Zen. 2014. "Why It's the Best Time in History to Be a Healthcare Entrepreneur." H@cking Medicine blog, February 14. Accessed May 10, 2016. hackingmedicine.mit.edu.

Clark, Mike, and Nick Goodwin. 2010. "Sustaining Innovation in Telehealth and Telecare." *Whole System Demonstrator Action Network (WSDAN) briefing paper.* Accessed May 10, 2016. www.kingsfund.org.uk.

Clarke, Adele E. 2010. "Epilogue." In *Biomedicalization: Technoscience and Transformations of Health and Illness in the U.S.*, edited by Adele E. Clarke, Janet K. Shim, Laura Mamo, Jennifer R. Fosket, and Jennifer R. Fishman, 380–405. Durham, NC: Duke University Press.

Clarke, Adele E., Janet K. Shim, Laura Mamo, Jennifer R. Fosket, and Jennifer R. Fishman. 2003. "Biomedicalization: Technoscientific Transformations of Health, Illness and U.S. Biomedicine." *American Sociological Review* 68: 161–194.

Clarke, Adele E., Janet K. Shim, Laura Mamo, Jennifer R. Fosket, and Jennifer R. Fishman, eds. 2010a. *Biomedicalization: Technoscience and Transformations of Health and Illness in the U.S.* Durham, NC: Duke University Press.

Clarke, Adele E., Janet K. Shim, Laura Mamo, Jennifer R. Fosket, and Jennifer R. Fishman. 2010b. "Biomedicalization: A Theoretical and Substantive Introduction." In *Biomedicalization: Technoscience and Transformations of Health and Illness in the U.S.*, edited by Adele E. Clarke, Janet K. Shim, Laura Mamo, Jennifer R. Fosket, and Jennifer R. Fishman, 1–44. Durham, NC: Duke University Press.

Clarke, Adele E., Janet K. Shim, Laura Mamo, Jennifer R. Fosket, and Jennifer R. Fishman. 2010c. "Biomedicalization." In *Biomedicalization: Technoscience and Transformations of Health and Illness in the U.S.*, edited by Adele E. Clarke, Janet K. Shim, Laura Mamo, Jennifer R. Fosket, and Jennifer R. Fishman, 47–87. Durham, NC: Duke University Press.

Cline, Rebecca J., and Katie M. Haynes. 2001. "Consumer Health Information Seeking on the Internet: The State of the Art." *Health Education Research* 16 (6): 671–692.

Cohen, G. A. 1995. *Self-Ownership, Freedom, and Equality.* Cambridge, UK: Cambridge University Press.

Cohen, Glenn, Ruben Amarasingham, Anand Shah, Bin Xie, and Bernard Lo. 2014. "The Legal and Ethical Concerns That Arise from Using Complex Predictive Analytics in Health Care." *Health Affairs* 33 (7): 1139–1147.

Cohen, I. Glenn, Holly Fernandez Lynch, and Christopher T. Robertson. 2016. *Nudging Health.* Baltimore, MD: Johns Hopkins University Press.

Cohen, Julie E. 2012. *Configuring the Networked Self: Law, Code, and the Play of Everyday Practice.* New Haven, CT: Yale University Press.

Colagiuri, Stephen, Crystal M. Lee, Ruth Colagiuri, Dianna Magliano, Jonathan E. Shaw, Paul Z. Zimmet, and Ian D. Caterson. 2010. "The Cost of Overweight and Obesity in Australia." *Medical Journal of Australia* 192 (5): 260–264.

Comor, Edward. 2011. "Contextualizing and Critiquing the Fantastic Prosumer: Power, Alienation and Hegemony." *Critical Sociology* 37 (3): 309–327.

Cook, S. D. Noam 2005. "That Which Governs Best: Ethics, Leadership and Human Systems." In *The Quest for Moral Leaders: Essays in Leadership Ethics,* edited by Joanne B. Ciulla, Terry L. Price, and Susan E. Murphy, 131–143. Northampton, MA: Edward Elgar.

Cooper, Melinda, and Catherine Waldby. 2014. *Clinical Labor: Human Research Subjects and Tissue Donors in the Global Bioeconomy.* Durham, NC: Duke University Press.

Corkery, Michael, and Jessica Silver-Greenberg. 2014. "Miss a Payment? Good Luck Moving That Car." *New York Times,* September 24. www.nytimes.com.

Cribb, Alan. In press. *Healthcare in Transition.* Bristol: Policy Press.

Crisis Mappers. n.d. "CrisisMappers: The Humanitarian Technology Network." Accessed May 10, 2016. www.crisismappers.net.

Crompton, Susan, Jonathan Ellison, and Kathryn Stevenson. 2002. "Better Things to Do or Dealt Out of the Game? Internet Dropouts and Infrequent Users." *Canadian Social Trends* 65: 2–5.

Crowdrise. 2016. "Crowdrise: if You Don't Give Back No One Will Like You." Accessed May 10, 2016. www.crowdrise.com.

CureTogether. 2016. "The Smarter Way to Find the Best Treatments." Accessed May 10, 2016. www.curetogether.com.

Curit BV. n.d. "CurIt Disease Management and Telemedicine." Accessed May 10, 2016. www.curit.com.

Dahl, Robert A. 1957. "The Concept of Power." *Behavioral Science* 2 (3): 201–215.

DataKind. 2015. "Harnessing the Power of Data Science in the Service of Humanity." Accessed May 10, 2016. www.datakind.org.

Davies, Kevin. 2009. "Exclusive: Stephen Friend on the Road from Merck to Sage." *BioITWorld,* May 28. Accessed May 10, 2016. www.bio-itworld.com.

Davis, Karen, Kristof Stremikis, David Squires, and Cathy Schoen. 2014. *Mirror, Mirror on the Wall, 2014 Update: How the U.S. Health Care System Compares Internationally.* New York: The Commonwealth Fund. Accessed May 10, 2016. www.commonwealthfund.org.

Davis, Kathy. 2008. *The Making of Our Bodies, Ourselves: How Feminism Travels Across Borders.* Durham, NC: Duke University Press.

Dawson, J., I. Boller, H. Doll, G. Lavis, R. Sharp, P. Cooke, and C. Jenkinson. 2011. "The MOXFQ Patient-Reported Questionnaire: Assessment of Data Quality, Reliability and Validity in Relation to Foot and Ankle Surgery." *The Foot* 21 (2): 92–102.

Dean, Jodi. 2014. "Big Data: Accumulation and Enclosure." Public Lecture at Carleton University, Ottawa, Candada, November 27. Accessed May 10, 2016, www.academia.edu/7125387/Big_data_accumulation_and_enclosure.

Dean, Kathryn. 1989. "Conceptual, Theoretical and Methodological Issues in Self-Care Research." *Social Science & Medicine* 29 (2): 117–123.

De Craemer, Willy. 1983. "A Cross-Cultural Perspective on Personhood." *The Milbank Memorial Fund Quarterley. Health and Society* 61 (1): 19–34.

DeFriese, Gordon H., Alison Woomert, Priscilla A. Guild, Allan B. Steckler, and Thomas R. Konrad. 1989. "From Activated Patient to Pacified Activist: A Study of the Self-Care Movement in the United States." *Social Science & Medicine* 29 (2): 195–204.

Deleuze, Gilles, and Félix Guatarri. 1987. *A Thousand Plateaus: Capitalism and Schizophrenia.* Minneapolis: University of Minnesota Press.

Delfanti, Alessandro. 2013. *Biohackers: The Politics of Open Science.* London: Pluto Press.

Del Savio, Lorenzo, Alena Buyx, and Barbara Prainsack. 2016. "Opening the Black Box of Participation in Medicine and Healthcare." *ITA-manuscript* 16/01. Accessed May 10. 2016. epub.oeaw.ac.at.

Delude, Cathryn M. 2015. "Deep Phenotyping: The Details of Disease." *Nature* 527 (7576): S14-S15.

Denison, D.C. 2013. "The Examined Life of Rachel Kalmar: Data Scientist." *Make Magazine,* May 8. Accessed May 10, 2016: www.makezine.com.

Dennis, Carina. 2012. "The Rise of the 'Narciss-ome.'" *Nature News,* March 16. Accessed 10 April 2017: http://www.nature.com/news/the-rise-of-the-narciss-ome-1.10240.

[U.S.] Department of Health and Human Services [HHS]. 2014. "Your Health Records." HealthIT.gov. Accessed April 14, 2017. https://www.healthit.gov/patients-families/blue-button/about-blue-button.

[U.S.] Department of Health and Human Services [HHS]. 2016. "Organ Procurement and Transplantation Network." Accessed April 18, 2017. https://optn.transplant.hrsa.gov.

Derrida, Jacques. 1992. *Given Time: I. Counterfeit Money.* Chicago: University of Chicago Press.

de Vries, Arjen E. 2013. "Telemonitoring: Weinig Effect, Toch Niet Meer te Stoppen (telemonitoring: Little Effect, But Impossible to Stop)." Webcast from the Dutch National Heart Failure Day, September 27. Accessed May 10, 2016. www.cvgk.nl/d/1415/telemonitoring-weinig-effect-toch-niet-meer-te-stoppen (in Dutch).

de Vries, Arjen E., Martie H. L. van der Wal, Wendy Bedijn, Richard M. de Jong, Rene B. van Dijk, Hans L. Hillege, and Tiny Jaarsma. 2011. "Follow-Up and Treatment of an Instable Patient With Heart Failure Using Telemonitoring and a Computerised Disease Management System: A Case Report." *European Journal of Cardiovascular Nursing* 11 (4): 432–438.

Dickenson, Donna. 2013. *Me Medicine vs. We Medicine: Reclaiming Biotechnology for the Common Good.* New York: Columbia University Press.

Dierckx, Riet, Pierpaolo Pellicori, J.G.F. Cleland, and Andrew L. Clark. 2015. "Telemonitoring in Heart Failure: Big Brother Watching *Over* You." *Heart Failure Review* 20: 107–116.

Digeser, Peter. 1992. "The Fourth Face of Power." *Journal of Politics* 54 (4): 977–1007.

Dixon, Pam, and Bob Gellman. 2014. "The Scoring of America: How Secret Consumer Scores Threaten Your Privacy and Your Future." *World Privacy Forum,* April 2. Accessed May 10, 2016. www.pogowasright.org.

DNAland. 2015. "Know Your Genome: Help Science." Accessed May 10, 2016. dna.land.

Dodds, Susan. 2000. "Choice and Control in Feminist Bioethics." In *Relational Autonomy: Feminist Perspectives on Autonomy, Agency, and the Social Self,* edited by Catriona Mackenzie and Natalie Stoljar, 213–235. Oxford: Oxford University Press.

Doerr, Megan, Chritine Suver, and John Wilbanks. 2016. "Developing a Transparent, Participant-Navigated Electronic Informed Consent for Mobile-Mediated Research." White paper, April. Accessed April 23, 2017: https://ssrn.com/abstract=2769129.

Dolgin, Elie. 2014a. "New Platforms Aim to Obliterate Silos of Participatory Science." *Nature Medicine* 20 (6): 565–566.

Dolgin, Elie. 2014b. "Patent-Free Pact Pushes the Boundaries of Precompetitive Research." *Nature Medicine* 20 (6): 564–565.

Donders, Yvonne. 2011. "The Right to Enjoy the Benefits of Scientific Progress: In Search of State Obligations in Relation to Health." *Medicine, Health Care and Philosophy* 14 (4): 371–381.

Doods, Justin, Kirstin Holzapfel, Martin Dugas, and Fleur Fritz. 2012. "Development of Best Practice Principles for Simplifying Eligibility Criteria." *Studies in Health Technology and Informatics* 192: 1153–1153.

Douzinas, Costas. 2000. *The End of Human Rights: Critical Legal Thought at the Turn of the Century.* Oxford: Hart Publishing.

Dove, Edward S. 2013. Review of *The Connected Self: The Ethics and Governance of the Genetic Individual*, by Heather Widdows. *New Genetics and Society* 32 (4): 448–451.

Dove, Edward S., Yann Joly, and Bartha M. Knoppers. 2011. "Power to the People: A Wiki-Governance Model for Biobanks." *Genome Biology* 13 (5): 158.

Downie, Jocelyn, and Jennifer J. Llewellyn, eds. 2011. *Being Relational: Reflections on Relational Theory and Health Law.* Vancouver: University of British Columbia Press.

Dryzek, John S. 1996. "Political Inclusion and the Dynamics of Democratization." *American Political Science Review* 90 (1): 475–487.

Dryzek, John S., David Downes, Christian Hunold, David Schlosberg, and Hans-Kristian Hernes. 2003. *Green States and Social Movements: Environmentalism in the United States, United Kingdom, Germany, and Norway.* Oxford: Oxford University Press.

Dryzek, John S., and Aviezer Tucker. 2008. "Deliberative Innovation to Different Effect: Consensus Conference in Denmark, France, and the United States." *Public Administration Review* 68 (5): 864–876.

Durkheim, Emile. 1969 [1898]. "Individualism and the Intellectuals." Translated and commented on by Steven Lukes. In Steven Lukes, "Durkheim's 'Individualism and the Intellectuals.'" *Political Studies* 17 (1): 1–27.

Duster, Troy. 2015. "A Post-Genomic Surprise: The Molecular Reinscription of Race in Science, Law, and Medicine." *British Journal of Sociology* 66 (1): 1–27.

Dyke, Stephanie O. M, Edward S. Dove, and Bartha M. Knoppers. 2016. "Sharing Health-Related Data: A Privacy Test?" *NPJ Genomic Medicine* 1:16024.

Eagle, Nathan, and Kate Greene. 2014. *Reality Mining: Using Big Data to Engineer a Better World.* Cambridge, MA: MIT Press.

Eggers, Dave. 2013. *The Circle.* London: Penguin.

Eggleson, Kathleen. 2014. "Transatlantic Divergences in Citizen Science Ethics— Comparative Analysis of the DIYbio Code of Ethics Drafts of 2011." *NanoEthics* 8 (2): 187–192.

Eisenberg, Richard. 2015. "Your Doctor Will Skype You Now." *Forbes*, September 27. Accessed May 10, 2016. www.forbes.com.

El Emam, Khaled, Sam Rodgers, and Bradley Malin. 2015. "Anonymising and Sharing Individual Patient Data." *British Medical Journal* 350:h1139.

Elliott, Carl. 2004. *Better Than Well: American Medicine Meets the American Dream.* London: W. W. Norton.

Elster, Jon. 1989. *The Cement of Society.* Cambridge, UK: Cambridge University Press.

Elwyn, Glyn, Paul James Barr, Stuart W. Grande, Rachel Thompson, Thom Walsh, and Elissa M. Ozanne. 2013. "Developing CollaboRATE: A Fast and Frugal Patient-Reported Measure of Shared Decision Making in Clinical Encounters." *Patient Education & Counseling* 356: 102–107.

Ely, Eleanor. 2008. "Volunteer Monitoring and the Democratization of Science." *Volunteer Monitor* 19 (1): 1–5.

Epstein, Charlotte. 2013. "Theorizing Agency in Hobbes's Wake: The Rational Actor, the Self, or the Speaking Subject?" *International Organization* 67 (2): 287–316.

Epstein, Steven. 1995. "The Construction of Lay Expertise: AIDS Activism and the Forging of Credibility in the Reform of Clinical Trials." *Science, Technology, & Human Values* 20 (4): 408–437.

Epstein, Steven. 1996. *Impure Science: AIDS, Activism, and the Politics of Knowledge.* Berkeley: University of California Press.

Ericson, Richard V., and Aaron Doyle. 2003. *Risk and Morality.* Toronto: University of Toronto Press.

European Commission. 2014. "Advice for 2016/2017 of the Horizon 2020 Advisory Group for Societal Challenge 1, 'Health, Demographic Change and Wellbeing.'" Brussels: European Commission. Accessed May 15, 2016. ec.europa.eu.

European Commission. 2016. "Reform of EU data Protection Rule." Accessed May 10, 2016. ec.europa.eu.

European Council. 2015. "EU Data Protection Reform: Council Confirms Agreement with the European Parliament." Press release, December 18. Accessed May 10, 2016. www.consilium.europa.eu.

European Parliament. 2016. "Data Protection Reform—Parliament Approves New Rules Fit for The Digital Era." Press release, April 14. Accessed May 10, 2016. www.europarl.europa.eu.

European Science Foundation [ESF]. 2012. *Personalised Medicine for the European Citizen—Towards More Precise Medicine for The Diagnosis, Treatment and Prevention of Disease.* Strasbourg: ESF.

European Society of Radiology [ESR]. 2011. "Medical Imaging in Personalised Medicine: A White Paper of the Research Committee of the European Society of Radiology." *Insights into Imaging* 2 (6): 621–630.

Evans, Barbara J. 2016. "Barbarians at the Gate: Consumer-Driven Health Data Commons and the Transformation of Citizen Science." *American Journal of Law and Medicine* 42 (4).

Explore Data Initiative. n.d. "Data Catalog." Accessed May 10, 2016. catalog.data.gov/dataset.

Eysenbach, Gunther. 2005. "The Law of Attrition." *Journal of Medical Internet Research* 7 (1): e11.

Facio, Flavia M., Stephanie Brooks, Johanna Loewenstein, Susannah Green, Leslie G. Biesecker, and Barbara B. Biesecker. 2011. "Motivators for Participation in a Whole-Genome Sequencing Study: Implications for Translational Genomics Research." *European Journal of Human Genetics* 19 (12): 1213–1217.

Fanning, Jason, and Edward McAuley. 2014. "A Comparison of Tablet Computer and Paper-Based Questionnaires in Healthy Aging Research." *Journal of Medical Internet Research* 3 (3): e38.

Federal Trade Commission [FTC]. 2000. "Privacy Online: Fair Information Practices in the Electronic Marketplace. A Report to Congress (May)." Accessed May 10, 2016, www.ftc.gov.

Fleming, Gina. 2015. "Data Digest: Announcing Our Annual Benchmark on the State of US Consumers and Technology in 2015." Forrester Research, September 28. Accessed August 22, 2016. blogs.forrester.com.

Food and Drug Administration [FDA]. 2009. "Guidance for Industry: Patient-Reported Outcome Measures: Use in Medicinal Product Development to Support Labeling Claims." Accessed May 10, 2016. www.fda.gov.

Fornai, Francesco, Patrizia Longone, Luisa Cafaro, Olga Kastsiuchenka, Michela Ferrucci, Maria L. Manca, Gloria Lazzeri, Alida Spalloni, Natascia Bellio, Paola Lenzi, Nicola Modugno, Gabriele Siciliano, Ciro Isidoro, Luigi Murri, Stefano Ruggieri, and Antonio Paparelli. 2008. "Lithium Delays Progression of Amyotrophic Lateral Sclerosis." *Proceedings of the National Academy of Sciences* 105 (6): 2052–2057.

Foucault, Michel. 1973 [French edition, 1963]. *The Birth of the Clinic: An Archaeology of Medical Perception.* Translated by A. M. Sheridan. London: Tavistock Publications.

Foucault, Michel. 1980 [1976]. *The History of Sexuality, Volume I: An Introduction.* Translated by R. Hurley. New York: Vintage Books.

Foucault, Michel. 1991 [1975]. *Discipline and Punish: The Birth of the Prison.* Translated by Alan Sheridan. Harmondsworth, UK: Penguin.

Fox, Renee C., and Judith P. Swazey. 2008. *Observing Bioethics.* New York: Oxford University Press.

Fox, Susannah. 2011. "The Social Life of Health Information." Pew Research Center, May 12. Accessed May 10, 2016. www.pewinternet.org.

Fox, Susannah. 2013. "After Dr Google: Peer-to-peer Health Care." *Pediatrics* 131 (Supplement 4): 224–225.

Fraser, Steve. 2015. *The Age of Acquiescence: The Life and Death of the American Resistance to Organized Wealth and Power.* New York: Little, Brown.

Frick, Andrea, Marie-Therese Bächtiger, and Ulf-Dietrich Reips. 2001. "Financial Incentives, Personal Information and Drop-Out in Online Studies." In *Dimensions of Internet Science,* edited by Ulf-Dietrich Reips, and Michael Bosnjak, 209–219. Lengerich, Germany: Pabst.

Frühwald, Thomas. 2013. "Eine Choosing Wisely Initiative für Österreich?" [A choosing wisely initiative for Austria?]. *Zeitschrift für Gerontologie und Geriatrie* [*Journal for Gerontology and Geriatrics*] 46 (6): 599–600.

Frydman, Gilles. 2013. "A Patient-Centric Definition of Participatory Medicine." *PatientDriven*, March 17, 2013. Accessed May 10, 2016. www.patientdriven.org.

Fuchs, Christian, Kees Boersma, Anders Albrechtslund, and Marisol Sandoval. 2012. "Introduction: Internet and Surveillance." In *Internet and Surveillance: The Challenges of Web 2.0 and Social Media,* edited by Christian Fuchs, Kees Boersma, Anders Albrechtslund, and Marisol Sandoval, 1–28. New York and London: Routledge.

Gallagher, Arlene M., Efrosini Setakis, Jonathan M. Plumb, Andreas Clemens, and Tjeerd-Pieter van Staa. 2011. "Risk of Stroke and Mortality Associated with Suboptimal Anticoagulation in Atrial Fibrillation Patients." *Thrombosis and Haemostatis* 6 (5): 968–977.

Gallarotti, Giulio M. 2011. "Soft Power: What It Is, Why It's Important, and the Condition for its Effective Use." *Journal of Political Power* 4 (1): 25–41.

Gawande, Atul. 2014. *Being Mortal: Medicine and What Matters in the End.* Toronto: Doubleday Canada.

Geppert, Cynthia, Philip Candilis, Stephen Baker, Charles Lidz, Paul Appelbaum, and Kenneth Fletcher. 2014. "Motivations of Patients with Diabetes to Participate in Research." *AJOB Empirical Bioethics* 5 (4): 14–21.

Gewin, Virginia. 2013. "Biotechnology: Independent Streak." *Nature* 499 (7459): 509–511.

Gibbs, Wayt W. 2004. "Biomarkers and Ageing: The Clock-Watcher." *Nature* 508 (7495): 168–170.

Gilleade, Kiel, and Stephen H. Fairclough. 2010. "Physiology as XP—Body Blogging to Victory." *BIOS-PLAY.* Accessed May 10, 2016. www.physiologicalcomputing.net.

Gilligan, Carol C. 1982. *In a Different Voice: Psychological Theory and Women's Development.* Cambridge, MA: Harvard University Press.

Glasziou, Paul, Ray Mynihan, Tessa Richards, and Fiona Godlee. 2013. "Too Much Medicine, Too Little Care." *British Medical Journal* 347: f4747.

Global Disaster Alert and Coordination System [GDACS]. 2014. "GDACS: Global Disaster Alert and Coordination System." Accessed May 10, 2016. portal.gdacs.org.

Goetz, Thomas. 2008. "Practicing Patients." *New York Times,* March 23. Accessed May 10, 2016, www.nytimes.com.

Gold, Ashley. 2014. "Global Healthcare IT Market Projected to Hit $66 by 2020." *FierceHealthIT,* April 1. Accessed May 10, 2016. www.fiercehealthit.com.

Goldacre, Ben. 2012. *Bad Pharma: How Drug Companies Mislead Doctors and Harm Patients.* London: Fourth Estate.

Good Stewardship Working Group. 2011. "The 'Top 5' Lists in Primary Care: Meeting the Responsibility of Professionalism." *Archives of Internal Medicine* 171 (15): 1385–1390.

Google DeepMind. 2016. "DeepMind Health: Clinician-Led Technology." Accessed May 10. 2016. deepmind.com/health.

Gottweis, Herbert. 1998. *Governing Molecules: The Discursive Politics of Genetic Engineering in Europe and the United States.* Cambridge, MA: MIT Press.

Goyal, Deepak, Jasmine Bhaskar, and Prashant Singh. 2012. "Designing the Low Cost Patient Monitoring Device (LCPMD) & Ubiquitous Based Remote Health Monitoring and Health Management System Using Tablet PC." Parallel Distributed and Grid Computing [PDGC], 2nd IEEE International Conference, Solan, India, December 6–8.

Graeber, David. 2001. *Toward an Anthropological Theory of Value: The False Coin of Our Own Dreams.* New York: Palgrave Macmillan.

Grand View Research. 2017. "Electronic Health Records Market Size Worth $33.41 Billion by 2025, April. Accessed April 17, 2017. http://www.grandviewresearch.com/press-release/global-electronic-health-records-market.

Greenhalgh, Hugo. 2015. "Sell Your Own Personal Data." *Financial Times,* October 16. Accessed May 15, 2016. www.ft.com.

Greenhalgh, Trisha, Jeremy Howick, Neal Maskrey, for the Evidence Based Medicine Renaissance Group. 2014. "Evidence Based Medicine: A Movement in Crisis?" *British Medical Journal* 348: g3725. doi: https://doi.org/10.1136/bmj.g3725.

Greysen, Scott R., Raman R. Khanna, Ronald Jacolbia, Herman M. Lee, and Andrew D. Auerbach. 2014. "Tablet Computers for Hospitalized Patients: A Pilot Study to Improve Patient Engagement." *Journal of Hospital Medicine* 9 (6): 296–399.

Griffith, Erin. 2014. "Why Big Health Insurance Is Pouring Money into Startups." *Fortune,* September 24. Accessed May 15, 2016. www.fortune.com.

Gromeier, Matthias. 2018. "Use of the Polio Virus to Treat Glioblastoma." *Annual Review of Medicine* 69. doi: 10.1146/annurev-med-050715-104655.

Gruessner, Vera. 2015. "These Wearable Devices Detect UV Radiation, Prevent Cancer." mHealthIntelligence.com, June 15. Accessed August 14, 2016. www.mhealthintelligence.com.

Gunaratnam, Yasmin. 2014. "Morbid Mixtures: Hybridity, Pain and Transnational Dying." *Subjectivity* 7 (1): 74–91.

Gunderman, Richard B., and Allison A. Tillack. 2012. "The Loneliness of the Long-Distance Radiologist." *Journal of the American College of Radiology* 9 (8): 530–533.

Gurwitz, David, Elena Milanesi, and Thomas Koenig. 2014. "Grant Application Review: The Case of Transparency." *PLoS Biology* 12 (12): e1002010.

Gymrek, Melissa, Amy L. McGuire, David Golan, Eran Halperin, and Yaniv Erlich. 2013. "Identifying Personal Genomes by Surname Inference." *Science* 339 (6117): 321–324.

Hafen, E., D. Kossmann, and A. Brand. 2014. "Health Data Cooperatives—Citizen Empowerment." *Methods of Information in Medicine* 53 (2): 82–86.

Haggerty, Kevin D. 2006. "Tear Down the Walls: On Demolishing the Panopticon." In *Theorizing Surveillance. The Panopticon and Beyond,* edited by David Lyon, 23–45. Uffculme, UK: Willan Publishing.

Haggerty, Kevin D., and Richard V. Ericson. 2000. "The Surveillant Assemblage." *British Journal of Sociology* 51 (4): 605–622.

Haig, Scott. 2007. "When the Patient is a Googler." *Time,* November 8. Accessed May 10, 2013. www.time.com.

Hakkarainen, Päivi. 2012. "'No Good for Shoveling Snow and Carrying Firewood': Social Representations of Computers and the Internet by Elderly Finnish Non-Users." *New Media and Society* 14 (7): 1198–1215.

Haklay, Muki. 2009. "The Digital Divide of OpenStreetMap." Povesham.Wordpress, December 28. Accessed May 10, 2016. povesham.wordpress.com.

Haraway, Donna. 1991. *Simians, Cyborgs, and Women: The Reinvention of Nature.* New York: Routledge.

Haraway, Donna. 2013 [1991]. "A Cyborg Manifesto: Science, Technology and Socialist-Feminism in the Late Twentieth Century." In *Simians, Cyborgs and Women: The Reinvention of Nature,* edited by Donna Haraway, 273–328. New York: Taylor and Francis.

Harris, Anna, Susan E. Kelly, and Sally Wyatt. 2016. *Cybergenetics. Health Genetics and the New Media.* London: Routledge.

Hartzband, Pamela, and Jerome Groopman. 2016. "Medical Taylorism." *New England Journal of Medicine* 374 (2): 106–108.

Harvey, Alison, Angela Brand, Stephen T. Holgate, Lars V. Kristiansen, Hans Lehrach, Aarno Palotie, and Barbara Prainsack. 2012. "The Future of Technologies for Personalised Medicine." *New Biotechnology* 29 (6): 625–633.

Haselton, Martie G., Daniel Nettle, and Paul W. Andrews. 2005. "The Evolution of Cognitive Bias." In *The Handbook of Evolutionary Psychology,* edited by David M. Buss, 724–746. Hoboken, NJ: John Wiley and Sons.

Hatch, Mark. 2013. *The Maker Movement Manifesto: Rules for Innovation in the New World of Crafters, Hackers, and Tinkerers.* New York: McGraw-Hill Professional.

Hatkoff, Craig, Irwin Kula, and Zach Levine. 2014. "How To Die In America: Welcome to La Crosse, Wisconsin." *Forbes,* April 23. www.forbes.com.

Hatt, Tim, Corina Gardner, Adam Wills, and Martin Harris. 2013. "Scaling Mobile for Development. Harness the Opportunity in the Developing World." *GSMA Intelligence,* April. Accessed May 10, 2016, www.gsmaintelligence.com.

Haugaard, Mark. 2012. "Rethinking the Four Dimensions of Power: Domination and Empowerment." *Journal of Political Power* 5 (1): 33–54.

Hawn, Carleen. 2009. "Take two aspirin and tweet me in the morning: how Twitter, Facebook, and othe social media are reshaping health care." *Health Affairs* 28 (2): 361–368.

Hayden, Cori. 2003. *When Nature Goes Public: The Making and Unmaking of Bioprospecting in Mexico.* Princeton, NJ: Princeton University Press.

Hayden, Cori. 2007. "Taking as Giving Bioscience, Exchange, and the Politics of Benefit-sharing." *Social Studies of Science* 37 (5): 729–758.

[U.K.] Health and Social Care Information Centre (HSCIC). 2015. "Letter from Dawn Monaghan, Information Commissioner's Office to Kingsley Manning, Health and Social Care Information Centre" See p. 74–76, December. Accessed April 14, 2017. https://www.gov.uk/government/uploads/system/uploads/attachment_data/file/478842/20151125_HSCICBoardpapers_Part1_Web.pdf.

"Healthcare Startup Boom: 2015 Could See More than $12B Invested into VC-Backed Companies." 2015. *CB Insights,* September 17. Accessed May 15, 2016: www.cbinsights.com.

Hedgecoe, Adam. 2004. *The Politics of Personalised Medicine: Pharmacogenetics in the Clinic.* Cambridge, UK: Cambridge University Press.

Hedgecoe, Adam, and Paul Martin. 2003. "The Drugs Don't Work: Expectations and the Shaping of Pharmacogenetics." *Social Studies of Science* 33 (3): 327–364.

Heidegger, Martin. 1996 [1927]. *Being and Time.* Translated by Joan Stambaugh. Albany: State University of New York Press.

Hein, Buster. 2015. "How Apple Watch Could Predict Heart Attacks in the Future." CultofMac, May 8. Accessed May 10, 2016. www.cultofmac.com.

Heiskala, Risto. 2001. "Theorizing Power: Weber, Parsons, Foucault and Neostructuralism." *Social Science Information* 41 (2): 241–264.

Hern, Alex. 2016. "Facebook's 'Ethnic Affinity' Advertising Sparks Concerns of Racial Profiling." *The Guardian,* March 22. Accessed November 6, 2016. www.theguardian.com.

Hicks, Jennifer. 2016. "Beyond Fitness Trackers at CES: Tiny Wearable Biosensor Continuously Monitors Your Body Chemistry." *Forbes,* January 7. Accessed May 10, 2016. www.forbes.stfi.re.

Hilbert, Martin. 2011. "Digital Gender Divide or Technologically Empowered Women in Developing Countries? A Typical Case of Lies, Damned Lies, and Statistics." *Women's Studies International Forum* 34 (6): 479–489.

Hill, Shirley. 2003. *Managing Sickle Cell Disease in Low-Income Families.* Philadelphia: Temple University Press.

Hiltzik, Michael. 2015. "Need Help Paying for Amgen's Repatha? Get Ready to Give up Your Privacy." *Los Angeles Times,* November 13. Accessed May 10, 2016. www.latimes.com

Hindmarsh, Richard, and Barbara Prainsack (eds). 2010. *Genetic Suspects: Global Governance of Forensic DNA Profiling and Databasing.* Cambridge, UK: Cambridge University Press.

Hobbes, Thomas. 1651. *Leviathan.* Full text available at: www.gutenberg.org/files/3207/3207-h/3207-h.htm. Accessed May 14, 2016.

Hobbs, Sarah J., and Piran C. L. White. 2012. "Motivations and Barriers in Relation to Community Participation in Biodiversity Recording." *Journal for Nature Conversation* 20 (6): 364–373.

Hochman, David. 2007. "Michael Hebberoy, a Food Provocateur, Moves His Feast to Seattle." *New York Times,* November 8. Accessed May 10, 2016, www.nytimes.com.

Hodson, Hal. 2016. "Revealed: Google AI Has Access to Huge Haul of NHS Patient Data." *New Scientist,* April 29. Accessed May 15, 2016. www.newscientist.com.

Hoffman, Sharona, Andy Podgurski. 2009. "E-Health Hazards: Provider Liability and Electronic Health Record Systems." *Berkeley Technology Law Review* 24 (4): 1523–1581.

Hogerzeil, Hans V. 2013. "Big Pharma and Social Responsibility—The Access to Medicine Index." *New England Journal of Medicine* 369 (10): 896–899.

Hood, Leroy. 2014. "Leroy Hood on Participatory Medicine: Future Benefits and Challenges Ahead." *Biome,* April 15. Accessed May 6, 2014.

Hood, Leroy, and Charles Auffray. 2013. "Participatory Medicine: A Driving Force for Revolutionizing Healthcare." *Genome Medicine* 5 (110). Accessed May 10, 2016. doi:10.1186/gm514.

Hood, Leroy, and Mauricio Flores. 2012. "A Personal View on Systems Medicine and the Emergence of Proactive P4 Medicine: Predictive, Preventive, Personalized and Participatory." *New Biotechnology* 29 (6): 613–624.

Horn, Paul S., and Amadeo J. Pesce. 2002. "Effect of Ethnicity on Reference Intervals." *Clinical Chemistry* 48 (10): 1802–1804.

Horner, Lisa. 2011. *A Human Rights Approach to the Mobile Internet.* Melville, South Africa: Association for Progressive Communications. Accessed May 10, 2016. www5.apc.org/es/system/files/LisaHorner_MobileInternet-ONLINE.pdf.

Horning, Reid. 2011. "Implementing an Electronic Medical Record With Computerized Prescriber Order Entry at a Critical Access Hospital." *American Journal of Health-System Pharmacy* 68 (23): 2288–2292.

Horrigan, Bryan. 2010. *Corporate Social Responsibility in the 21st Century: Debates, Models and Practices Across Government, Law and Business.* Cheltenham, UK: Edward Elgar Publishing.

Horvath, Steve. 2013. "DNA Methylation Age of Human Tissues and Cell Types." *Genome Biology* 14 (10): R115.

Howe, Daniel C., and Helen Nissenbaum. 2009. "Resisting Surveillance in Web Search." In *Lessons from the Identity Trail: Anonymity, Privacy and Identity in a Networked Society,* edited by Ian R. Kerr, Valerie M. Steeves, and Carole Lucock, 417–438. New York: Oxford University Press.

Howie, Lynn, Bradford Hirsch, Tracie Locklear, and Amy P. Abernethy. 2014. "Assessing the Value of Patient-Generated Data to Comparative Effectiveness Research." *Health Affairs* 33 (7): 1220–1228.

Huang, Bevan E., Widya Mulyasasmita, and Gunaretnam Rajagopal. 2016. "The Path from Big Data to Precision Medicine." *Expert Review of Precision Medicine and Drug Development* 1 (2): 129–143.

Hufstader Gabriel, M., Emily B. Jones, Leila K. Samy, and Jennifer King. 2014. "Progress and Challenges: Implementation and Use of Health Information Technology Among Critical-Access Hospitals." *Health Affairs* 33 (7): 1262–1270.

Hughes, Benjamin, Indra Joshi, and Jonathan Wareham. 2008. "Health 2.0 and Medicine 2.0: Tensions and Controversies in the Field." *Journal of Medical Internet Research* 10 (3): e23.

Humanitarian Kiosk. n.d. "What Is It?" Accessed May 10, 2016. www.humanitarianresponse.info.

Hunter, Kathryn M. 1991. *Doctors' Stories: The Narrative Structure of Medical Knowledge.* Princeton, NJ: Princeton University Press.

Insel, Thomas. 2011. "Director's Blog: Improving Diagnosis Through Precision Medicine." Director's Blog, National Institutes of Health, November 15. Accessed May 10, 2016. www.nimh.nih.gov.

InSTEDD. 2016. "InSTEDD Innovative Support to Emergencies Diseases and Disasters." Accessed May 10, 2016. www.instedd.org.

[U.S.] Institute of Medicine of the National Academies [IOM]. 2014. *Capturing Social and Behavioral Domains and Measures in Electronic Health Records: Phase 2.* Washington: National Academies Press.

[U.S.] Institute of Medicine of the National Academies [IOM]. 2015. *Dying in America: Improving Quality and Honoring Individual Preferences Near the End of Life.* Washington, D.C.: National Academies Press.

Jacob, Marie-Andrée. 2012. *Matching Organs with Donors: Legality and Kinship in Transplants.* Philadelphia: University of Pennsylvania Press.

Jasanoff, Sheila. 2004. "The Idiom of Co-Production." In *States of Knowledge: The Co-production of Science and the Social Order,* edited by Sheila Jasanoff, 1–12. London: Routledge.

Jensen, Peter B., Lars J. Jensen, and Søren Brunak. 2012. "Mining Electronic Health Records: Towards Better Research Applications and Clinical Care." *Nature Reviews Genetics* 13 (6): 395–405.

John, Nicholas A. 2012. "Sharing and Web 2.0: The Emergence of a Keyword." *New Media and Society* 15 (2): 167–182.

Jones, Kathryn. 2008. "In Whose Interest? Relationships Between Health Consumer Groups and the Pharmaceutical Industry in the UK." *Sociology of Health and Illness* 30 (6): 929–943.

Jotkowitz, A. B., and S. Glick. 2009. "Navigating the Chasm Between Religious and Secular Perspectives in Modern Bioethics." *Journal of Medical Ethics* 35 (6): 357–360.

Joyce, Kelly. 2008. *Magnetic Appeal: MRI and the Myth of Transparency.* Ithaca, NY: Cornell University Press.

Joyce, Kelly. 2010. "The Body as Image." In *Biomedicalization: Technoscience, Health, and Illness in the US,* edited by Adele E. Clarke, Janet K. Shim, Laura Mamo, Jennifer R. Fosket, and Jennifer R. Fishman, 197–217. Durham, NC: Duke University Press.

Juengst, Eric, Michelle L. McGowan, Jennifer R. Fishman, and Richard A. Settersten. 2016. "From 'Personalized' to 'Precision' Medicine: The Ethical and Social Implications of Rhetorical Reform in Genomic Medicine." *Hastings Center Report* 46 (5): 21–33.

Jutel, Annemarie, and Deborah Lupton. 2015. "Digitizing Diagnosis: A Review of Mobile Applications in the Diagnostic Process." *Diagnosis* 2 (2): 89–96.

Kahneman, Daniel. 2011. *Thinking Fast and Slow.* Basingstoke, UK: Macmillan.

Kahneman, Daniel, Jack L. Knetsch, and Richard H. Thaler. 1986. "Fairness and the Assumptions of Economics." *Journal of Business:* S285-S300.

Kai, Joe, J. Beavan, and C. Faull. 2011. "Challenges of Medicated Communication, Disclosure and Patient Autonomy in Cross-Cultural Cancer Care." *British Journal of Cancer* 105 (7): 918–924.

Kallinikos, Jannis. 2006. *Consequences of Information: Institutional Implications of Technological Change.* Northampton, MA: Edward Elgar Publishing.

Kallinikos, Jannis, and Niccolò Tempini. 2014. "Patient Data as Medical Facts: Social Media Practices as a Foundation For Medical Knowledge Creation." *Information Systems Research* 25 (4): 817–833.

Kang, Jerry, Katie Shilton, Deborah Estrin, Jeff Burke, and Mark Hansen. 2012. "Self-Surveillance Privacy." *Iowa Law Review* 97: 809–847.

Katz, Jay. 2002 [1984]. *The Silent World of Doctor and Patient.* Baltimore, MD: Johns Hopkins University Press.

Kaufman, Sharon R. 2005. *And a Time to Die: How American Hospitals Shape the End of Life.* New York: Simon and Schuster.

Kaufman, Sharon R. 2015. *Ordinary Medicine.* Durham, NC: Duke University Press.

Kaye, J., Edgar A. Whitley, Nadja Kanellopoulou, Sadie Creese, Kay J. Hughes, and David Lund. 2011. "Dynamic Consent: A Solution to a Perennial Problem?" *British Medical Journal* 343: d6900–d6900.

Kelly, S. E., T. D. Spector, L. F. Cherkas, B. Prainsack, and J. M. Harris. 2015. "Evaluating the Consent Preferences of UK Research Volunteers for Genetic and Clinical Studies." *PloS One* 10 (3): e0118027.

Kelty, Christopher, Aaron Panofsky, Morgan Currie, Roderic Crooks, Seth Erickson, Patricia Garcia, Michael Wartenbe, and Stacy Wood. 2015. "Seven Dimensions of Contemporary Participation Disentangled." *Journal of the Association for Information Science and Technology* 66 (3): 474–488.

Kerr, Anne, and Sarah Cunningham-Burley. 2000. "On Ambivalence and Risk: Reflexive Modernity and the New Genetics." *Sociology* 34 (2): 283–304.

Kerr, Anne, Sarah Cunningham-Burley, and Amanda Amos. 1998. "The New Genetics and Health: Mobilizing Lay Expertise." *Public Understanding of Science* 7 (1): 41–60.

Khoury, Muin J., and Sandro Galea. 2016. "Will Precision Medicine Improve Population Health?" *Journal of the American Medical Association* 316 (13): 1357–1358.

Khoury, Muin J., Tram K. Lam, John P. Ioannidis, Patricia Hartge, Margaret R. Spitz, Julie E. Buring, Stephen J. Chanock, Robert T. Croyle, Katrina A. Goddard, Geoffrey S. Ginsburg, Zdenko Herceg, Robert A. Hiatt, Robert N. Hoover, David J. Hunter, Barnet S. Kramer, Michael S. Lauer, Jeffrey A. Meyerhardt, Olufunmilayo I. Olopade, Julie R. Palmer, Thomas A. Sellers, Daniela Seminara, David F. Ransohoff, Timothy R. Rebbeck, Georgia Tourassi, Deborah M. Winn, Ann Zauber, and Sheri D. Schully. 2013. "Transforming Epidemiology for 21st Century Medicine and Public Health." *Cancer Epidemiology, Biomarkers and Prevention* 22 (4): 508–516.

Kickbusch, Ilona. 1989. "Self-Care in Health Promotion." *Social Science and Medicine* 29 (2): 125–130.

King, Rachael. 2015. "Analytics Predict Which Patients Will Suffer Post-Surgical Infections." *Wall Street Journal,* February 11. Accessed May 10, 2016, www.wsj.com.

Kinsella, Audrey. 1998. "Home Telecare in the United States." *Journal of Telemedicine and Telecare* 4 (4): 195–200.

Kirkpatrick, Robert. 2011. "Data Philanthropy Is Good for Business." *Forbes,* September 20. Accessed November 7, 2016. www.forbes.com.

Kirkpatrick, Robert. 2013. "Big Data for Development." *Big Data* 1 (1): 3–4.

Kish, Leonard J., and Eric J. Topol. 2015. "Unpatients—Why Patients Should Own Their Medical Data." *Nature Biotechnology* 33 (9): 921–924.

Klawiter, Maren. 2008. *The Biopolitics of Breast Cancer: Changing Cultures of Disease and Activism.* Minneapolis: University of Minnesota Press.

Knoppers, Bartha M., Jennifer R. Harris, Isabelle Budin-Ljøsne, and Edward S. Dove. 2014. "A Human Rights Approach to an International Code of Conduct for Genomic and Clinical Data Sharing." *Human Genetics* 133 (7): 895–903.

Knowledge@Wharton. 2012. "Why Companies Can No Longer Afford to Ignore Their Social Responsibilities." *Time,* May 28. Accessed May 10, 2016. business.time.com.

Koenig, Barbara A. 2014. "Have We Asked Too Much of Consent?" *Hastings Center Report* 44 (4): 33–34.

Koenig, Barbara A., and Jan Gates-Williams. 1995. "Understanding Cultural Difference in Caring for Dying Patients." *Western Journal of Medicine* 163 (3): 244–249.

Kohane, Isaac S. 2011. "Using Electronic Health Records to Drive Discovery in Disease Genomics." *Nature Reviews Genetics* 12 (6): 417–428.

Kontokosta, Constantine E. 2016. "The Quantified Community and Neighborhood Labs: A Framework for Computational Urban Science and Civic Technology Innovation." *Journal of Urban Technology* 23 (4): 67–84.

Koops, Bert-Jaap. 2013. "On Decision Transparency, or How to Enhance Data Protection After the Computational Turn." In *Privacy, Due Process and the Computational Turn. The philosophy of law meets the philosophy of technology,* edited by Mireille Hildebrandt, and Katja de Vries, 196–220. Abingdon, UK: Routledge.

Kristeva, Julia. 1980. *Desire in Language: A Semiotic Approach to Literature and Art.* New York: Columbia University Press.

Kruse, Corinna. 2016. *The Social Life of Forensic Evidence.* Berkeley: University of California Press.

Kusch, Maren. 1991. *Foucault's Strata and Fields. An Investigation into Archaeological and Genealogical Science Studies.* Dordrecht, Netherlands: Kluwer Academic Publishers.

Lacan, Jacques. 1977 [1966]. *Ecrits: A Selection.* Translated by A. Sheridan. London: Tavistock.

Lacan, Jacques. 2002 [1966]. *Ecrits: A Selection.* Translated by Bruce Fink. New York: W. W. Norton.

Lakoff, George, and Mark Johnson. 1980. *Metaphors We Live By.* Chicago: University of Chicago Press.

Lareau, David. 2012. "The Data Tsunami." *Healthcare IT News,* May 3. Accessed May 10, 2016. www.healthcareitnews.com.

Latimer, Joanna. 2007. "Becoming In-Formed: Genetic Counselling, Ambiguity and Choice." *Health Care Analysis* 15 (1): 13–23.

Laurent, M. 2000. "Office Parlementaire d'Evaluation des Choix Scientifiques et Technologiques" [Parliamentary Office for the Evaluation of Scientific and Technological Choices]. In *Parliaments and Technology: The Development of Technology Assessment in Europe,* edited by Norman J. Vig, and Herbert Paschen, 125–146. Albany: State University of New York Press.

Laurie, Graeme. 2002. *Genetic Privacy: A Challenge to Medico-Legal Norms.* Cambridge, UK: Cambridge University Press.

Lavee, Jakob, Tamar Ashkenazi, Avraham Stoler, Jonathan Cohen, and Rafael Beyar. 2013. "Preliminary Marked Increase in the National Organ Donation Rate in Israel Following Implementation of a New Organ Transplantation Law." *American Journal of Transplantation* 13 (3): 780–785.

Laverack, Glenn. 2009. *Public Health: Power, Empowerment and Professional Practice.* New York: Palgrave Macmillan.

Leber, Jessica. 2014. "Beyond the Quantified Self: The World's Largest Quantified Community." *Fast Company,* April 22. www.fastcoexist.com.

Leisinger, Klaus M. 2005. "The Corporate Social Responsibility of the Pharmaceutical Industry: Idealism Without Illusion and Realism Without Resignation." *Business Ethics Quarterly* 15 (4): 577–594.

Le Métayer, Daniel, and Shara Monteleone. 2009. "Automated Consent Through Privacy Agents: Legal Requirements and Technical Architecture." *Computer Law and Security* Review 25 (2): 136–144.

Lemke, Thomas. 2001. "The Birth of Bio-Politics: Michael Foucault's Lectures at the College de France on Neo-Liberal Governmentality." *Economy and Society* 30 (2): 190–207.

Lemke, Thomas. 2011. *Biopolitics: An Advanced Introduction.* New York: New York University Press.

Leonelli, Sabina. 2014. "Data Interpretation in the Digital Age." *Perspectives on Science* 22 (3): 397–417.

Leonelli, Sabina. 2016. *Data-Centric Biology: A Philosophical Study.* Chicago: Chicago University Press.

Leonelli, Sabina, Daniel Spichtinger, and Barbara Prainsack. 2015. "Sticks and Carrots: Encouraging Open Science at its Source." *GEO Geography and Environment* 2 (1): 12–16.

Lerman, J. 2013. "Big Data and Its Exclusions." *Stanford Law Review Online* 66 (55): 55–63.

Levinson, Wendy, Marjon Kallewaard, R. Sacha Bhatia, Daniel Wolfson, Sam Shortt, and Eve A. Kerr, on behalf of the Choosing Wisely International Working Group. 2015. "'Choosing Wisely': A Growing International Campaign." *British Medical Journal Quality and Safety* 24 (2), 167–174.

Levitsky, Sandra R. 2014. *Caring for Our Own: Why There Is No Political Demand for New American Social Welfare Rights.* Oxford, UK: Oxford University Press.

Levy, E., P. Levy, C. Le Pen, and A. Basdevant. 1995. "The Economic Cost of Obesity: The French Situation." *International Journal of Obesity* 19 (11): 788–792.

Lidsky, David. 2015. "Inventure: For Introducing Trust to an Unsteady Economy. *Fast-Company,* September 2. Accessed May 10, 2016. www.fastcompany.com.

Lillie, Elizabeth O., Bradley Patay, Joel Diamant, Brian Issell, Eric J. Topol, and Nicholas J. Schork. 2011. "The N-of-1 Clinical Trial: The Ultimate Strategy for Individualizing Medicine?" *Personalized Medic*ine 8 (2), 161–173.

Lluch, Maria. 2011. "Healthcare Professionals' Organisational Barriers to Health Information Technologies—A Literature Review." *International Journal of Medical Informatics* 80 (12): 849–862.

Lobstein, Tim. 2015. "Prevalence and Costs of Obesity." *Medicine* 43 (2): 77–79.

Lock, Margaret. 2013. *The Alzheimer Conundrum: Entanglements of Dementia and Aging.* Princeton, NJ: Princeton University Press.

Locke, John. 1988 [1689]. *Two Treatises of Government.* Edited by Peter Laslett. Cambridge, UK: Cambridge University Press.

Lohr, Steve. 2013. "Searching Big Data for 'Digital Smoke Signals.'" *New York Times,* August 7. Accessed May 10, 2016. www.nytimes.com.

Longhurst, Christopher A., Robert Harrington, and Nigam H. Shah. 2014. "A 'Green Button' For Using Aggregate Patient Data at the Point of Care." *Health Affairs* 33 (7): 1229–1235.

Loukides, Mike. 2014. "Academic Biology and Its Discontents." *O'Reilly Radar,* February 6. Accessed May 10, 2016. radar.oreilly.com.

Lown, Beth A., and Dayron Rodriguez. 2012. "Lost in Translation? How Electronic Health Records Structure Communication, Relationships and Meaning." *Academic Medicine* 87 (4): 392–394.

Lucivero, Federica, and Lucie Dalibert. 2013. "Should I Trust My Gut Feelings or Keep Them at a Distance? A Prospective Analysis of Point-Of-Care Diagnostic Practices." In *Bridging Distance in Technology and Regulation,* edited by Ronald E. Leenes, and Eleni Kosta, 151–163. Oisterwijk, Netherlands: Wolff Legal Publishers.

Lucivero, Federica, and Barbara Prainsack. 2015. "The Lifestylisation of Healthcare? 'Consumer Genomics' and Mobile Health as Technologies for Healthy Lifestyle." *Applied and Translational Genomics* 4: 44–49.

Lukes, Steven. 1974. *Power: A Radical View.* Houndmills, UK: Macmillan Education.

Lunshof, Jeantine E., Ruth Chadwick, Daniel B. Vorhaus, and George M. Church. 2008. "From Genetic Privacy to Open Consent." *Nature Reviews Genetics* 9 (5): 406–411.

Lunshof, Jeantine E., George Church, and Barbara Prainsack. 2014. "Raw Personal Data: Providing Access." *Science* 343 (6169): 373–374.

Lupton, Deborah. 2013. "Watery Metaphors: Swimming or Drowning in the Data Ocean." Sociological Life blog, October 29. Accessed May 10, 2016. www.simplysociology.wordpress.com.

Lupton, Deborah. 2014. "The Commodification of Patient Opinion: The Digital Patient Experience Economy in the Age of Digital Data." *Sociology of Health and Illness* 36 (6): 856–869.

Lupton, Deborah, and Annemarie Jutel. 2015. "'It's Like Having a Physician in Your Pocket!' A Critical Analysis of Self-Diagnosis Smartphone Apps." *Social Science and Medicine* 133: 128–135.

Lupton, Michelle K., Lachlan Strike, Narelle K. Hansell, Wei Wen, Karen A. Mather, Nicola J. Armstrong, Anbupalam Thalamuthu, Katie L. McMahon, Greig I. de Zubicaray, Amelia A. Assareh, Andrew Simmons, Petroula Proitsi, John F. Powell, Grant W. Montgomery, Derrek P. Hibar, Eric Westman, Magda Tsolaki, Iwona Kloszewska, Hilkka Soininen, Patrizia Mecocci, Bruno Velas, Simon Lovestone, the Alzheimer's Disease Neuroimaging Initiative, Henry Brodaty, and David Ames. 2016. "The Effect of Increased Genetic Risk for Alzheimer's Disease on Hippocampal and Amygdala Volume." *Neurobiology of Aging* 40 (April): 68–77.

Lynch, Michael, Simon A. Cole, Ruth McNally, and Kathleen Jordan. 2008. *Truth Machine: The Contentious History of DNA Fingerprinting.* Chicago: University of Chicago Press.

MacAskill, William. 2015. *Doing Good Better: How Effective Altruism Can Help You Make a Difference.* New York: Random House.

Machado, Helena, and Barbara Prainsack. 2012. *Tracing Technologies: Prisoners' Views in the Era of CSI.* Farnham, UK: Ashgate.

Mackenzie, Catriona, and Natalie Stoljar, eds. 2000. *Relational Autonomy: Feminist Perspectives on Autonomy, Agency, and the Social Self.* Oxford: Oxford University Press.

Macpherson, C. B. 1962. *The Political Theory of Possessive Individualism: Locke to Hobbes.* Toronto: Oxford University Press.

Majone, Giandomenico. 1997. "From the Positive to the Regulatory State—Causes and Consequences from Changes in the Modes of Governance" *Public Policy* 17 (2): 139–67

Manson, Neil C., and Onora O'Neill. 2007. *Rethinking Informed Consent in Bioethics.* Cambridge, UK: Cambridge University Press.

Marcantonio, E. R., J. Aneja, R. N. Jones, D. C. Alsop, T. G. Fong, G. J. Crosby, D. J. Culley, L. A. Cupples, and S. K. Inouye. 2008. "Maximizing Clinical Research Participation in Vulnerable Older Persons: Identification of Barriers and Motivators." *Journal of the American Geriatrics Society* 56 (8): 1522–1527.

Markens, Susan, C. H. Browner, and Nancy Press. 1999. "'Because of the Risks': How U.S. Pregnang Women Account for Refusing Prenatal Screening." *Social Science & Medicine* 49 (3): 359–369.

Marmot, Michael. 2005. "Social Determinants of Health Inequalities." *Lancet* 365: 1099–1104.

Marmot, Michael. 2015. *The Health Gap: The Challenge of an Unequal World.* London: Bloomsbury.

Marris, Claire. 2015. "The Construction of Imaginaries of the Public as a Threat to Synthetic Biology." *Science as Culture* 24 (1): 83–98.

Marteau, Theresa M., David Ogilvie, Martin Roland, Marc Suhrcke, and Michael P. Kelly. 2011. "Judging Nudging: Can Nudging Improve Population Health?" *British Medical Journal* 342: 263–265.

Martin, Chuck. 2014. "What the Shopper Gets Out of Being Tracked." *MediaPost,* May 28. Accessed May 10, 2016, www.mediapost.com.

Marvin, Carolyn. 1988. *When Old Technologies Were New: Thinking About Electric Communication in the Late Nineteenth Century.* New York: Oxford University Press.

Massachusetts General Hospital. 2016. "Center for Assessment Technology and Continuous Health." www.massgeneral.org/catch.

Masum, Hassan. 2012. "Insider Views of Collaborative R&D for Health: Q&A With Matt Todd." *Center for Global Health R&D,* September 13. Accessed May 10, 2016. www.healthresearchpolicy.org/blog.

Matthew, Dayna Bowen. 2015. *Just Medicine: A Cure for Racial Inequality in American Health Care.* New York: New York University Press.

Mauss, Marcel. 1966 [1925]. *The Gift.* London: Routledge and Kegan Paul.

Maust, Dawn. 2012. "Implementation of an Electronic Medical Record in a Health System." *Journal of Nursing Staff Development* 28 (1): E11-E15.

Maybury, Rick. 2013. "Should I Leave My iPad Switched On?" *Telegraph,* June 29. Accessed May 10, 2016, www.telegraph.co.uk.

Mayer-Schönberger, Viktor, and Kenneth Cukier. 2013. *Big Data.* London: John Murray Publishers.

McGoey, Linsey. 2012. "Philanthrocapitalism and its Critics." *Poetics* 40 (2): 185–199.

McGoey, Linsey. 2014. "The Philanthropic State: Market-State Hybrids in the Philanthrocapitalist Turn." *Third World Quarterly* 35 (1): 109–125.

McGoey, Linsey. 2015. *No Such Thing as a Free Gift. The Gates Foundation and the Price of Philanthropy.* London: Verso.

McGowan, Michelle L., Suparna Choudhury, Eric T. Juengst, Marcie Lambrix, Richard A. Settersten Jr., and Jennifer R. Fishman. 2017. "'Let's Pull These Technologies out of the Ivory Tower': The Politics, Ethos, and Ironies of Participant-Driven Genomic Research." *Biosocieties.* doi: 10.1057/s41292-017-0043-6.

McGowan, Michelle L., Jennifer R. Fishman, and Marcie A. Lambrix. 2010. "Personal Genomics and Individual Identities: Motivations and Moral Imperatives of Early Users." *New Genetics and Society* 29 (3): 261–290.

McGowan, Michelle L., Richard A. Settersten Jr., Eric T. Juengst, and Jennifer R. Fishman. 2014. "Integrating Genomics Into Clinical Oncology: Ethical and Social Challenges From Proponents of Personalized Medicine." *Urologic Oncology: Seminars and Original Investigations* 32 (2): 187–192.

McMahon, Aisling, Alena Buyx, and Barbara Prainsack. Work in progress. "Big Data Needs Harm Mitigation Strategies: The Role of Harm Mitigation Funds in the Governance of Data-Rich Projects."

Menke, Andy, Trevor J. Orchard, Giuseppina Imperatore, Kay M. Bullard, Elizabeth Mayer-Davis, and Catherine C. Cowie. 2013. "The Prevalence of Type 1 Diabetes in the United States." *Epidemiology* 24 (5): 773–774.

Merchant, Brian. 2015. "Looking Up Symptoms Online? These Companies Are Tracking You." *Motherboard,* February 23. Accessed May 10, 2016. motherboard.vice.com.

Meskó, Bertalan. 2014. *The Guide to the Future of Medicine: Technology and the Human Touch.* n.p.: Webicina.

Metzler, Ingrid. 2010. "Biomarkers and Their Consequences for the Biomedical Profession: A Social Science Perspective." *Personalized Medicine* 7 (4): 407–420.

Meyers, Diana. 1994. *Subjection and Subjectivity*. New York: Routledge.

Michie, Susan, and Robert West. 2013. "Behaviour Change Theory and Evidence: A Presentation to Government." *Health Psychology Review* 7 (1): 1–22.

Milberry, Kate. 2014. "(Re)making the Internet: Free Software and the Social Factory Hack." In: *DIY Citizenship. Critical Making and Social Media*, edited by Matt Ratto, and Megan Boler, 53–63. Cambridge, MA.: MIT Press.

Miller, Lisa. 2014. "The Google of Spit." *New York Times*, April 22. Accessed May 10, 2016. www.nymag.com.

Mills, C. 2011. *Futures of Reproduction: Bioethics and Biopolitics*. Dordrecht, Netherlands: Springer.

Mills, Troy R., Jared Vavroch, James A. Bahensky, and Marcie M. Ward. 2010. "Electronic Medical Record Systems in Critical Access Hospitals: Leadership Perspectives on Anticipated and Realized Benefits." *Perspectives in Health Information Management* 7:1c.

Mirowski, Philip. 2014. *Never Let a Serious Crisis Go to Waste: How Neoliberalism Survived the Financial Meltdown*. London: Verso.

Mister Jalopy. n.d. "Owner's Manifesto." *Make 04*. Accessed December 6, 2013. www.makezine.com.

Mockford, Carole, Sophie Staniszewska, France Griffiths, and Sandra Herron-Marx. 2012. "The Impact of Patient and Public Involvement on UK NHS Health Care: A Systematic Review." *International Journal for Quality in Health Care* 24 (1): 28–38.

Mol, Annemarie. 2000. "What Diagnostic Devices Do: The Case of Blood Sugar Measurement." *Theoretical Medicine and Bioethics* 21 (1): 9–22.

Moloney, Rachael M., Ellis S. Tambor, and Sean R. Tunis. 2016. "Patient and Clinician Support for the Learning Healthcare System: Recommendations for Enhancing Value." *Journal of Comparative Effectiveness Research* 5 (2): 123–128.

Moore, Gordon E. 1965. "Cramming More Components onto Integrated Circuits." *Electronics* 38 (8): 114–117.

Moore, Phoebe, and Andrew Robinson. 2016. "The Quantified Self: What Counts in the Neoliberal Workplace." *New Media and Society*. 18 (11): 2774–2792.

Moore, Sarah E. H. 2010. "Is the Healthy Body Gendered? Towards a Feminist Critique of the New Paradigm of Health." *Body and Society* 16 (2): 95–118.

Moran, Michael. 2001. "The Rise of the Regulatory State in Britain." *Parliamentary Affairs* 54 (1): 19–34.

Morden, Nancy E., Carie H. Colla, Thomas D. Sequist, and Meredith B. Rosenthal. 2014. "The Politics and Economics of Labeling Low-Value Services." *New England Journal of Medicine* 370 (7): 589–592.

Morozov, Evgeny. 2011. *The Net Delusion: How Not to Liberate the World*. London: Penguin.

Morozov, Evgeny. 2013. *To Save Everything, Click Here: The Folly of Technological Solu-tionism*. New York: Public Affairs.

Morrison, Kathleen. 2012. "Patient Utilization of ODLs and Insights Related to ODLs in Chronology." Project Health Design Blog, May 29. Accessed May 10, 2016. www.projecthealthdesign.typepad.com.

Morrison, Stacey, and Ricardo Gomez. 2014. "Pushback: Expressions of Resistance to the 'Evertime' of Constant Online Connectivity." *First Monday* 19 (8). Accessed May 10. 2016. www.firstmonday.org.

Moynihan, Ray, Jenny Doust, and David Henry. 2012. "Preventing Overdiagnosis: How to Stop Harming the Healthy." *British Medical Journal* 344: e3502.

Mul, Jos de. 1999. "The Informatization of the Worldview." *Information, Communication and Society* 2 (1): 69–94.

Muller, Mike. 2013. "Nestlé Baby Milk Scandal Has Grown Up But Not Gone Away." *The Guardian*, February 13. Accessed May 10, 2016. www.theguardian.com.

Mulley, Albert, Angela Coulter, Miranda Wolpert, Tessa Richards, and Kamran Ab-basi. 2017. "New Approaches to Measurement and Management for High Integrity Health Systems." *British Medical Journal* 356: j1401.

Murdoch, Iris. 1992. *Metaphysics as a Guide to Morals*. London: Chatto and Windus.

Murdoch, Travis B., and Allan S. Detsky. 2013. "The Inevitable Application of Big Data to Health Care." *Journal of the American Medical Association* 309 (13): 1351–1352.

My Cleveland Clinic. 2016. "My Chart." Accessed May 10, 2016. my.clevelandclinic.org/.

Napoli, Philip M., and Jonathan A. Obar. 2013. "Mobile Leapfrogging and Digital Divide Policy: Assessing the Limitations of Mobile Internet Access." New America Foundation, May 12. Accessed May 10, 2016. www.ssrn.com/abstract=2263800.

Napoli, Philip M., and Jonathan A. Obar. 2014. "The Emerging Internet Underclass: A Critique of Mobile Internet Access." *Information Society* 30 (5): 223–234.

Napoli, Philip M., and Jonathan A. Obar. 2015. "The Mobile Conversion, Internet Regression, and the 'Re-Passification' of the Media Audience." In *Producing Theory 2.0: The Intersection of Audiences and Production in a Digital World*, vol. 2), edited by Rebecca A. Lind, 125–140. New York: Peter Lang.

National Health Service [NHS] England. 2012. "The Power of Informa-tion." May 21. Accessed April 9, 2017. https://www.england.nhs.uk/2012/05/the-power-of-information/.

National Health Service [NHS] England. 2014. "Five Year Forward View." October. Ac-cessed April 9, 2017. https://www.england.nhs.uk/wp-content/uploads/2014/10/5yfv-web.pdf.

National Health Service [NHS] England. 2015. "Your Health and Care Records." March 7. Accessed April 9, 2017. http://www.nhs.uk/NHSEngland/thenhs/records/healthrecords/Pages/overview.aspx.

National Health Service [NHS] Scotland. 2016. "Realising Realistic Medicine: Chief Medical Officer's Annual Report 2015–2016." Accessed April 15, 2017. http://www.gov.scot/Resource/0051/00514513.pdf.

[U.S.] National Human Genome Research Institute [NHGRI]. 2014. "DNA Sequencing Costs" National Human Genome Research Institute, April 8. Accessed May 10, 2016. www.genome.gov.

[U.S.] National Institutes of Health [NIH]. 2016a. "All of Us Research Program Stakeholder Briefing." Accessed November 22, 2016. videocast.nih.gov.

[U.S.] National Institutes of Health [NIH]. 2016b. "PMI Cohort Program Announces a New Name: The All of Us Research Program." Accessed April 15, 2017. https://www.nih.gov/allofus-research-program/pmi-cohort-program-announces-new-name-all-us-research-program.

[U.S.] National Research Council of the Academies [NRC]. 2011. *Toward Precision Medicine: Building a Knowledge Network for Biomedical Research and a New Taxonomy of Disease*. Washington, DC: NAS.

Neal, Patrick. 1988. "Hobbes and Rational Choice Theory." *Western Political Quarterly* 41 (4): 635–652.

Nedelsky, Jennifer. 1990. "Law, Boundaries and the Bounded Self." *Representations* 30:162–189.

Nedelsky, Jennifer. 2011. *Law's Relations: A Relational Theory of Self, Autonomy, and Law*. New York: Oxford University Press.

Neff, Gina. 2014. "Data Empathy: Learning From Healthcare." *Medium,* September 5. Accessed May 10, 2016. www.medium.com.

Nelson, Eugene C., Elena Eftimovska, Cristin Lind, Andreas Hager, John H. Wasson, and Staffan Lindblad. 2015. "Patient Reported Outcome Measures in Practice." *British Medical Journal* 356:g7818.

Nelson, Julie A., and Marianne A. Ferber. 1993. *Beyond Economic Man: Feminist Theory and Economics*. Chicago: University of Chicago Press.

Nettleton, Sarah. 2004. "The Emergence of E-Scaped Medicine?" *Sociology* 38 (4): 661–679.

Nicolini, Davide. 2007. "Stretching Out and Expanding Work Practices in Time and Space: The Case of Telemedicine." *Human Relations* 60 (6): 889–920.

Nielsen, Nielsen. 2011. *Reinventing Discovery: The New Era of Networked Science*. Princeton, NJ: Princeton University Press.

Nietzsche, Friedrich W. 2011 [1886]. *Beyond Good and Evil. Unter Mitarbeit von Steven Crossley*. Old Saybrook, CT: Tantor Media.

Nike. 2012. "Nike Digital Privacy Policy." Accessed May 10, 2016. www.nike.com

Nike. 2014. "Check Out Your NikeFuel Story From 2013." Accessed February 2 2014. www.yearinnikefuel.com [user login required].

Nike. 2015. "Game On, World." Accessed May 10, 2016. www.nike.com

Nissenbaum, Helen. 2004. "Privacy as Contextual Integrity." *Washington Law Review* 79 (1): 119–158.

Noury, Mathieu, and José López. 2016. "Nanomedicine and Personalised Medicine: Understanding the Personalisation of Health Care in the Molecular Era." *Sociology of Health & Illness*. doi: 10.1111/1467-9566]

Nov, Oded. 2007. "What Motivates Wikipedians?" *Communications of the ACM* 50 (11): 60–64.

Nowotny, Helga. 2016. *The Cunning of Uncertainty*. Cambridge, UK: Polity.

Nuffield Council on Bioethics [NCOB]. 2010. *Medical Profiling and Online Medicine: The Ethics of "Personalised Healthcare" in a Consumer Age*. London: Nuffield Council on Bioethics.

N.V. 2013. "The Difference Engine: Pay Up or Shut Up." *Economist*, September 27. www.economist.com.

Nye, Joseph S., Jr. 1990. "Soft Power." *Foreign Policy* 80:157–171.

Nye, Joseph S., Jr. 2004. *Soft Power: The Means to Success in World Politics*. New York: Public Affairs.

Ohnsorge, Kathrin, Heike R. Gudat Keller, Guy A. M. Widdershoven, and Christoph Rehmann-Sutter. 2012. "'Ambivalence' at the End of Life: How to Understand Patients' Wishes Ethically." *Nursing Ethics* 19 (5): 629–641.

Olesen, Virginia, and Ellen Lewin. 1985. "Women, Health and Healing: A Theoretical Introduction." In *Women, Health and Healing: Toward a new perspective*, edited by Virginia Olesen, and Ellen Lewin, 1–24. London: Tavistock.

Oliver, Eric J. 2006. *Fat Politics: The Real Story Behind America's Obesity Epidemic*. New York: Oxford University Press.

Oliver, Kelly. 1998. *Subjectivity Without Subjects: From Abject Fathers to Desiring Mothers*. Lanham, MD: Rowman and Littlefield.

O'Neill, Onora. 2003. "Some Limits of Informed Consent." *Journal of Medical Ethics* 29 (1): 4–7.

Open FDA. n.d. "Open-Source APIs for FDA Drug, Device, and Food Data." Accessed May 10, 2016. https://open.fda.gov.

Openhumans. n.d. "Open Humans: Awesome Studies, Your Data, Advancing Research." Accessed May 10, 2016. www.openhumans.org.

OpenSNP. n.d. "Welcome to openSNP." Accessed May 10, 2016. www.opensnp.org.

Organisation for Economic Co-Operation and Development [OECD]. 2017. "Tackling Wasteful Spending on Health." January. Accessed April 20, 2007. http://www.oecd.org/health/tackling-wasteful-spending-on-health-9789264266414-en.htm.

Oudshoorn, Nelly. 2009. "Physical and Digital Proximity: Emerging Ways of Health Care in Face-To-Face and Telemonitoring of Heart-Failure Patients." *Sociology of Health and Illness* 31 (3): 390–405.

Oudshoorn, Nelly. 2011. *Telecare Technologies and the Transformation of Healthcare*. New York: Palgrave Macmillan.

Oudshoorn, Nelly. 2012. "How Places Matter: Telecare Technologies and the Changing Spatial Dimensions of Healthcare." *Social Studies of Science* 42 (1): 121–142.

Oudshoorn, Nelly, and Trevor Pinch. 2003. "How Users and Non-Users Matter." In *How Users Matter. The Co-Construction of Users and Technology*, edited by Nelly Oudshoorn, and Trevor J. Pinch, 1–29. Cambridge, MA: MIT Press.

Özdemir, Vural, Eugene Kolker, Peter J. Hotez, Sophie Mohin, Barbara Prainsack, Brian Wynne, Effy Vayena, Yavuz Coşkun, Türkay Dereli, Farah Huzair, Alexander Borda-Rodriguez, Luigi N. Bragazzi, Jack Faris, Raj Ramesar, Ambroise Wonkam, Collet Dandara, Bipin Nair, Adrián LLerena, Koray Kılıç, Rekha Jain, Jaipal P.

Reddy, Kishore Gollapalli, Sanjeeva Srivastava, and Ilona Kickbusch. 2014. "Ready to Put Metadata on the Post-2015 Development Agenda?" *OMICS: A Journal of Integrative Biology* 18 (1): 1–9.

Pálsson, Gísli. 2009. "Biosocial Relations of Production." *Comparative Studies in Society and History* 51 (2): 288–313.

Paras, Eric. 2006. *Foucault 2.0: Beyond Power and Knowledge.* New York: Other Press.

Pariser, Eli. 2012. *The Filter Bubble: What the Internet Is Hiding from You.* New York: Penguin.

Parrott, Emma. 2014. "Social Responsibility—The New Buzzword for Tech Investment?" Fieldhouse Blog, April 4. Accessed May 10, 2016. www.fieldhouseassociates.com.

Parry, Bronwyn. 2004. *Trading the Genome: Investigating the Commodification of Bio-Information.* New York: Columbia University Press.

Parsons, Talcott. 1951. "Illness and the Role of the Physician: A Sociological Perspective." *American Journal of Orthopsychiatry* 21 (3): 452–460.

Pasquale, Frank. 2015. *The Black Box Society: The Secret Algorithms That Control Money and Information.* Cambridge, MA: Harvard University Press.

PatientsLikeMe. 2014a. "How Does PatientsLikeMe Make Money?" Accessed May 10, 2016. www.patientslikeme.com

PatientsLikeMe. 2014b. "Genentech and PatientsLikeMe Enter Patient-Centric Research Collaboration." Accessed May 10, 2016. www.patientslikeme.com.

PatientsLikeMe. 2016. "Live Better, Together: Making Healthcare Better for Everyone Through Sharing, Support and Research." Accessed May 10, 2016. www.patientslikeme.com.

Patsakis, Constantinos, and Augusti Solanas. 2013. "Privacy as a Product: A Case Study in the M-Health Sector." Information, Intelligence, Systems, and Applications [IILS], 4th IEEE International Conference, Piraeus, Greece, July 10–12. *Information, Intelligence, Systems and Applications. Fourth International Conference,* 1–6.

Patterson, Christopher C., Gisela G. Dahlquist, Eva Gyürüs, Anders Green, and Gyula Soltész—the EURODIAB Study Group. 2009. "Incidence Trends for Childhood Type 1 Diabetes in Europe During 1989–2003 and Predicted New Cases 2005–20: A Multicentre Prospective Registration Study." *Lancet* 373 (9680): 2027–2033.

Peppet, Scott. 2012. "Privacy & the Personal Prospectus: Should We Introduce Privacy Agents or Regulate Privacy Intermediaries?" *Iowa Law Review Bulletin* 97: 77–93.

PerMed Consortium. 2015. *Shaping Europe's Vision for Personalised Medicine: Strategic Research and Innovation Agenda.* Cologne: Deutsches Zentrum für Luft- und Raumfahrt. Accessed May 10, 2016, www.permed2020.eu.

Petersen, Alan. 1996. "Risk and the Regulated Self: The Discourse of Health Promotion as Politics of Uncertainty." *Australian and New Zealand Journal of Sociology* 31 (1): 44–57.

Petersen, Alan, and Robin Bunton. 2002. *The New Genetics and the Public's Health.* London: Routledge.

Petersen, Alan, and Deborah Lupton. 1996. *The New Public Health: Health and Self in the Age of Risk.* London: Sage.

Pew Research Center. 2011. "Health Information is a Popular Pursuit Online." Pew Research Center, February 1. Accessed May 10, 2016. www.pewinternet.org.

Pew Research Center. 2015. "Health Fact Sheet." Pew Research Center, December 16. Accessed May 10, 2016. www.pewinternet.org.

Philippakis, Anthony A., Danielle R. Azzariti, Sergi Beltran, Anthony J. Brookes, Catherine A. Brownstein, Michael Brudno, Han G. Brunner, Orion J. Buske, Knox Carey, Cassie Doll, Sergiu Dumitriu, Stephanie O. M. Dyke, Johan T. den Dunnen, Helen V. Firth, Richard A. Gibbs, Marta Girdea, Michael Gonzalez, Melissa A. Haendel, Ada Hamosh, Ingrid A. Holm, Lijia Huang, Matthew E. Hurles, Ben Hutto, Joel B. Krier, Andriy Misyura, Christopher J. Mungall, Justin Paschall, Benedict Paten, Peter N. Robinson, François Schiettecatte, Nara L. Sobreira, Ganesh J. Swaminathan, Peter E. Tascher, Sharon F. Terry, Nicole L. Washington, Stephan Züchner, Kym M. Boycott, and Heidi L. Rehm. 2015. "The Matchmaker Exchange: A Platform for Rare Disease Gene Discovery." *Human Mutation* 36 (10): 915–921.

Pitkin, Hanna F. 1993. *Wittgenstein and Justice: On the Significance of Ludwig Wittgenstein for Social and Political Thought.* Berkeley: University of California Press.

Piwek, Lukasz, David A. Ellis, Sally Andrews, and Adam Joinson. 2016. "The Rise of Consumer Health Wearables: Promises and Barriers." *PLoS Medicine* 13/2:e1001953.

Popejoy, Alice B., and Stephanie M. Fullerton. 2016. "Genomics Is Failing on Diversity." *Nature* 538 (7624): 161.

Powles, Julia, and Hal Hodson. 2017. "Google DeepMind and Healthcare in an Age of Algorithms." *Health and Technology.* doi 10.1007/s12553-017-0179-1.

Prainsack, Barbara. 2006. "Negotiating Life: The Regulation of Embryonic Stem Cell Research and Human Cloning in Israel." *Social Studies of Science* 36 (2): 173–205.

Prainsack, Barbara. 2007. "Research Populations: Biobanks in Israel." *New Genetics and Society* 26 (1): 85–103.

Prainsack, Barbara. 2011a. "The Power of Prediction: How Personal Genomics Became a Policy Challenge." *Österreichische Zeitschrift für Politikwissenschaft* [Austrian Political Science Journal] 40 (4): 401–415.

Prainsack, Barbara. 2011b. "Voting with Their Mice: Personal Genome Testing and the 'Participatory Turn' in Disease Research." *Accountability in Research* 18 (3): 132–147.

Prainsack, Barbara. 2013. "Let's Get Real About Virtual: Online Health Is Here to Stay." *Genetics Research* 95 (4): 111–113.

Prainsack, Barbara. 2014a. "Understanding Participation: The 'Citizen Science' of Genetics." In *Genetics as Social Practice: Transdisciplinary Views on Science and Culture,* edited by Barbara Prainsack, Silke Schicktanz, and Gabriele Werner-Felmayer, 147–164. Farnham, UK: Ashgate.

Prainsack, Barbara. 2014b. "The Powers of Participatory Medicine." *PLoS Biology* 12 (4): e1001837.

Prainsack, Barbara. 2014c. "Personhood and Solidarity: What Kind of Personalized Medicine Do We Want?" *Personalized Medicine* 11 (7): 651–657.

Prainsack, Barbara. 2015a. "Is Personalized Medicine Different? (Reinscription: The Sequel). Response to Troy Duster." *British Journal of Sociology* 66 (1): 28–35.

Prainsack, Barbara. 2015b. "Three 'H's for Health—The Darker Side of Big Data." *Bioethica Forum* 8 (2): 4–5.

Prainsack, Barbara. 2015c. "Why We Should Stop Talking about Data 'Sharing.'" DNAdigest Blog, December 1. Accessed May 10, 2016. www.dnadigest.org.

Prainsack, Barbara. 2016. "How to Avoid Selling Out—Public Attitudes to Commercial Access to Health Data." *BioNews*, April 25. Accessed May 10, 2016. www.bionews.org.uk.

Prainsack, Barbara, and Alena Buyx. 2011. *Solidarity: Reflections on an Emerging Concept in Bioethics.* London: Nuffield Council on Bioethics.

Prainsack, Barbara, and Alena Buyx. 2013. "A Solidarity-Based Approach to the Governance of Research Biobanks." *Medical Law Review* 21 (1): 71–91.

Prainsack, Barbara, and Alena Buyx. 2017. *Solidarity in Bioethics and Beyond.* Cambridge, UK: Cambridge University Press.

Prainsack, Barbara, and David Gurwitz. 2007. "'Public Fears in Private Places?' Ethical and Regulatory Concerns Regarding Human Genomic Databases." Special issue of *Personalized Medicine* 4 (4): 447–505.

Prainsack, Barbara, and Martin Kitzberger. 2009. "DNA Behind Bars: 'Other' Ways of Knowing Forensic DNA Evidence." *Social Studies of Science* 39 (1): 51–79.

Prainsack, Barbara, and Ursula Naue. 2006. "Relocating Health Governance: Personalized Medicine in Times of 'Global Genes.'" *Personalized Medicine* 3 (3): 349–355.

Prainsack, Barbara, and Hauke Riesch. 2016. "Interdisciplinarity Reloaded? Drawing Lessons From 'Citizen Science.'" In *Investigating Interdisciplinary Collaboration: Theory and Practice Across Disciplines,* edited by S. Frickel, M. Albert, and B. Prainsack, 194–212. New Brunswick, NJ: Rutgers University Press.

Prainsack, Barbara, and Tim D. Spector. 2006. "Twins: A Cloning Experience." *Social Science & Medicine* 63 (10): 2739–2752.

Prainsack, Barbara, and Victor Toom. 2010. "The Prüm Regime: Situated Dis/Empowerment in Transnational DNA Profile Exchange." *British Journal of Criminology* 50 (6): 1117–1135.

Prainsack, Barbara, and Effy Vayena. 2013. "Beyond the Clinic: 'Direct-To-Consumer' Genomic Profiling Services and Pharmacogenomics." *Pharmacogenomics* 14 (4): 403–412.

Preventing Overdiagnosis. 2016. "Preventing Overdiagnosis: Winding Back the Harms of Too Much Medicine." Accessed May 10, 2016. www.preventingoverdiagnosis.net.

Priaulx, Nicky, and Anthony Wrigley. 2013. *Ethics, Law and Society*, vol. 5. Farnham, UK: Ashgate.

Price, Lloyd. 2014. "An Insider's View of Health Tech." KPMG, n.d. Accessed May 15, 2016. www.kpmgtechgrowth.co.uk.

PR Newswire. 2010. "Responsible Science for Do-It-Yourself Biologists." Accessed May 10, 2016. www.prnewswire.com.

Purtova, Nadezhda. 2015. "The Illusion of Personal Data as No One's Property." *Law, Innovation and Technology* 7 (1): 83–111.

Quigley, Muireann. 2012. "Nudging for Health: On Public Policy and Designing Choice Architecture." *Medical Law Review* 21 (4): 588–621.

Rabeharisoa, Vololona, and Michel Callon. 2002. "The Involvement of Patients' Associations in Research." *International Social Science Journal* 54 (171): 57–63.

Rabeharisoa, Vololona, Tiago Moreira, and Madeleine Akrich. 2014. "Evidence-Based Activism: Patients', Users', and Activists' Groups in Knowledge Society." *BioSocieties* 9 (2): 111–128.

Raddick, Jordan M., Georgia Bracey, Pamela L. Gay, Chris J. Lintott, Phil Murray, Kevin Schawinski, Alexander S. Szalay, and Jan Valdenberg. 2010. "Galaxy Zoo: Exploring the Motivations of Citizen Science Volunteers." *Astronomy Education Review* 9 (1): 010103.

Ratto, Matt, and Megan Boler. 2014. *DIY Citizenship: Critical Making and Social Media.* Cambridge, MA: MIT Press.

Reardon, Jenny. 2011. "The 'Persons' and 'Genomics' of Personal Genomics." *Personalized Medicine* 8c(1): 95–107.

Reed, Jason, Jordan M. Raddick, Andrea Lardner, and Karen Carney. 2013. "An Exploratory Factor Analysis of Motivations for Participating in Zooniverse, a Collection of Virtual Citizen Science Projects." *Proceedings of the Annual Hawaii International Conference on System Sciences,* 610–619.

Reips, Ulf-Dietrich. 2002. "Standards for Internet-Based Experimenting." *Experimental Psychology* 49 (4): 243–256.

Relman, Arnold. 2014. "A Challenge to American Doctors." *New York Review of Books* 61 (13): 32–33.

Reuters. 2014. "23andMe Lands $1.4 Million Grant from NIH to Detect Genetic Roots for Disease." Reuters, July 29. Accessed May 10, 2016. www.reuters.com.

Rheingold, Howard. 2002. *Smart Mobs: The Next Social Revolution.* Cambridge: MA: Perseus Publishing.

Rhodes, R. A. William. 1997. *Understanding Governance.* Buckingham, UK: Open University Press.

Richardson, Janice. 2007. "The Law and the Sublime: Rethinking the Self and its Boundaries." *Law and Critique* 18 (2): 229–252.

Ridderikhoff, Jacobus, and Bart van Herk. 1999. "Who Is Afraid of the System? Doctors' Attitude Towards Diagnostic Systems." *International Journal of Medical Informatics* 53 (1): 91–100.

Riesch, Hauke, Clive Potter, and Linda Davies. 2013. "Combining Citizen Science and Public Engagement: The Open Air Laboratories Programme." *Journal of Science Communication* 12 (3): 1–19.

Rimmer, Matthew. 2012. "23andMe Inc.: Patent Law and Lifestyle Genetics." *Journal of Law, Information and Science* 22 (1): 132–164.

Rise. 2015. "Rise." Accessed May 10, 2016. www.rise.us.

Riska, Elianne. 2010. "Gender and Medicalization and Biomedicalization Theories." In *Biomedicalization: Technoscience and Transformations of Health and Illness in the U.S.*, edited by Adele E. Clarke, Janet K. Shim, Laura Mamo, Jennifer R. Fosket, and Jennifer R. Fishman, 147–170. Durham, NC: Duke University Press.

Ritzer, George, Paul Dean, and Nathan Jurgenson. 2012. "The Coming of Age of the Prosumer." *American Behavioral Scientist* 56 (4): 379–398.

Robbins, Rebecca. 2015. "At Walgreens and CVS, a Push to Collect Customer Health Data by Dangling Discounts." *STAT,* November 23. Accessed May 10, 2016. www.statnews.com.

Roberts, Dorothy. 2011. *Fatal Invention: How Science, Politics and Big Business Re-Create Race in the Twenty-First Century.* New York: The New Press.

Robertson, Tony, David G. Batty, Geoff Der, Candida Fenton, Paul G. Shiels, and Michaela Benzeval. 2013. "Is Socioeconomic Status Associated with Biological Aging as Measured by Telomere Length?" *Epidemiologic Reviews* 35 (1): 98–111.

Robert Wood Johnson Foundation. n.d. "Project HealthDesign: Rethinking the Power and Potential of Personal Health Records." Accessed May 10, 2016. www.rwjf.org.

Robinson, Laura, Shelia R. Cotton, Hiroshi Ono, Anabel Quan-Haase, Gustavo Mesch, Wenhong Chen, Jeremy Schulz, Timothy M. Hale, and Michael J. Stern. 2015. "Digital Inequalities and Why They Matter." *Information, Communication and Society* 18 (5): 569–582.

Robinson, Peter N. 2012. "Deep Phenotyping for Precision Medicine." *Human Mutation* 33 (5): 777–780.

Rorty, Richard. 1989. *Contingency, Irony, and Solidarity.* Cambridge, UK: Cambridge University Press.

Rose, Nikolas. 1999. *Powers of Freedom: Reframing Political Thought.* Cambridge, UK: Cambridge University Press.

Rose, Nikolas. 2007. *The Politics of Life Itself: Biomedicine, Power, and Subjectivity in the Twenty-First Century.* Princeton, NJ: Princeton University Press.

Roski, Joachim, George W. Bo-Linn, and Timothy A. Andrews. 2014. "Creating Value in Health Care Through Big Data: Opportunities and Policy Implications." *Health Affairs* 33 (7): 1115–1122.

Sage Bionetworks. 2014a. "History." Accessed September 22, 2014. www.sagebase.org.

Sage Bionetworks. 2014b. "Portable Legal Consent—About Informed Consent." Accessed September 22, 2014. www.sagebase.org.

Salesforce Foundation. 2014. "The 1/1/1/ Model. Salesforce Foundation Homepage." Accessed May 10, 2016. www.salesforcefoundation.org.

Sandel, Michael. 2012. *What Money Can't Buy: The Moral Limits of Markets.* London: Allen Lane.

Sawers, Paul. 2012. "Despite Record Donations, Half of Wikipedia Users Don't Know It's Not-for-Profit." *TheNextWeb,* February 5. Accessed May 10, 2016. thenextweb.com.

Schaffer, Rebecca, Kristine Kuczynski, and Debra Skinner. 2008. "Producing Genetic Knowledge and Citizenship through the Internet: Mothers, Pediatric Genetics, and Cybermedicine." *Sociology of Health and Illness* 30 (1): 145–159.

Schatz, Bruce R. 2015. "National Surveys of Population Health: Big Data Analytics for Mobile Health Monitors." *Big Data* 3 (4): 219–229.

Schmier, Jordana K., Mechelle L. Jones, and Michael T. Halpern. 2006. "Cost of Obesity in the Workplace." *Scandinavian Journal of Work, Environment and Health* 32 (1): 5–11.

Schork, Nicholas J. 2015. "Personalized Medicine: Time for One-Person Trials." *Nature* 520 (7549): 609–611.

Schradie, Jen. 2015. "The Gendered Digital Production Gap: Inequalities of Affluence." *Communication and Information Technologies Annual (Studies in Media and Communications)* 9:185–213.

Schreiber, Monika. 2014. *The Comfort of Kin: Samaritan Community, Kinship, and Marriage*. Leiden: Brill.

Science Europe. 2013. Position Statement on the Proposed European General Data Protection Regulation. *Science Europe*, Brussels. Accessed May 15, 2016. www.scienceeurope.org.

Scott, John. 2000. "Rational Choice Theory." In *Understanding Contemporary Society: Theories of the Present*, edited by Gary Browning, Abigail Halcli, and Frank Webster, 126–138. London: Sage.

Searight, Russell H., and Jennifer Gafford. 2005. "Cultural Diversity at the End of Life: Issues and Guidelines for Family Physicians." *American Family Physician* 71 (3): 515–522.

Selkirk, Christina G., Scott M. Weissman, Andy Anderson, and Peter J. Hulick. 2013. "Physicians' Preparedness for Integration of Genomic and Pharmacogenetic Testing Into Practice Within a Major Healthcare System." *Genetic Testing and Molecular Biomarkers* 17 (3): 219–225.

Serres, Michel. 1994. *Atlas*. Paris: Juilliard [in French].

Shams, Issac, Saeede Ajorlou, and Kai Yang. 2015. "A Predictive Analytics Approach to Reducing 30-Day Avoidable Readmissions Among Patients with Heart Failure, Acute Myocardial Infarction, Pneumonia, or COPD." *Health Care Management Science* 18 (1): 19–34.

Sharon, Tamar. 2014. *Human Nature in an Age of Biotechnology*. Dordrecht, Netherlands: Springer.

Sharon, Tamar. 2016. "The Googlization of Health Research: From disruptive innovation to disruptive ethics." *Personalized Medicine* 13 (6): 563–574.

Shirk, Jennifer L., Heidi L. Ballard, Candie C. Wilderman, Tina Philips, Andrea Wiggins, Rebecca Jordan, Ellen McCallie, Matthew Minarchek, Bruce V. Lewenstein, Marianne E. Krasny, and Rick Bonney. 2012. "Public Participation in Scientific Research: A Framework for Deliberate Design." *Ecology and Society* 17 (2): 29. Accessed May 10, 2016. www.ecologyandsociety.org.

Shirky, Clay. 2008. *Here Comes Everybody: The Power of Organizing Without Organizations*. New York: Penguin.

Shirts, Brian H., Andrew R. Wilson, and Brian R. Jackson. 2011. "Partitioning Reference Intervals by Use of Genetic Information." *Clinical Chemistry* 57 (3): 475–481.

Siedentop, Larry. 2014. *Inventing the Individual: The Origins of Western Liberalism*. Cambridge, M.A.: Harvard University Press.

Siegal, Gil. 2014. "Making the Case for Directed Organ Donation to Registered Donors in Israel." *Israel Journal of Health Policy Research* 3 (1). doi: 10.1186/2045-4015-3-1.

Siest, Gerard, Joseph Henny, Ralph Gräsbeck, Peter Wilding, Claude Petitclerc, Josep M. Queralto, and Peter H. Petersen. 2013. "The Theory of Reference Values: An Unfinished Symphony." *Clinical Chemistry and Laboratory Medicine* 51 (1): 47–64.

Sikweyiya, Yandisa, and Rachel Jewkes. 2013. "Potential Motivations for and Perceived Risks in Research Participation: Ethics in Health Research." *Qualitative Health Research* 23 (7): 999–1009.

Slavkovic, Aleksandra, and Fei Yu. 2015. "O Privacy, Where Art Thou? Genomics and Privacy." *Chance* 28 (2): 37–39.

Sleepio. 2016. "Let's Build Your Sleep Improvement Program." Accessed May 10, 2016. www.sleepio.com.

Smith, Adam. 1976 [1759]. *The Theory of Moral Sentiments*. Indianapolis: Liberty Classics.

Smith, Adam. 1976 [1776]. *An Inquiry into the Nature and Causes of the Wealth of Nations*. London: Everyman's Library.

Smith, Barry, Michael Ashburner, Cornelius Rosse, Jonathan Bard, William Bug, Werner Ceusters, Louis J. Goldberg, Karen Eilbeck, Amelia Ireland, Christopher J. Mungall, The OBI Consortium, Neocles Leontis, Philippe Rocca-Serra, Alan Ruttenberg, Susanna-Assunta Sansone, Richard H. Scheuermann, Nigam Shah, Patricia L Whetzel and Suzanna Lewis. 2007. "The OBO Foundry: Coordinated Evolution of Ontologies to Support Biomedical Data Integration." *Nature Biotechnology* 25: 1251–1255.

Sorell, Tom, and Heather Draper. 2012. "Telecare, Surveillance, and the Welfare State." *American Journal of Bioethics* 12 (9): 36–44.

Spreckley, Freer. 1981. *Social Audit—A Management Tool for Co-operative Working*. Leeds, UK: Beechwood College.

Stacey, Clare. 2011. *The Caring Self: The Work Experiences of Home Care Aides*. Ithaca, NY: Cornell University Press.

Stacey, Margaret. 1984. "Who Are the Health Workers? Patients and Other Unpaid Workers in Health Care." *Economic and Industrial Democracy* 5 (2): 157–184.

Stalder, Felix. 2009. "Privacy Is Not the Antidote to Surveillance." *Surveillance & Society* 1 (1): 120–124.

Stalder, Felix, and Wolfgang Sützl, eds. 2011. "Ethics of Sharing." Special issue, *Ethics* 15 (9).

Statista. 2016. "Forecast Unit Sales of Health and Fitness Trackers Worldwide from 2014 to 2015 (in millions), by Region." Accessed November 28, 2016. www.statista. com.

Stephens, Monica. 2013. "Gender and the GeoWeb: Divisions in the Production of User-Generated Cartographic Information." *GeoJournal* 78 (6): 981–996.

Sterckx, Sigrid, and Julian Cockbain. 2014. "The Ethics of Patenting in Genetics—A Second Enclosure of the Commons?" In *Genetics as Social Practice: Transdisciplinary Views on Science and Culture*, edited by Barbara Prainsack, Silke Schicktanz, and Gabriele Werner-Felmayer, 129–144. Farnham, UK: Ashgate.

Sterckx, Sigrid, Julian Cockbain, Heidi C. Howard, and Pascal Borry. 2013. "'I Prefer a Child With . . .' Designer Babies, Another Controversial Patent in the Arena of Direct-To-Consumer Genomics." *Genetics in Medicine* 15 (12): 923–924.

Stewart, Ellen. 2016. *Publics and Their Health Systems: Rethinking Participation.* Wiesbaden, Germany: Springer.

Strathern, Marilyn. 1988. *The Gender of the Gift: Problems With Women and Problems With Society in Melanesia.* Berkeley: University of California Press.

Strauss, Anselm L., Shizuko Fagerhaugh, Barbara Suczek, and Carolyn Wiener. 1982. "The Work of Hospitalized Patients." *Social Science and Medicine* 16:977–986.

Strauss, Anselm L., Shizuko Fagerhaugh, Barbara Suczek, and Carolyn Wiener. 1997. *Social Organization of Medical Work.* New Brunswick, NJ: Transaction Publishers.

Stresman, G. H., J. C. Stevenson, C. Owaga, E. Marube, C. Anyango, C. Drakeley, T. Bousema, and J. Cox. 2014. "Validation of Three Geolocation Strategies for Health-Facility Attendees for Research and Public Health Surveillance in a Rural Setting in Western Kenya." *Epidemiology and Infection* 142 (9): 1978–1989.

Strimbu, Kyle, and Jorge A. Tavel. 2010. "What are Biomarkers?" *Current Opinion in HIV and AIDS* 5 (6): 463–466.

Suber, Peter. 2012. *Open Access.* Cambridge, MA: MIT Press.

Suhrcke, Marc, Martin McKee, Regina Sauto Arce, Svetla Tsolova, and Jørgen Mortensen. 2006. "Investment in Health Could Be Good for Europe's Economies." *British Medical Journal* 333 (7576): 1017–1019.

Surden, Harry. 2007. "Structural Rights in Privacy." *SMU Law Review* 60: 1605–1629.

Swan, Melanie. 2012. "Crowdsourced Health Research Studies: An Important Emerging Complement to Clinical Trials in the Public Health Research Ecosystem." *Journal of Medical Internet Research* 14 (6): e46.

symptoms.webmd.com. 2011. "WebMD Symptom Checker." Accessed May 10, 2016. symptoms.webmd.com.

Szoka, Berin. 2013. "FDA Just Banned 23andMe's DNA Testing Kits, and Users Are Fighting Back." *Huffington Post,* November 26. Accessed May 10, 2016. www.huffingtonpost.com.

Tapscott, Don. 1997. *The Digital Economy: Promise and Peril in the Age of Networked Intelligence.* New York: McGraw-Hill.

Taweel, Adel, Stuart Speedie, Gareth Tyson, Abdel R. H. Tawil, Kevin Peterson, and Brendan Delaney. 2011. "Service and Model-Driven Dynamic Integration of Health Data." 20th ACM Conference on Information and Knowledge Management Proceedings, Glasgow, UK, October 24–28. *International Conference on Information and Knowledge Management Proceedings,* 11–17.

Taylor, Astra. 2014. *The People's Platform: Taking Back Power and Culture in the Digital Age.* New York: Picador.

Taylor, Charles. 1985a. "The Person." In *The Category of the Person: Anthropology, Philosophy, History,* edited by Michael Carrithers, Steven Collins, and Steven Lukes, 257–281. Cambridge, UK: Cambridge University Press.

Taylor, Charles. 1985b. *Philosophy and the Human Sciences: Philosophical Papers,* vol. 2. Cambridge, UK: Cambridge University Press.

Taylor, Charles. 1989. *Sources of the Self: The Making of Modern Identity.* Cambridge, MA: Harvard University Press.

Taylor, Mark. 2013. *Genetic Data and the Law. A Critical Perspective on Privacy Protection.* Cambridge, U.K.: Cambridge University Press.

Tempini, Niccolò. 2015. "Governing PatientsLikeMe: Information Production and Research Through an Open, Distributed, and Data-Based Social Media Network." *Information Society* 31 (2): 193–211.

Thaler, Richard H., and Cass R. Sunstein. 2008. *Nudge: Improving Decisions About Health, Wealth, and Happiness.* New Haven, CT: Yale University Press.

Thomas, Graham, and Sally Wyatt. 2000. "Access is Not the Only Problem: Using and Controlling the Internet." In *Technology and In/Equality: Questioning the Information Society,* edited by Sally Wyatt, Flis Henwood, and Peter Senker, 21–45. London: Routledge.

Thorpe, Charles. 2010. "Participation as Post-Fordist Politics: Demos, New Labour, and Science Policy." *Minerva* 48 (4): 389–411.

Till, Chris. 2014. "Exercise as Labour: Quantified Self and the Transformation of Exercise into Labour." *Societies* 4 (3): 446–462.

Timmermans, Stefan, and Marc Berg. 2003a. "The Practice of Medical Technology." *Sociology of Health and Illness* 25 (3): 97–114.

Timmermans, Stefan, and Marc Berg. 2003b. *The Gold Standard: The Challenge of Evidence-Based Medicine and Standardization in Health Care.* Philadelphia: Temple University Press.

Timmermans, Stefan, and Mara Buchbinder. 2010. "Patients-In-Waiting Living Between Sickness and Health in the Genomics Era." *Journal of Health and Social Behavior* 51 (4): 408–423.

Timmermans, Stefan, and Aaron Mauck. 2005. "The Promises and Pitfalls of Evidence-Based-Medicine." *Health Affairs* 24 (1): 18–28.

Titmuss, Richard. 1970. *The Gift Relationship: From Human Blood to Social Policy.* London: Allen and Unwin.

Tkacz, Nathaniel. 2015. *Wikipedia and the Politics of Openness.* Chicago: University of Chicago Press.

Tocchetti, Sara. 2012. "DIYbiologists as 'Makers' of Personal Biologies: How MAKE Magazine and Maker Faires Contribute in Constituting Biology as a Personal Technology." *Journal of Peer Production* 2:1–9.

Tocchetti, Sara. 2014. "How Did DNA Become Hackable and Biology Personal? Tracing the Self-Fashioning of the DYIbio Network." PhD thesis, London School of Economics and Political Science.

Tocchetti, Sara, and Sara A. Aguiton. 2015. "Is an FBI Agent a DIY Biologist Like Any Other? A Cultural Analysis of a Biosecurity Risk." *Science, Technology and Human Values* 40 (5): 825–853.

Toffler, Alvin. 1980. *The Third Wave: The Classic Study of Tomorrow.* New York: Bantam.

Topol, Eric. 2012. *The Creative Destruction of Medicine: How the Digital Revolution Will Create Better Health Care.* New York: Basic Books.

Topol, Eric. 2015. *The Patient Will See You Now: The Future of Medicine is in Your Hands.* New York: Basic Books.

Transplant Procurement Management [TPM]. 2010. "Donation and Transplantation Institute." Accessed May 10, 2016. www.tpm-dti.com.

Trevena, Lyndal J. 2011. "PatientsLikeMe and the Tale of Three Brothers." *Medical Journal of Australia* 195 (5): 258–259.

Trevor, Hughes J. 2016. "General Data Protection Regulation: A Milestone Of The Digital Age" Techcrunch, January 10. Accessed May 10, 2016. www.techcrunch.com.

Tsai, Adam G., David F. Williamson, and Henry A. Glick. 2011. "Direct Medical Cost of Overweight and Obesity in the USA: A Quantitative Systematic Review." *Obesity Reviews* 12 (1): 50–61.

Tsai, Daniel Fu-Chang. 2001. "How Should Doctors Approach Patients? A Confucian Reflection on Personhood." *Journal of Medical Ethics* 27 (1): 44–50.

Turner, Fred. 2010. *From Counterculture to Cyberculture: Stewart Brand, the Whole Earth Network, and the Rise of Digital Utopianism.* Chicago: University of Chicago Press.

Turow, Joseph, Michael Hennessy, and Nora Draper. 2015. "The Tradeoff fallacy: How Marketers Are Misrepresenting American Consumers and Opening Them up to Exploitation." A Report from the Annenberg School for Communication, University of Pennsylvania. Accessed December 1, 2016. www.asc.upenn.edu.

Turrini, Mauro, and Barbara Prainsack. 2016. "Beyond Clinical Utility: The Multiple Values of DTC Genetics." *Applied and Translational Genomics* 8:4–8.

Tutt, Andrew. 2016. "An FDA for Algorithms." Social Science Research Network. Accessed May 10, 2016. ssrn.com/abstract=2747994.

Tutton, Richard. 2012. "Personalizing Medicine: Futures Present and Past." *Sociology of Health and Illness* 75 (10): 1721–1728.

Tutton, Richard. 2014. *Genomics and the Reimagining of Personalized Medicine.* Farnham, UK: Ashgate.

Tutton, Richard, and Barbara Prainsack. 2011. "Enterprising or Altruistic Selves? Making up Research Subjects in Genetics Research." *Sociology of Health and Illness* 33 (7): 1081–1095.

Tyfield, D. 2012. *The Economics of Science: A Critical Realist Overview.* London: Routledge.

UBiome. 2016. Explore Your Microbiome." Accessed May 10, 2016. http://ubiome.com/.

United Nations. 1966. "International Convenant on Economic, Social and Cultural Rights." Accessed May 10, 2016. www.ohchr.org.

United Nations Global Pulse. 2014. "About Global Pulse." Accessed May 10, 2016. www.unglobalpulse.org.

University of California. 2014. "Personal Data for the Public Good." Robert Wood Johnson Foundation, March. Accessed May 10, 2016. www.rwjf.org.

Ushahidi. 2015. "Raise Your Voice." Accessed May 10, 2016. www.ushahidi.com.

Valentine, Christine. 2008. *Bereavement Narratives: Continuing Bonds in the Twenty-First Century.* London: Routledge.

van Deursen, Alexander J. A. M, and Jan A. G. M. van Dijk. 2014. "The Digital Divide Shifts to Differences in Usage." *New Media and Society* 16 (3): 507–526.

Van Dijck, José, and David Nieborg. 2009. "Wikinomics and Its Discontents: A Critical Analysis of Web 2.0 Business Manifestos." *New Media and Society* 11 (5): 855–874.

Vayena, Effy, E. Gourna, J. Streuli, E. Hafen, and B. Prainsack. 2012. "Experiences of Early Users of Direct-To-Consumer Genomic Testing in Switzerland; an Exploratory Study." *Public Health Genomics* 15 (6): 352–362.

Venco, Selma. 2012. "The Emergence of a New Medical Model: The International Division of Labour and the Formation of an International Outsourcing Chain in Teleradiology." *Work Organisation, Labour and Globalisation* 6 (2): 45–57.

Vicdan, Handan, and Nikhilesh Dholakia. 2013. "Medicine 2.0 and Beyond: From Information Seeking to Knowledge Creation in Virtual Health Communities." In *The Routledge Companion to Digital Consumption,* edited by Russell W. Belk and Rosa Llamas, 197–207. New York: Routledge.

Vickers, Geoffrey. 1983. *Human Systems Are Different.* London: Harper and Row.

Vitores, Anna. 2002. "From Hospital to Community: Case Management and the Virtualization of Institutions." *Athenea Digital.* Accessed May 10, 2016. www.atheneadigital.net.

Vogt, Henrik, Bjørn Hofmann, and Linn Getz. 2016. "The New Holism: P4 Systems Medicine and the Medicalization of Health and Life Itself." *Medicine, Health Care and Philosophy* 19 (2): 307–323.

Wachter, Robert M. 2015a. "How Medical Tech Gave a Patient a Massive Overdose." *Backchannel,* March 30. Accessed November 24, 2016. backchannel.com.

Wachter, Robert M. 2015b. *The Digital Doctor: Hope, Hype, and Harm at the Dawn of Medicine's Computer Age.* New York: McGraw-Hill Education.

Wagenaar, Hendrik. 2004. "'Knowing' the Rules: Administrative Work as Practice." *Public Administration Review* 64 (6): 643–656.

Wagenaar, Hendrik. 2011. *Meaning in Action. Interpretation and Dialogue in Policy Analysis.* Armonk, NY: M. E. Sharp.

Wagner, Jennifer K. 2013. "The Sky is Falling for Personal Genomics! Oh, Nevermind. It's Just a Cease & Desist Letter from the FDA to 23andMe." *Genomics Law Report,* December 3. Accessed May 10, 2016. www.genomicslawreport.com.

Watson, Sara M. 2013. "You Are Your Data." *Slate,* November 12. Accessed: May 10, 2016. www.slate.com.

Weaver, Matthew. 2014. "NHS Admits it Should Have Been Clearer Over Medical Records-Sharing Scheme." *The Guardian,* February 4. Accessed May 10, 2016. www.theguardian.com.

Weber, Griffin M., Kenneth D. Mandl, and Isaac S. Kohane. 2014. "Finding the Missing Link for Big Biomedical Data." *Journal of the American Medical Association* 331 (24): 2479–2480.

Webster, Andrew. 2002. "Innovative Health Technologies and the Social: Redefining Health, Medicine and the Body." *Current Sociology* 50 (3): 443–457.

Weeden, Curt. 1998. *Corporate Social Investing: The Breakthrough Strategy for Giving and Getting Corporate Contributions.* Oakland, CA: Berrett-Koehler.

Wehrlen, Leslie, Mike Krumlauf, Elizabeth Ness, Damiana Maloof, and Margaret Bevans. 2016. "Systematic Collection of Patient Reported Outcome Research Data: A Checklist for Clinical Research Professionals." *Contemporary Clinical Trials* 48:21–29.

Wei, Lu. 2012. "Number Matters: The Multimodality of Internet Use as an Indicator of the Digital Inequalities." *Journal of Computer-Mediated Communication* 17 (3): 303–318.

Welch, H. Gilbert, Lisa Schwartz, and Steve Woloshin. 2011. *Overdiangosed: Making People Sick in the Pursuit of Health.* Boston, MA: Beacon Press.

Wellcome Trust. 2016. "The One-Way Mirror: Public Attitudes to Commercial Access to Health Care." Ipsos MORI Social Research Institute." Accessed May 10, 2016. www.wellcome.ac.uk

Wesolowski, Amy, Nathan Eagle, Andrew J. Tatem, David L. Smith, Abdisalan M. Noor, Robert W. Snow, and Caroline O. Buckee. 2012. "Quantifying the Impact of Human Mobility on Malaria." *Science* 338 (6104): 267–270.

Wheeler, Deborah L. 2001. "The Internet and Public Culture in Kuwait." *International Communication Gazette* 63 (2–3): 187–201.

Wheeler, Deborah L. 2003. "The Internet and Youth Subculture in Kuwait." *Journal of Computer-Mediated Communication.* 8 (2). doi:10.1111/j.1083–6101.2003.tb00207.x.

White House. 2015. "Factsheet: President Obama's Precision Medicine Initiative" Press release, January 30. Accessed May 10, 2016. https://www.whitehouse.gov/the-press-office/2015/01/30/fact-sheet-president-obama-s-precision-medicine-initiative.

Whitten, Pamela, and Lorraine Buis. 2007. "Private Payer Reimbursement for Telemedicine Services in the United States." *Telemedicine and e-Health* 13 (1): 15–24.

Wicks, Paul, Timothy E. Vaughan, Michael P. Massagli, and James Heywood. 2011. "Accelerated Clinical Discovery Using Self-Reported Patient Data Collected Online and a Patient-Matching Algorithm." *Nature Biotechnology* 29 (5): 411–414.

Widdows, Heather. 2013. *The Connected Self: The Ethics and Governance of the Genetic Individual.* Cambridge, UK: Cambridge University Press.

Wilbanks, J. 2013. "Informed consent for online health research features PLC." *Sage Bionetworks,* March 3. Accessed March 22, 2014. www.sagebase.org.

Williams, Brian, Vikki Entwistle, Gill Haddow, and Mary Wells. 2008. "Promoting Research Participation: Why Not Advertise Altruism?" *Social Science and Medicine* 66 (7): 1451–1456.

Wilson, James. 2016. "The Right to Public Health." *Journal of Medical Ethics.* 42: 367–375.

Wolf, Anne M., and Graham A. Colditz. 1998. "Current Estimates of the Economic Cost of Obesity in the United States." *Obesity Research* 6 (2): 97–106.

Wolf, Joan B. 2010. *Is Breast Best? Taking on the Breastfeeding Experts and the New High Stakes of Motherhood.* New York: New York University Press.

Wolfson, Daniel, John Santa, and Lorie Slass. 2014. "Engaging Physicians and Consumers in Conversations About Treatment Overuse and Waste: A Short History of the Choosing Wisely Campaign." *Academic Medicine* 89 (7): 990–995.

Woolgar, Steve, and Daniel Neyland. 2013. *Mundane Governance: Ontology and Accountability.* Oxford: Oxford University Press.

World Bank. 2015. "Internet Users (per 100 people)." Accessed May 10, 2016. http://data.worldbank.org/indicator/IT.NET.USER.P2.

Wright, David. 2011. "Should Privacy Impact Assessments Be Mandatory?" *Communications of the ACM* 54 (8): 121–131.

Wu, Robert C., Diego Delgado, Jeannine Costigan, Jane Maciver, and Heather Ross. 2005. "Pilot Study of an Internet Patient-Physician Communication Tool for Heart Failure Disease Management." *Journal of Medical Internet Research* 7 (1): e8.

Yang, Jing, PingLei Pan, Wei Song, Rui Huang, JianPeng Li, Ke Chen, QiYong Gong, JianGuo Zhong, HaiChun Shi, and HuiFang Shang. 2012. "Voxelwise Meta-Analysis of Gray Matter Anomalies in Alzheimer's Disease and Mild Cognitive Impairment Using Anatomic Likelihood Estimation." *Journal of the Neurological Sciences* 316 (1): 21–29.

Zapata, Heidi. J., and Vincent J. Quagliarello. 2015. "The Microbiota and Microbiome in Aging: Potential Implications in Health and Age-Related Diseases." *Journal of the American Geriatrics Society* 63 (4): 776–781.

Ziebland, Sue, and Sally Wyke. 2012. "Health and Illness in a Connected World: How Might Sharing Experiences on the Internet Affect People's Health?" *Milbank Quarterly* 90 (2): 219–249.

Žižek, Slavoj. 2006. "Nobody Has to Be Vile." *London Review of Books* 28 (7): 10.

Zuboff, Shoshana. 2015. "Big Other: Surveillance Capitalism and the Prospects of an Information Civilization." *Journal of Information Technology* 30: 75–89.

# INDEX

ABIMF. *See* American Board of Internal Medicine Foundation

ACA. *See* Affordable Care Act

accountability, 183–84

activated patients, 15–17, 37

active participation, 68, *69*

activity trackers: Fitbit, 56, 61–62, 65; FuelBand, 55–58, 61, 63–65, 211nn5–6, 212nn10–11; telemonitoring compared with, 61–62

adult onset diabetes. *See* Type-2 diabetes

Affordable Care Act (ACA), 107–8

agenda setting, 26–27

aging, somatic biomarkers and, 102–4, 178

Aguiton, Sara, 124

algorithm-based predictive modeling, 180–83

All of Us Research Program, 3, 5, 7, 10, 79

Alphabet, 108, 127. *See also* Google

ALS. *See* amyotrophic lateral sclerosis

altruism: in organ donation, 140, 143–47; self-interest *vs.*, 135–36, 140, 142–47, 152–54, 213n5

amateurs, quality control and, 31

American Board of Internal Medicine Foundation (ABIMF), 171

Amgen, 121

amygdala, xiii, 102

amyotrophic lateral sclerosis (ALS), xiii, 22–23, 28

Apixio, 167

Apple, 20, 47, 55–56, 108, 134

Arendt, Hannah, 138

assisted reproduction, 103–4

atomistic individualism, 135–36, 142, 150, 190, 199

Ausiello, Dennis, 58–59

automation, 99–100, *100*

autonomy, 142–43, 189–91, 197

Bachrach, Peter, 83

Bainbridge, Lisanne, 99

Baratz, Morton S., 83

Bates, David, 180

battery-powered devices, 33

Baylis, Francoise, 142

BD2K. *See* Big Data to Knowledge

bedside medicine, 3

behavioral economics, 138–39

behavior change, 81–82, 84–87

Berger, Peter, 3–4

Berwick, Don, 185–86

big data analytics, 131–32, 155, 157

Big Data to Knowledge (BD2K), 79

biohacking, 124–25

biomarkerization, 3, 97–99

biomarkers: defined, 97; imaging, 97–102, 104–5; inequality and, 105–6; power and, 97–106; social, xv, 143, 154, 156, 165–66; somatic, 102–4, 178

biomedicalization (Clarke et al.), 11, 84, 115; exclusionary disciplining as part of biomedicalization, 38–39; stratified, 209n1

Birch, Kean, 94

blockbuster medicine, 1

Blue Button initiative, 168–69

Bobe, Jason, 125

Boero, Natalie, 85
Boler, Megan, 130
"Bottom of Pyramid" (BOP) consumers, xiii, 121
brain tumors, 2, 9
Brake, David, 36
breast cancer, 2, 76–77
Britnell, Mark, 15
Brunton, Finn, 126–27
Buyx, Alena, 152

Calderwood, Catherine, 163–64
cancer, xiv, 2, 9, 76–77, 101
Canguilhem, Georges, 102
capitalism, 112–15. *See also* commercial interests
CardioConsult HF, 51–55, 61–63
care.data, xiii, 123, 127, *128–29*, 132
caregiving, 197
Carmichael, Alexandra, 24
Casilli, Antonio A., 117–18
cell phones, 33, 41–42, 48, 109–10. *See also* smartphones
Center for Medicare and Medicaid, U.S. (CMS), 163, 182
Center for Urban Science and Progress, NYU, 49–50
change, behavior, 81–82, 84–87
Chiapperino, Luca, 190
choice, 189–92
Choosing Wisely, 171–74
chronic health problems, 24, 34–35, 102, 177, 204
Chu, Zen, 175
*The Circle* (Eggers), 46–47
citizen scientists, 26, 31, 210n4
Clarke, Adele, 38–39, 209n1
clinic, evidence in, 158–63
clinical reference values, 37
clinical validity and utility, 90, 213n7
CMS. *See* Center for Medicare and Medicaid, U.S.
Cohen, Glenn, 184

Cohen, Julie, 124, 131
command power, 82
commercial interests: commodification of privacy and, 130–31; CSR and, xiii, 113–14, 116–18, 213n4; data protection and, 107–8, 130–33; health activism entangled with, 26, 45, 106–11, 123, 133–34; health entrepreneurism and, 107–10; introduction to, 107–8; opting out of, 126–30, *128–29*; of PatientsLikeMe, 108–9, 123; prosumption and, 117–26; "sharing" and, 122–27. *See also* profit
Committee on a Framework for Developing a New Taxonomy of Disease, 5
communication, web-based tools for, 116
community: in categories of participation, 27–29; maker, 72; personhood and, 141; quantified, 49–50
computed tomography (CT), xiii, 97
conscious participation, 68, *69*
consent: informed, 140–41, 143, 146; instrument of, 63–65, 68, 164, 203; Portable Legal Consent, 169–70, 216n7
Consumer Reports, 171
continuous health, 73
control groups, 49
co-optive power, 82
coordination, in categories of participation, 26–27
corporate social responsibility (CSR), xiii, 113–14, 116–18, 213n4
corporate wellness programs, 58
corporations: multinational, 43, 96, 151, 206; pharmaceutical, 18, 42, 114, 121. *See also* commercial interests
cost: containment, 156–57, 177–80; of personalized medicine, 11, 42, 102, 106, 156–57, 172; of technologies, 11, 102
country doctor, 3–4
crowdsourcing, xiii, 23, 116
CSR. *See* corporate social responsibility
CT. *See* computed tomography
Cukier, Kenneth, 7, 22

CureTogether: filter bubble in, 38; as lean-forward technology, 19, 21, 24–26, 45; 23andMe acquiring, 25, 39–40, 45, 133
Curit BV, 51
*Cyborg Manifesto* (Haraway), 210n2

data: big data analytics, 131–32, 155, 157; doubles, 51, 55; drug safety, 60; entre-preneurism, 109–10; flow, 51, 66–67, 157, 204, 213n1; "Google Maps" of, 5–7, 6, 59, 187; governance, 140, 147–52, 204–5, 205; interpretation, as luxury item, 176–77; obfuscation, 130–31; observational, xv, 160–62, 180; patients as gatekeepers to, 166–68; philan-thropy, 111, 115; power asymmetries in, 43, 72, 74, 94, 124, 126–27, 150, 183, 189, 206; quality, 31, 59–60; reidentification and, 71, 170, 203; rethinking, 202–5; "sharing," 11, 67, 122–27, 123, 132–33; subjects, primary and secondary, 148; travel, 66–67; use, new understanding of, 67–73, 69; utility hierarchy of, 188; water metaphor for, 157–58. *See also* protection
data collection: from activated patients, 15–17, 37; challenges of, 59–62, 210n7; from citizen scientists, 26, 31, 210n4; conscious and/or active participation in, 68, 69; consent to, 63–65; crowd-sourcing of, 23; hypercollection, 40–41, 49, 71; inequality influencing, 37–38, 78; opting out of, 126–30, 128–29; overview of, 6–7, 10, 12–14; patient work 2.0 and, 188, 201–5, 205; public scrutiny of, 117; resistance to, 130–31; rethinking, 203–4; transparency of, 32, 39, 64. *See also* digital surveillance; transmitting patient
datafication, 7, 22, 62–65, 206
Data Protection Regulation. *See* General Data Protection Regulation, EU
Death over Dinner, 172–74

decision making. *See* personal decision making
Deleuze, Gilles, 138
dementia, 102
democratic empowerment, 191, *192*, 193, 201
democratic value, of participation, 26, 40, 44–45, 74, 94
Dennis, Carina, 202
devices, making of, 72–73
de Vries, Arjen, 52–54
diabetes, 1–2, 9
Dickenson, Donna, 8, 136
Digeser, Peter, 82–85, 87, 89, 104
digital health divide, 32–36
digital home assistants, 41–42
digital surveillance: with activity trackers, 58, 62; expansion of, in home, 50–58; participatory design of, 117–18; privacy influenced by, 42, 50, 63–65; surveil-lant assemblage and, 51–55, 57, 60; three "H"s of, 40–43; by transmitting patients, 48
direct-to-consumer (DTC), xiii, 90–96, 104–5, 212n1
discipline, 80
discrimination, 148–49, 151, 182; age, 104; racial, 10, 18–19, 86, 207; redlining, xv, 18–19
discursive meaning, 14
disempowerment: by biomarkerization, 99; by digital surveillance, 53; by DTC genetics, 96; by personalized medi-cine, 16, 18–19, 53, 79, 96, 99, 101, 106, 192, 194
DIY biology. *See* Do-It-Yourself biology
DNA databases, 95–96, 189
DNAland, 133, 170
DNA testing, 47, 75–78
Do-It-Yourself (DIY) biology, 124–26
*Downton Abbey*, 113
Draper, Heather, 53
drug safety data, 60

DTC. *See* direct-to-consumer
dualism, 136–38
Durkheim, Emile, 137–39

Eagle, Nathan, 109–10
economics: behavioral, 138–39; of partici-
    patory projects, 31–39; transparency
    of, 32
education, digital divide and, 35–36
Effective Altruism movement, 114–15
Eggers, Dave, 46–47
Eggleson, Kathleen, 125
e-health filter bubble, 37–39
elderly patients, 32
electronic health records, 78, 216n10; in
    clinic, 160–62; global market for, 107;
    patients as gatekeepers to, 166–68;
    portability of, 59
emancipatory empowerment, 191–92, *192*,
    195–98, 200–201
empowerment: concerns about, 7–11, 16,
    18–19, 44, 62, 190, 200; democratic,
    191, *192*, 193, 201; emancipatory, 191–
    92, *192*, 195–98, 200–201; fresh look
    at, 189–90, *192*; genome testing and,
    89–96; individualistic, 191–92, *192*;
    instrumental, 191, *192*, 193, 196, 200;
    research and, 18–19; self-monitoring
    and, 73–74, 198
end-of-life decision making, 140–43, 152,
    172–74
entrepreneurism, 27, 30, 107–10
epigenetics, xiii, 103
Epstein, Charlotte, 137
Ericson, Richard, 51
ESF. *See* European Science Foundation
ethnicity, 19
EU. *See* European Union
European Science Foundation (ESF), xiv,
    13
European Union (EU), xiv, 210n8. *See also*
    General Data Protection Regulation

evaluation, in categories of participation,
    27, 29
evertime, 49
evidence: accountability vacuum and,
    183–84; in clinic, 158–63; hard, 158–59;
    high-touch medicine and, 155–57,
    174–77; meaning and, 155–57; patients
    as gatekeepers and, 166–68; patients'
    experience and knowledge, 163–65;
    personal decision making and, 171–75,
    185; predictive analytics and, 180–84;
    research and, 169–70; social biomark-
    ers, xv, 143, 154, 156, 165–66; social
    life of, 154–56, 158–70, 184–86, 188;
    solidarity and, 177–80; understanding
    of, 154–55, 187–88
exclusion: new patterns of, 32–39, 188–89,
    200, 207; rationing and, 178–79
exclusionary disciplining, 38–39
Explore Data initiative, 213n1
external validity problem, 160
extitutionalization, 211n3

Facebook, 19, 21, 123
fair information practice, 131
*Fat Politics* (Oliver), 85–86
FDA. *See* Food and Drug Administration,
    U.S.
Federal Trade Commission, U.S. (FTC),
    xiv, 131
feminist scholarship, 138–39, 142
filter bubble, e-health, 37–39
Fishman, Jennifer, 31
Fitbit, 56, 61–62, 65
flow, 51, 66–67, 157, 204, 213n1
flow metric, 66–67
Food and Drug Administration, U.S.
    (FDA), xiv, 92, 95, 164, 213n1
for-profit *vs.* nonprofit distinction, 107–8,
    117, 119, 123, 133
*Forward Look on Personalised Medicine
    for the European Citizen*, 13

Foucault, Michel, 80–83, 87–88, 138, 212nn2–3
"The Fourth Face of Power" (Digeser), 82–85
Friend, Stephen, 169
Frydman, Gilles, 44
FTC. See Federal Trade Commission, U.S.
FuelBand: activity tracking with, 55–58, 61, 63–65, 211nn5–6, 212nn10–11; customer service, 65, 212nn10–11

Gallagher, Arlene, 163
Gates-Williams, Jan, 141
Gattaca, 46, 210n1
Gawande, Atul, 156
GBM. See glioblastoma multiforme
General Data Protection Regulation, EU, 62, 71–72, 130, 212n3
General Practice Research Database, 162
Genetic Data and the Law (Taylor, M.), 148
genetic risk, 76–77, 91–93, 95
genome testing: criticism of, 90–93; DTC, 90–96, 104–5, 212n1; motivations for, 31–32; power and, 89–96, 104–5; 23andMe, 75–78, 90, 94–95, 110, 189. See also DNA testing
Genomics England, 150
glioblastoma multiforme (GBM), xiv, 2
Global Pulse, 111
glucose monitoring, 1–2
Gomez, Ricardo, 36, 49
Google, 31, 134; Glass, 175; Maps, 5–7, 6, 59, 187; NHS collaborating with, 96, 108; 23andMe backed by, 95–96
Graeber, David, 58
Green Button initiative, 160–61, 168
Greene, Kate, 110
Greenhalgh, Trisha, 158–59
group-based solidarity, 152
Guattari, Félix, 138
Gunderman, Richard, 100

Haggerty, Kevin, 51
Hannan, Amir, 216n5
Haraway, Donna, 210n2
hard evidence, 158–59
hard power, 82, 189
harm, of digital surveillance, 41–42
harm mitigation: enhancement of, 43, 150; funds, 150–52, 183, 204–5, 205
HCC Profiler. See Hierarchical Condition Category Profiler
health: activism, commercial interest entangled with, 26, 45, 106–11, 123, 133–34; chronic problems with, 24, 34–35, 102, 177, 204; continuous, 73; digital, divide in, 32–36; e-health filter bubble and, 37–39; goals, 87; idealism, 108–11; public, ethics of, 214n2; risk and, 81–82; social determinants of, 82; value of, 121–22
Health and Social Care Information Centre, 127
health care: access to, 86–87; atomistic individualism in, 135–36, 142, 150, 190, 199; at end of life, 140–43, 152, 172–74; function creep of, 116–17; rationing, 177–80; universal, 162–63, 177–80, 185, 207. See also personalized medicine
Health Data Exploration Project, 122
Health Insurance Portability and Accountability Act (HIPAA), xiv, 61–62, 161
health records. See electronic health records
heart disease, 76, 98–100, 100
heart failure (HF), 51–55
Hebb, Michael, 172–73
hedonistic prosumption, 119–20, 120
Heidegger, Martin, 137
Heywood, James, 23
HF. See heart failure
Hierarchical Condition Category (HCC) Profiler, 167

high-throughput technologies, xiv, 4
high-touch medicine, 155–57, 174–77
HIPAA. *See* Health Insurance Portability and Accountability Act
hippocampus, xiv, 102
Hobbes, Thomas, 137
home assistants, digital, 41–42
Horner, Lisa, 36
Horvath, Steve, 103
Howie, Lynn, 164
Hudson Yards, 49–50
humiliation, of digital surveillance, 42–43
hypercollection, 40–41, 49, 71

IBM, 167
idealistic capitalism, 112–15
idealistic prosumption, 119–20, *120*
imaging, medical, 97–102, 104–5
impact investing, 213n2
incomplete patients, 59–62
individual autonomy, 189–91, 197
individualism: atomistic, 135–36, 142, 150, 190, 199; solidarity and, 140. *See also* personhood
individualistic empowerment, 191–92, *192*
individual risk, 82, 102, 205–6
inequality: biomarkers and, 105–6; data collection influenced by, 37–38, 78; in digital divide, 32–36; in e-health filter bubble, 37; exacerbated, 9–10; observational data and, 162; social determinants and, 86–87. *See also* exclusion
inflammation, 103
information commons, 6, 43, 207
informed consent, 140–41, 143, 146
Institute of Medicine (IOM), xiv
institutions, trustworthiness of, 132
instrumental empowerment, 191, *192*, 193, 196, 200
insulin treatment, 1–2
intellectual property rights, 11, 40
*International Covenant on Economic, Social and Cultural Rights*, 158

Internet, 209n2; access, 33–37; changing role of, 6–7, 19–22, 47–48; early days of, 209n1; e-health filter bubble and, 37–39; non-use, 34–44
Internet of Things (IoT), xiv, 49
Internet Protocol address. *See* IP address
interpretation, as luxury item, 176–77
IOM. *See* Institute of Medicine
IoT. *See* Internet of Things
iPad, 20, 48
IP (Internet Protocol) address, xiv, 71
Israel, organ donation in, 143–47, 215nn6–7

Jacob, Marie-Andrée, 144–47, 153
Jana, 109–10
Johnson, Mark, 158
journeys, 145, 187
Judaism, Orthodox, 144

Kahneman, Daniel, 100
Kalmar, Rachel, 55
Kang, Jerry, 43, 66
Kant, Immanuel, 136–37
Katz, Jay, 199
Kirkpatrick, Robert, 111, 115
Koenig, Barbara, 141
Kohane, Isaac, 161

Lacan, Jacques, 138
Lakoff, George, 158
laptops, 34, 48
Laurie, Graeme, 204
laws, 40, 43, 61–62, 131. *See also* regulations
lean-back digital technologies, 20, 209n1
lean-forward digital technologies: CureTogether, 19, 21, 24–26, 45; digital divide and, 35; emergence of, 16, 20–21; patient researcher and, 16, 19, 20–26, 35, 45; PatientsLikeMe, 19, 21–26, 45; trend toward, 209n1
Le Métayer, Daniel, 72

Leonelli, Sabina, 66–67
Levitsky, Sandra, 197
lithium carbonate study, 23, 26, 28–31, 59
Locke, John, 136–37
Longhurst, Christopher, 160
long-term care, 197
Lou Gehrig's disease. *See* amyotrophic lateral sclerosis
Lukes, Steven, 83
Lupton, Deborah, 157

Mackenzie, Catriona, 142
magnetic resonance imaging (MRI), xiv, 47, 97–98
Majone, Giandomenico, 81
maker community, devices made by, 72
marketing tools, web-based, 116
Marmot, Michael, 86
Mauss, Marcel, 139
Mayer-Schönberger, Viktor, 7, 22
McGoey, Linsey, 111, 112, 114, 214n5
McGowan, Michelle, 31, 45, 106
meaning: discursive, 14; evidence and, 155–57; in participation, 198–201; in personal decision making, 171–75, 185, 199; of personalized medicine, 1–5, 199–201, 207–8; of personhood, 135, 147–48
medical imaging, 97–102, 104–5
*Me Medicine vs. We Medicine* (Dickenson), 8
methodology, 13–14
metrics: flow, 66–67; ODL, xv, 180; PROM, xv, 30, 60, 164–65
microbiomes, 115, 214n6
Mijnzorgnet.nl ("My care network"), 167–68
mobile leapfrogging, 33–34
Monteleone, Shara, 72
Moore's Law, 4
Morozov, Evgeny, 212n9
Morrison, Stacey, 36, 49

motor neuron disease. *See* amyotrophic lateral sclerosis
MRI. *See* magnetic resonance imaging
MS. *See* multiple sclerosis
multimorbidity, 159
multinational corporations, 43, 96, 151, 206
multiple sclerosis (MS), xiv, 162–63
"My care network" (Mijnzorgnet.nl), 167–68
MyChart, 166–68

Napoli, Philip, 35
National Academies of Science, Engineering, and Medicine, U.S. (NAS), xiv, 5, 59
National Center of Health Statistics, 216n2
National Health Service (NHS), xiv, 167, 177–78, 216n1; care.data initiative, xiii, 123, 127, 128–29, 132; Google collaborating with, 96, 108
National Institutes of Health, U.S. (NIH), xv, 79
National Security Agency, U.S. (NSA), 132
N=1 studies, 202
newborn screening, 47
New York University (NYU), 49–50
NHS. *See* National Health Service
Nielsen, Jakob, 209n1
Nietzsche, Friedrich, 138
NIH. *See* National Institutes of Health, U.S.
Nike, 114. *See also* FuelBand
Nissenbaum, Helen, 63, 126–27
nonprofit *vs.* for-profit distinction, 107–8, 117, 119, 123, 133
nonproprietary devices, 73
Nowotny, Helga, 41
NSA. *See* National Security Agency, U.S.
nudge, 87, 213n5
Nye, Joseph, 82
NYU. *See* New York University

Obama, Barack, 5, 7, 10, 15

Obar, Jonathan, 35

obesity epidemic, 85–87

observational data, xv, 160–62, 180

ODL (observations of daily living) metrics, xv, 180

OECD. *See* Organisation for Economic Co-Operation and Development

Ohnsorge, Kathrin, 141–42

Oliver, Eric, 85–86

Omics research, xv, 87

1/1/1/ model, 114

Open FDA initiative, 213n1

Openhumans, 133

openness: in categories of participation, 27, 29–30; obligation toward, 158

Open Science movement, 94, 123–26

OpenSNP, 92, 170

opting out, 126–30, *128–29*, 215n1

organ donation, 140, 143–47, 152–53, 215nn4–7

Organisation for Economic Co-Operation and Development (OECD), 173

Orthodox Judaism, 144

Oudshoorn, Nelly, 50

overdiagnosis, 173–74

ownership, privacy and, 64–65, 67, 213n9

Parkinson's disease, 76–77

Parsons, Talcott, 88

participation: active, 68, *69*; commercial and societal value connected in, 117–18; concerns about, 39–45; conscious, 68, *69*; democratic value of, 26, 40, 44–45, 74, 94; digital surveillance design and, 117–18; discourse, 192–201; disempowerment by, 16, 18–19, 53, 194; economic dimensions of, 31–39; forms of, 19, 26–30, 62, *69*, 73; goalposts of, 189; meaningful, characteristics of, 198–201; political dimensions of, 31–39, 198; power of, 87–89; public, 26–30; in Web 2.0

enterprises, 31, 122. *See also* data collection; patient work

participatory medicine, 44, 209n3

participatory turn, 16–18

Pasquale, Frank, 183

patient-centered medicine, 163–66, 185–86

patient-reported outcome measures (PROM), xv, 30, 60, 164–65

patient researcher: activated patient as, 15–17, 37; contributions from, 15–23; downsides of being, 39–45; lean-forward digital technologies and, 16, 19, 20–26, 35, 45; as permanent contributor, 45

patients: activated, 15–17, 37; agency of, 10–11, 44, 70, 79–80; elderly, 32; experience and knowledge of, 163–65; as gatekeepers to data, 166–68; incomplete, 59–62; risky, 42; role of, 3, 7, 10–12, 15–16; standard, fiction of, 8. *See also* empowerment; transmitting patient

PatientsLikeMe, 210n7; commercial interests and health idealism in, 108–9, 123; as lean-forward digital technology, 19, 21–26, 45; research by, 23, 26, 28–31, 39, 59

patient work: at home, 50–58; personalized medicine requiring, 11, 15–16, 50–58, 185, 187–208; prosumption and, 121; during "radical difference," 205–8; 2.0, 188, 201–5, *205*; visibility of, 188

Patsakis, Constantinos, 130

Peppet, Scott, 64

Personal Data Guardians, 72

Personal Data Vaults, 72

personal decision making: end-of-life, 140–43, 152, 172–74; meaning in, 171–75, 185, 199; on therapies and treatments, 140–43, 152, 171–75

personalization from below, 11–12

personalized medicine: changing meaning of, 1–5, 155–57, 184–86, 199–201, 207–8; defined, 4–5. *See also specific topics*

personhood: community-based understandings of, 141; data governance
and, 140, 147–51; end-of-life decision
making and, 140–43, 152; meaning of,
135, 147–48; organ donation and, 140,
143–47, 152–53, 215nn4–7; personalization and, 12–13; as rational actor,
136–40, 214n1

pharmaceutical companies, 18, 42, 114,
121

philanthrocapitalism, 214n5

philanthropy, 111, 115, 213n4, 214n5

philosophy, 137–39

physical labor, gender and, 58

politics: democratization and, 191; of participation, 31–39, 198; of personalized
medicine, 8–9, 31–39

Portable Legal Consent, 169–70, 216n7

postmodern philosophy, 138

poverty, humiliation and, 42–43

power: asymmetries, 43, 72, 74, 94, 124,
126–27, 150, 183, 189, 206; behavior
change and, 81–82, 84–87; biomarkers
and, 97–106; DNA analysis and, 75–78;
faces of, 82–85, 87, 89, 92–93, 96, 99,
104; Foucault on, 80–83, 87–88, 138,
212nn2–3; genome testing and, 89–96,
104–5; hard, 82, 189; of participation,
87–89; risk linked to, 81–82; soft,
82–84, 189; sovereign, 80; technology
shifting, 74, 79–80, 89–106; transmitting patient and, 79; understanding
of, 75–85. See also disempowerment;
empowerment

PPI. See public and patient involvement

precision medicine, 1, 3, 5, 7, 10, 79. See
also personalized medicine

Precision Medicine Initiative. See All of
Us Research Program

predictive analytics, 42, 151, 180–84

Preventing Overdiagnosis, 173–74

prevention, risk reduced by, 81–82, 102

primary data subjects, 148

privacy: challenges, 70–73; as collective
concern, 206–7; commodification
of, 130–31; conceptualized, 66–67;
control-based view of, 65–67; in
datafication era, 62–65; data governance and, 147–51; defined, 63; digital
surveillance influencing, 42, 50, 63–65;
electronic health records and, 161–62;
humiliation and, 42–43; ownership
and, 64–65, 67, 213n9; reidentification and, 71, 170, 203; ryanairation
of, 212n9; structural, 62; transmitting
patient and, 62–67; utility and, 61

Privacy-by-Default, xv, 71

Privacy-by-Design, xv, 71, 130

productivity, activity trackers and, 57–58

profit: in nonprofit vs. for-profit distinction, 107–8, 117, 119, 123, 133; from
research, 110–11; social responsibility
converging with, 116–18

PROM. See patient-reported outcome
measures

prosumption: commercial interests and,
117–26; defined, xv, 21; DIY biology
and, 124–26; Open Science and, 123–
24; personalized medicine and, 118–26,
120; types of, 118–20, 120

protection: as collective concern, 132, 202,
206–8; commercial interests and, 107–
8, 130–33; in datafication era, 63–65;
laws, 40, 43, 61–62, 131; Personal Data
Guardians and Vaults for, 72; personhood and, 140, 147–51; regulations,
43, 62, 71–72, 130, 212n13; rethinking,
204–5, 205

public and patient involvement (PPI), 189,
216n1

public health ethics, 214n2

public participation, 26–30

public-private partnerships, 110

quality control, 31

quantified community, 49–50

racial discrimination, 10, 18–19, 86, 207
"radical difference," 205–8
radiologists, 99–101, 213n10
randomized controlled trials, 159–60, 201
rational actor paradigm, 136–40, 214n1
rationing, 177–80
Ratto, Matt, 130
Realistic Medicine, 163–64, 216n3
*Reality Mining: Using Big Data to Engineer a Better World* (Eagle and Greene), 110
Reda, Daniel, 24
redlining, xv, 18–19
regulations: General Data Protection Regulation, 62, 71–72, 130, 212n13; multinational corporations and, 43
regulatory state, 81
Rehmann Sutter, Christoph, 214n1
reidentification, 71, 170, 203
relational autonomy, 142–43
repassification, by mobile web-based services, 35–36
research: coordination, 26; data use rethought for, 202–5; drop-out rates in, 28, 210n5; methods, 13–14; N=1 studies, 202; Omics, xv, 87; patient-reported outcomes, 30, 60, 164–65; Patients-LikeMe, 23, 26, 28–31, 39, 59; profits from, 110–11; randomized controlled trials, 159–60, 201; risk in, 149–50; social evidence and, 169–70. *See also* patient researcher
risk: data governance and, 204–5, *205*; genetic, 76–77, 91–93, 95; individual, 82, 102, 205–6; power linked to, 81–82; in research, 149–50
risky patients, 42
Rose, Nikolas, 84
ryanairation, of privacy, 212n9

Sage Bionetworks, 169
Salesforce Foundation, 114
sanctioned deviance, 88

scalable medicine, 175
Science and Technology Studies (STS), xvi, 14
secondary data subjects, 148
security systems, 51
self, technologies of, 80–81
self-care, 17–18
self-interest: altruism *vs.*, 135–36, 140, 142–47, 152–54; rational choice and, 136–40, 214n1; research risk and, 149–50; role of, 139
self-monitoring: challenges of, 59–62; empowerment and, 73–74, 198; in expansion of digital surveillance, 50–58; as fun, 60–61
self-optimization, 205–6
self-ownership, 136–37
self-tracking, 24–25, 61, 210n3. *See also* self-monitoring
semantic web, 59
sensitive, label of, 70–72
shared history (*historia meshutefet*), 146–47
"sharing": commercial interests and, 122–27; data, 11, 67, 122–27, 123, 132–33
Sharon, Tamar, 74, 108, 134
Shaw, Stanley, 58–59
sick role, 88
single nucleotide polymorphism. *See* SNP
Sleepio, 116
smart glasses, xv, 48, 175–76
smartphones, 21, 33–36
smart socks, 2
smart watches, 21
Smith, Adam, 112–13
SNP (single nucleotide polymorphism), 92–93, 213n6
social biomarkers, xv, 143, 154, 156, 165–66
social determinants, behavior change *vs.*, 82, 85–87
social isolation, telemonitoring and, 53–54

social media, 17, 19, 32; in *The Circle*, 46–47; user-generated content on, 20–21, 123

social responsibility. *See* corporate social responsibility

soft power, 82–84, 189

Solanas, Agusti, 130

solidarity: governance based on, 152; individualism and, 140; personalized medicine and, 140, 152–54, 177–80, 207

somatic biomarkers, 102–4, 178

Sorell, Tom, 53

sovereign power, 80

standard patient, fiction of, 8

start-ups, 107–8

state of nature, 137

Stoljar, Natalie, 142

stratified medicine, 5, 209n1

Strauss, Anselm, 15–16

stroke diagnosis, 97, 162

structural privacy, 62

STS. *See* Science and Technology Studies

subgroup analyses, 37

surveillance. *See* digital surveillance

surveillant assemblage, 51–55, 57, 60

tablet computers: access to, 32–34; always on, 48–49; iPad, 20, 48

Taylor, Astra, 94

Taylor, Charles, 214n1

Taylor, Mark, 63, 148–49, 204

technologies: access to, 94; cost of, 11, 102; disruptive, 78, 96; high-throughput, xiv, 4; high-touch medicine and, 155–57, 174–77; inequalities exacerbated by, 9–10; lean-back, 20, 209n1; power shifted by, 74, 79–80, 89–106; progress of, 1–4; reliance on, 12–13; of self, 80–81; undesirable effects of, 78–79; utility of, 61. *See also* lean-forward digital technologies

technology-in-practice, 91, 95

telemedicine, 12, 51, 73–74

telemonitoring: activity trackers compared with, 61–62; with CardioConsult HF, 51–55, 61–63; purpose of, 54

telephone communication, 175–76. *See also* cell phones; smartphones

Tempini, Niccolo, 116

*Theory of Moral Sentiments* (Smith), 112

theranostics, xvi, 101

Tillack, Allison, 100

Titmuss, Richard, 139

Tocchetti, Sara, 124

Topol, Eric, 6

transmitting patient: with CardioConsult HF, 51–55, 61–63; default state of, 48–50; with FuelBand, 55–58, 61, 63–65, 211nn5–6, 212nn10–11; incomplete, 59–62; new understanding of data use from, 67–73, 69; overview of, 46–48, 73–74; patient work at home by, 50–58; power and, 79; privacy and, 62–67

transnational corporations. *See* multinational corporations

tumors, molecular classification of, 2, 9

Tutton, Richard, 8

23andMe: CureTogether acquired by, 25, 39–40, 45, 133; genome testing by, 75–78, 90, 94–95, 110, 189; Google backing, 95–96

Twitter, 21

Type-1 diabetes, 1–2, 9

Type-2 diabetes, 1

United Kingdom (UK), 162, 211n4. *See also* National Health Service

United States (U.S.): All of Us Research Program in, 3, 5, 7, 10, 79; CMS, 163, 182; FDA, xiv, 92, 95, 164, 213n1; FTC, xiv, 131; HIPAA in, xiv, 61–62, 161; long-term care in, 197; MyChart in, 166–68; NAS, xiv, 5, 59; NIH, xv, 79; NSA, 132 universal health care, 162–63, 177–80, 185, 207

U.S. *See* United States

user-generated content, 20–21, 123

utilitaristic prosumption, 119–20, *120*

value creation, 119

Wachter, Robert, 99–100

Wagenaar, Hendrik, 14

waste reduction, 157, 173

water metaphor, 157–58

Watson, IBM, 167

Watson, Sara, 66–67

*The Wealth of Nations* (Smith), 112

Web 2.0, 31, 122

web-based tools, 209n1; communication and marketing, 116; exclusion in, 32–38; reliance on, 12, 19; repassification by, 35–36; research contributions and, 19–22

Weber, Max, 212n2

Western dualism, 136–38

*The West Wing*, 113

We-Think, 122

Widdows, Heather, 204

Wikimedia, 119–20

Wojcicki, Anne, 94

women: in digital divide, 33–35; long-term care by, 197; physical labor of, 58

Žižek, Slavoj, 112, 115

## ABOUT THE AUTHOR

Barbara Prainsack is Professor in the Department of Political Science at the University of Vienna, and in the Department of Global Health and Social Medicine at King's College London.